YOUR
HEALTH
HAS BEEN
HIJACKED

AND IT'S HIGH TIME TO TAKE IT BACK!

DR. TOM REED
DPM, DAPBS, DABPM, FACFAS

There are an estimated 50 trillion cells in the human body. Each cell is a perfectly orchestrated symphony in design - a masterpiece of miniaturized complexity so astounding that even the most sophisticated icons in science can't help from being humbled by the miracle set before them.

Dr. Tom Reed

Reed Between The Lines Publishing
www.DrTomReed.com

Your Health Has Been Hijacked
Copyright © 2019 by Dr. Tom Reed All Rights Reserved.

Disclaimer

This book contains the opinions and ideas of the author. Its purpose is to be educational and informative on the subjects that it addresses. It is not in any way a substitute for the advice of the reader's own physician*(s)* or other medical professionals based on the reader's own individual condition, symptoms, or concerns. If the reader needs personal medical, health, dietary, or other assistance, the reader should consult a competent physician or other qualified health care provider. The author specifically disclaims any liability, loss, or risk, personal or otherwise, that is incurred as a consequence, directly or indirectly, of following any directions or suggestions, or application of any of the contents of this book.

ISBN 978-1-7324002-2-1

This book may be purchased in bulk for promotional, educational, or business use.

Visit www.DrTomReed.com for information on ordering this and other educational materials.

Editor's Commentary

I'm a skeptic at heart. I don't ride too far from the middle of the road in most areas of life. I'm not a fad chaser nor a bandwagon rider. I take everything with a grain of salt. If you want me to believe what you have to say, you better have some proof to back it up. I mean real proof. Not fabricated stories, or false inferences, or junk science. In part, it's how I'm wired, and in part, my experiences in life have trained me to be this way.

Working on this book has been a bit unsettling for me. If I'm honest, it's made me a little unsure about how I feel about the medical profession as a whole, and it has certainly raised some red flags about the pharmaceutical industry. The notion that people do unscrupulous things for the sake of a buck is not a foreign concept, but the realization that it is so widespread among industries who are supposed to be for my good, that's mind-blowing.

I have not been the same since working on this book. I can't walk through the grocery store without seeing labels meant to convince me something is healthy when it isn't. I can't watch the news without hearing "facts" about some new drug or "safe" vaccine without rolling my eyes because I know they aren't telling the whole story. I look around my home, and I see toxins everywhere.

If you're ready to pull your head out of the sand and have your eyes opened, then open the pages of this book and get started. But be prepared for it to change the way you shop, and eat, and clean, and care for your body. Your health HAS been hijacked. You better believe it.

Carol Jones
Editor of Your Health Has Been Hijacked

Praises for Your Health Has Been Hijacked

Reading the tome of this 35-year-practicing doctor feels like having a fireside chat with your neighbor. There is none of the usual medical doublespeak and hyperbole, just a straight forward, honest presentation of the facts, supported by clinical research and statistics, that any layman can understand, and any medical professional should appreciate. However, the author doesn't sugar coat the severity of our circumstances. Our toxic, chemical-laden environs comprise a monumental assault even on the healthiest immune system, impacting brain function and overall longevity. The "better living through chemistry" experiment has created a sicker population than ever recorded in recent history. The good news is, one can only conclude that the human body is an amazing organic creation that, given the right care and support, can overcome anything...

Gwen Olsen
Author of Confessions of an Rx Drug Pusher

This book is a must for every home library, in fact every medical library as well. It takes the reader through not just the big picture of living a natural lifestyle, but also the nitty gritty for those that want a deeper understanding of our bodies. Dr. Reed makes it easy to walk into a better life and have healthier emotions. He connects the dots completely! Give this book as a gift to everyone you love as well as every skeptic. His knowledge and wisdom stands the test of time and is a movement for change towards living with awareness and using our own God-given voices.

Jodie Meschuk
Author of Speak Up Buttercup
Authority on autism recovery and a mom who will never stop until every child is healed!

The world needs to know the information in this book. We CAN combat and adapt! Knowledge and awareness are the keys to better health.

Deborah Warner
Ph.D. in Nutritional Science, Clinic Solutions-Houston

Angels Sing to You in The Wind, All You Have to Do is Listen.

This book is dedicated to my sweet wife Angel *(Evangeline).*

Thank you for always being there for me,
especially through life's many trials.
Your love is as sweet and fresh as a new spring's morn.
Always willing to share in my dreams,
And yet you stand alone in your uniqueness
that has blessed so many since you were created.

CONTENTS

PREFACE

---

*"The further a society drifts from the truth, the
more it will hate those that speak it."*

George Orwell

In 1983, my mom committed suicide, drowned in the bathtub of her own home. I was in my surgical residency at the time when I received a phone call from my brother, Jerry, telling me the devastating news. My stepdad found her after returning from an errand. He called 911, and the closest fire department rescue team responded, just a couple of minutes away. Jerry was a firefighter and paramedic at the time of my mother's death and happened to be on the truck that responded. He heard the call and the address and said, *"Hey, That's my house!"* Professional firefighters and paramedics *(EMS)* don't ask what or why in the moment - they hear the firehouse alarm, the adrenalin kicks in, and they go. In the moment, as the fire truck raced toward our parents' home, he thought that perhaps the person reported dead at the residence was the renter who lived upstairs. The possibility of his own mother lying dead in a bathtub never occurred to him.

Imagine the trauma of walking into your parents' house and seeing your own mother dead in a tub of water. Under normal circumstances, this would be such a devastating experience; to function in any semblance of normalcy would be nearly impossible. But Jerry, as any other trained emergency professional would do, responded in the most professional way. He dragged her out of the tub and into the bedroom where he started CPR *(Cardiopulmonary Resuscitation)*. His efforts were futile - she was gone long before he started.

After I hung up with Jerry, I rushed out of the hospital clinic and drove the forty-five minutes to her house. By the time I got there, she had already been taken away. I can't even remember who was there at the time; everything was so surreal. I do remember very vividly walking into her bedroom and seeing an unopened envelope on her bed addressed to me. I was bawling as I opened it. This was the last communication she had with anyone before she went into the bathroom to end her life. She sent her husband to the store and then took several sleeping pills to make the process easier.

I opened the folded note and read. *"Dear Tommy, I just can't take this depression any longer. Please forgive me. Love, Mother."* That note was much more than a final goodbye. You see, that was the first time I remember my mother ever saying she loved me. Behind all of the tears, all I could think was that I wanted to say back to her, *"I love you too, Mom."*

Years later, while visiting with my brother Jerry, he told my new wife, Evangeline *(Angel)*, about a picture of me that was found next to the note. Apparently, it was removed by someone before I got there, and I didn't know anything about it. He felt it was best that I knew about it and that she should tell me in her own timing. Angel and I were driving around town not too long after that visit when she told me about the picture. I pulled over to the side of the road and broke down in tears. Emotional wounds, freshly opened, provided a necessary release, and my real healing started that day.

I just didn't know that my mom loved me that much. Not only words in a note, and a first and final, I love you, but to know that mine was the last face she would look at brought forth an intense emotional response that connected me to my mom in a way that even years of a healthy relationship could not produce. In a way, it was like her spirit passed through me in the moment, and I felt her essence inside of me.

Looking back, I realize my mom died at the hands of the pharmaceutical profiteers and a doctor who *(in my professional opinion)* was negligently prescribing her four very toxic antipsychotic medications. The side effects were many and were spelled out on the package inserts. She became disoriented, slurred her speech, developed Parkinson's syndrome, and cardiac arrhythmias, and became even more depressed. The combined effects of these medications just amplified the side effects. The profiteers were happy to line their pockets with cash at the expense of my mom's health until she overdosed with their poisons and drowned herself to end the misery.

Even before I wrote this book, I had a longstanding and compelling desire to somehow step into the gap for my mom and others like her, people whose lives and families have been maimed by the pharmaceutical industry and other chemical manufacturers interested only in money. Over the years, I have spoken at many health-related events, and this book represents the culmination of that experience, as well as years of research. To give you a better understanding of my calling and my heart in writing this book, though, I need to set the stage with a little more background.

Days Of Future Passed

I grew up in a relationally challenged *(code word for dysfunctional)* family in Washington DC during the 1950s and '60s, at the height of racial tensions between blacks and whites, nationally. I was the youngest of four boys. My parents were alcoholics, heavy smokers, and argued incessantly - sadly, a typical and emerging post-WWII family model. I remember my next oldest brother and me sitting at the top of the stairs of our family home, yelling down to my parents over and over again to stop arguing.

As a teen, I walked the streets of northeast DC in fear, playing out scenarios of how I would escape the increasing assaults on me from the local thugs. The fear was so profound that when most people went into their homes and locked the doors, I left the doors open so I could get away quickly if someone tried to get into the house when I was alone after school.

I have only scattered memories of my childhood, some good, mostly not so good, and certainly not the endearing, fun, and readily accessible memories that most families seem to have. My dad died from a heart attack when I was sixteen years old. I never really knew him. He was reserved, and I don't remember ever actually having a conversation with him. He took me to grade school sports events, played catch with me once or twice that I remember, and apparently everyone at his work really liked him. But his personal relationship with his four boys was very distant.

The night that he died, I remember my mom screaming for my brother and me. I remember saying to myself, *"Oh no, it has finally happened."* I can't explain why, but I had a premonition of my father's death. I ran into their bedroom only to find him lying face up in the bed, lifeless. My mom was crying and, in my panic, I tried CPR, something new I'd heard about on the news. I really didn't know what I was doing, but I tried to blow life back into his lungs and pound on his chest to get his heart started again. It didn't work, and his body just flopped around as we tried to shake life into him. His brown eyes, just like mine, were staring at me, open but completely lifeless. Anyone who has seen another family member dead but with open eyes staring back - it's just beyond explanation and cuts deep into your DNA. I still remember that look in his eyes as if it were yesterday.

I was a junior in high school at the time, and my mom decided to move out of DC and into the Maryland suburbs, not five minutes away. She met a nice man within a year of my father's death, and they were married not too long after. He was a *"caretaker"* personality, which is what my mother needed at the time.

Still experiencing the aftershock of my father's death, and with no moral compass to keep me grounded, I rebelled against most everything and everybody, including my mom's new husband, and as soon as I finished high school, I was promptly kicked out of the house. I entered an adult world confused and morally bankrupt, with no place to go and no plans for the future. I did manage to find work fairly quickly, and a place to live in a DC boarding house. I was introduced to the recreational drugs of the time and managed to quell the pain from the emptiness I felt inside.

At age 24, after a two-year failed marriage, several job terminations, recreational drug abuse, and a morally bankrupt life, I decided to do something that my family and friends thought was even more crazy - I decided to go to college and then to med school to become a doctor. The response from them was predictable - *"YOU ARE GOING TO DO WHAT?"* Their disbelief was not surprising; after all, I had been only a C student in high school, and I was giving up a decent job with the US Postal Service. In their minds, I must have been on drugs to entertain such a fantasy. But my heart was set, and there was no turning back.

The pre-med curriculum was predictably grueling, especially for me, since I was never taught nor had I developed the necessary study skills to survive the academic challenges of college. I did have an advantage in that I was now twenty-four: my head was showing signs of being screwed on right, and a newly emerging tenacity was developing, something that would carry me through many years, even to the present.

I was self-supporting in a very unforgiving world, climbing a steep mountain of unknowns, with everyone back home waiting for me to fail - waiting for their moment to say, *"I told you so."* That's how it was in the neighborhood where I grew up; the people there took any opportunity to tear you down and keep you in your place.

In addition to the pre-med academic rigors, I was a double major and worked twenty-four to thirty hours a week to support myself. I did pretty well, maintaining a decent enough GPA to get several academic scholarships and admission to podiatry medical school. I was off to Cleveland, Ohio for my medical school training. I had never really traveled much beyond my DC stomping grounds, so this was another new adventure.

The academic requirements of medical school were so much more demanding than college. My financial needs were still the same, and I had to work as well to pay the bills. After med school, I was accepted into a surgical residency program at the Veteran's Hospital in Baltimore, Maryland, which was under the auspices of Johns Hopkins University. After my mom died, it took a while to recover and return to my residency duties, but eventually I finished the program and opened my medical practice in Conroe, Texas, facing over two hundred and fifty thousand dollars in school debt and other practice loans.

Within my first year of practice, I met my soon-to-be wife. A colleague and I went to lunch at a local restaurant in Conroe where our waitress came to greet us and asked for our beverage order. The name on her tag read *"Angel,"* and she was! When she walked away from our table, I turned to my friend and said, *"Hey, that's the girl I'm going to marry."* He looked at me bewildered and then sarcastically responded, *"Oh, right, why would SHE want to marry YOU,"* insinuating that I wouldn't measure up to a beautiful woman like that. For a year, she would not go out with me - because she was already involved with someone else. But I just kept popping my head in and sitting at her tables. One evening, in January of 1985, I asked her if she would have dinner with me after she got off work. She said yes, and six months later we were married.

Angel also had a very troubled childhood, but we managed to grow together as a couple and as parents despite the emotional challenges of our upbringings. We stumbled along the way, laughing and crying together, seeking counsel from others to heal the wounds of our childhoods, always with the loving intent of trying to make a better life for our children. In the process, we made many mistakes. But, we always forgave each other and our children, and we taught them to do the same. Not that we were a perfect family, but we were a far cry from our roots. And one thing was for sure, my children never went to bed or left the house without Angel and me saying that we loved them. It was very routine for them. If they only knew how special that really was. If they had walked in our shoes and experienced some of the pain and hardship that we experienced, it wouldn't have seemed so routine. Looking back, I can see that my mom and dad, while not perfect, did the best they knew how to do in raising four boys. It took many years of raising my own children for me to come to terms with that. I love my parents despite my childhood. What I went through prepared me for the road I now travel, and I am thankful!

Not too long after Angel and I were married, my new mother-in-law gave me a book to read. On the inset title page, she wrote the following: *"To Thomas, Seeker of Truth."* I didn't much see myself that way at the time *(our perceptions are our reality)* and passed it off as a fanciful maneuver to encourage me to read the book, which of course, I did. I mean, really, how could I not? Offending my new mother-in-law was a bad idea! Besides, the title of the book, *"Creation and Time"* was intriguing, and appealed to my sense of adventure. In the years to follow however, her words, as simple of a compliment as I thought they were at the time, were full of an elder's wisdom and provided insight into the man she knew I would become.

Our perceptions are indeed our reality, our moment-by-moment truth; it's that simple. Life's journey seeks to impose its own symphony of especially created experiences that form the basis of our perceptions. They unveil truths about the world in which we live and breathe. But whose truth is being unveiled? Should we accept our perceptions of truth at face value? Determining truth in a complex world is perhaps not as simple as in times past. In today's twenty-four-hour news cycle, multimedia-driven, sleight-of-hand world, truth seems more relative that at any time in history. Truth becomes what someone can make you believe, an imposed illusion of perception. Anymore, to be *"street wise"* about such matters is not just an urban colloquialism, but a necessary skill to develop if we are to read between the lines of life and find real truth to survive the journey without too many dings, dents, or worse - a *"crash-and- burn"* experience.

My purpose in writing this book is to help provide you with enough useful knowledge that you can, with power, finesse, and confidence, find the truths in life that will lead you to wellness, purpose, and longevity. When we discover measurable truth, we need not worry about what others think, and we need not defend it. Real truth will always defend itself.

This book represents a new adventure in my life. One filled with passion, a desire to love others and share in ways that I am gifted, and even a self-serving desire to help myself continue to heal from the many wounds I have sustained over the years. I am not ashamed of those hurts and scars - they make me who I am; nor am I hesitant to share truth, as best as I can determine it. We live in a post-truth world where even the objective facts are less influential in shaping public opinion than are appeals to emotion and personal belief. So, while the facts may be true, interpretation may be relative, based on how someone feels about the facts, instead of on what the facts actually tell us.

There are many ways in which our health is being affected everyday by toxic chemicals that come into contact with us, through all sectors of our lives. You will learn the related facts in this book, along with the research to back it up. We hear so much from marketers about how this product cleans your counters, or gives a fresh smell to the laundry, how this one is best for shampooing your baby's hair, and this one will help you see butter-flies as you drift off to sleep at night. We are told how this medication will cure your diabetes and make you think you are healthy and that you can't survive without it, and then shamed into believing these seventy vaccines are necessary if our children are to survive to adulthood. These are the appeals to make us feel that we need those products or medications. But the fact of the matter, which is hidden, is that these products are laced with toxic chemicals that are inherently harmful. We are inundated from the time we wake with messages that are designed to manipulate our minds and shape our behaviors. The truth is that there are very few safe products out there available to the average consumer shopping at the grocery store or online.

Your health has been hijacked, and it's high time to take it back! Armed with solid research and my evidence-based observations and solutions *(from over thirty-five years as a medical/surgical specialist and health and nutrition specialist),* you will be well-prepared to move forward with a life-changing plan. I believe that by reading this book, you will find hope for your future.

CHAPTER 1

The Killing Fields
A Crisis Of Human Suffering

Throughout recorded history, humans have encountered horrific, large-scale tragedies ending in the loss or maiming of hundreds of millions of people. Plagues and other bacterial and viral infections, wars, famine, natural disasters, and mass exterminations have wiped out entire generations, cultures, and families who couldn't have imagined such devastation. Most of them were innocent bystanders who happened to be swept up and out of existence in the whirlwinds of human happenstance or design. It comes and then goes, leaving a trail of destruction behind. As we consider history, we engage our ingenuity, trying to improve what we can, hoping to avoid similar disasters in the future.

Over the course of the last three hundred years, mankind has faced challenges of a different kind: challenges brought on in the name of progress. The Industrial Revolution, for starters, birthed in Great Britain around 1760, marked a turning point in history. Almost every aspect of human life was influenced in some way by the emerging industrial technologies. [1] And by the mid 1800s, the industrialization of the world was well under way. [2]

Many of us picture this time in history very fondly, with sun umbrellas, ladies in long flowing dresses, carriage rides in the country on a beautiful spring day, and as fashion promenaded into the Romantic Era, gentlemen were impeccably dressed in the new tux look of the day. They were opening doors for the ladies, conversing with each other in a fancy ballroom about the latest innovation or the next play production coming to the local theatre.

But, when we take a closer look at that time in history, a different picture emerges. This was a time in history when there was a mass exodus of people from the quaint countryside into the city in hopes of finding work opportunities in the new world of urban mechanization. By 1760 at the latest, agricultural, rural textile operations, and other small businesses had greatly reduced available jobs, causing unemployed workers to move to the cities where ill-prepared housing and living accommodations greeted them. This resulted in wretched living conditions aggravated by profit-driven builders and landlords. [3]

The workplaces and housing conditions of the urban poor were deplorable and had no health or safety codes. Men and women worked twelve-to-six-teen- hour workdays. Children either roamed the streets while their parents worked, or they were coerced into child labor by parents or unscrupulous factory and mill owners. Their work frequently involved dangerous and demoralizing activities for up to eighteen hours a day.[4]

Entire cities like New York were surrounded by garbage dumps and shanty-towns where animals including hogs, horses, and dogs roamed the streets. Human and animal excrement were everywhere. Runoff from raw sewage mixed readily with sources of drinking water. Carcasses of dead and diseased animals found in the streets were used to make sausage that was sold to the unsuspecting public. Rats infested the cities of Boston and New York, causing widespread and severe public health problems. Infectious diseases were spreading. Tuberculosis, cholera, typhoid fever, dysentery, diphtheria, measles, smallpox, and pertussis were rampant at varying times in over-crowded, nutritionally deficient communities with no clean running water and no concept of hygiene or basic sanitation practices. [5]

What made all these diseases subside? After Louis Pasteur and others promoted the idea of *The Germ Theory of Disease*, it was thought that infections could develop mostly from poor nutrition and hygiene, and inadequate living conditions. These infections also typically run their course and historically subside on their own. Improving living conditions, including clean and running city water treated with chlorine as a disinfectant, better nutrition, water closets *(toilets)*, health and hygiene education, and time, were the main factors contributing to the decline in these diseases. While the search was on to develop antibiotics, antitoxins, toxoids, and vaccines, essentially all of these diseases were declining or nearly gone by the time the medications were made available to the public. Some antigerm preparations developed during that time actually made things worse, introducing new variants into the population that caused mutant strains to develop.

Now, in the last one hundred years, there have been new threats to human health, arguably more dreadful than any disease we have faced in the past. And, as profound as it may seem, indicators reflect the overall health of Americans is declining so rapidly, there is a very real possibility that we will never recover. Chronic diseases, genetic mutations, and the poisoning of every known person and animal on the face of the Earth is a result of this threat. The cause is not a viral or bacterial plague, nor some strange mutation that threatens our survival. Its face and effects are much more sinister and covert. And it is not just you who is being targeted - the damage that slowly ravishes the body is after your family and friends and can be passed down for generations to come.

What are these threats to our very existence? Toxic, man-made chemicals, and they are everywhere. They're in the food we eat, the water we drink, the air we breathe, the soil we use to grow our food, personal care products that we put on our bodies and in our mouths, the household products we use in our homes, yards, gardens, and the environment, and medications. Our food, water, and air are being systematically poisoned with harmful chemicals. Over time, the toxic burden of these chemicals builds up and accumulates in our brains and other organ systems, affecting how we feel, function, think, perform, and look. Infants, children, babies in-utero, and pregnant women are especially vulnerable to toxic chemicals, which are passed from the mother to child through the umbilical cord and breast milk. [7]

These chemicals are literally poisoning the entire world's population, from humans to wildlife to insects. There are more than 80,000 chemicals registered for use today, most of which *(approximately 60,000)* have not been studied for safety by any government agency, nor have they been studied for toxicity in synergy with each other. [8, 9]

Research and testing have shown that many of these chemicals are indeed harmful, and are known to kill, maim, and otherwise destroy the lives of innocent people, causing cancer, birth defects, and the vast majority of chronic diseases, including mental health disorders. Dr. Paula Baillie-Hamilton, an Oxford-educated physician in Britain and one of the leading authorities on food borne toxins, states, *"We are so contaminated that if we were cannibals, our meat would be banned for human consumption."* [10]

The killing fields in which we walk, talk, and have our existence, are saturated with observable evidence of harm and devastation, primarily at the hands of the industrial and pharmaceutical profiteers who develop toxic designer chemicals. Some chemicals are openly and heavily marketed to the general public in food, cleaning, and personal care products. Some are marketed to a specific industry like pest control, and still others make their way into our lives hidden in the recesses of everyday products, in the air, and in our drinking water though the guise of trade secrets *(the fragrance industry is a great example of this).* [11]

Not unlike the people who lived in the deplorable conditions in the 1800s, we are surrounded by toxic refuse - invisible synthetic chemicals - and our bodies absorb them until we are overloaded, and our organ systems begin to fail. They affect every sector of our lives, harming our children and us in the most appalling and permanent ways. The resulting physical, emotional, environmental, and economic damage over the past century is incalculable, and the alarms that should move us to take note and do something are ringing loudly.

No one is immune. Not even wildlife in the most environmentally pristine places on Earth - which says a lot about what is happening to the rest of us. Some may wonder, *"If our health is so bad, then why are we living longer?"* That's a fair question. The truth is, yes, we are living longer in terms of median survival age, but we are not living healthier, not by a long shot.

From conception to the moment we take our last breath, we are inundated with toxic, cancer-causing, and DNA-altering chemicals that are stealing our health, our longevity, our purpose, and the future of our children.

We line up every morning and await our daily dose of poisons from industries that claim to be giving us better lives, but in reality, are destroying the lives of millions of innocent men, women, and children daily. From the moment we awaken, we are exposed to hundreds and even thousands of toxic chemicals. The Environmental Working Group *(EWG),* a nonprofit research group, after an extensive year of reviewing more than one thousand biomonitoring studies, found over 420 chemicals in blood, urine, hair, and other human samples, known to or likely to cause cancer. They also conducted and published the results of an earlier 2005 study, identifying toxic chemicals, and other pollutants in the umbilical cord blood of 10 babies. It was the first test of its kind to ever be performed. What they found was shocking. Two hundred and eighty-seven industrial chemicals, some which are banned, were identified in the cord blood samples.

Of the chemicals detected, 180 are known to cause cancer in humans or animals, 217 are toxic to the brain and nervous system, and 208 cause birth defects or abnormal development in animal tests. On average, they found that each of the babies had been exposed to 200 chemicals and pollutants. A spokesperson for EWG commented, *"Had we tested for a broader array of chemicals, we would almost certainly have detected far more than 287."* Since then, other similar studies of umbilical cord blood have been published, confirming the results and identifying even hundreds more harmful chemicals embedded in our organ systems. [12]

The chemicals that rightly deserve the highest priority are those that contaminate the blood of babies before they are born - babies who are called pre-polluted by the EWG. There is an emerging consensus within scientific and medical communities that the most critical chemical exposures occur before birth, when the brain and other organs are exquisitely sensitive to trace changes in blood chemistry. But certainly, the rest of us are profoundly affected as well.

Approximately 100,000 synthetic chemicals have been unleashed on this planet worldwide with more than 1000 new chemicals entering the market-place every year. No one knows how these chemicals interact with each other. Sheldon Krimsky, Professor of Urban and Environmental Policy and Planning and adjunct professor in the Department of Family Medicine and Community Health at Tufts University School of Medicine wrote in 2008, *"[...] with up to 100,000 synthetic chemicals (approved for consumer use), the potential number of synergistic combinations becomes mind-boggling. It could take over 1000 years to complete a chemical by chemical testing program [...]"* [13]

Until recently, we were told by the mainstream media and the scientific and medical communities that we shouldn't be concerned about our toxic bioburden because, as they say *"The poison is in the dose,"* a mantra that is the foundation of our public health standards. However, many synthetic chemicals are biologically active at incredibly low levels and the combined effects have never been studied. In addition, the bioburden is cumulative. The liver is the primary filter for toxins in the body. When we are exposed to toxic chemicals, it is the liver that detoxifies and removes them into the body's elimination portals - the intestines, bladder, and skin. When the liver is overly stressed or overworked trying to remove those chemicals, it can't be as efficient detoxifying the body. The toxins then spill over into the body, circulating through the various organ systems, eventually being stored in fat and liver tissues.

Harmful effects are occurring in the human body even when the dose seems to be far below what is considered the threshold. With PCBs *(polychlori-nated biphenyl)* for instance, a known carcinogen, it only takes five parts per billion *(ppb)* in the mother's blood, the equivalent of one drop of water in 9,440 gallons of water *(118 bathtubs full)*, to cause permanent brain damage to a fetus in the womb. Even though production was banned in the United States in 1978, it is estimated that 40% of the PCB production is still in use in some capacity. [14]

In my youth, I remember seeing a commercial produced by DuPont touting *"better things for better living, through chemistry."* The idea of this new technology was exciting, and many people, including me, bought into it. But while the promise of DuPont's commercial was true, there was *(and is)* a dark side that is just as true, and certainly more important. In a landmark alliance known as project TENDR [15], forty-seven leaders and fifteen professional health organizations of various disciplines have come together in support of a consensus statement to say that many of the chemicals found in everyday products can result in neurodevelopmental disorders, including autism and attention-deficit disorders among others. *"Ten years ago, this consensus wouldn't have been possible, but the research is abundantly clear,"* said Irva Hertz-Piccioto, an environmental epidemiologist at the University of California, Davis, and co-chairwoman of Project TENDR. Many other concerned researchers, scientists, physicians, moms, dads, and children have voiced the same concerns. [16] Something must be done to solve this problem.

Better life through chemistry at its core is simply about money and power. And, the profiteers and scientists that are paid to develop chemicals often know how harmful those chemicals are, but don't seem to care about their impact on the lives of innocent people, most of whom are just trying to live a decent and productive life and raise a healthy family.

The health challenges we face are intimately connected with the toxic chemicals we interact with every day. These health challenges include cancer, chronic diseases, and unnecessary surgeries, especially removal of female reproductive organs and the thyroid. The chance to have healthy children is stolen from parents because of unnecessary and harmful vaccine mandates that are permanently disabling many children with diseases such as ASD *(Autism Spectrum Disorder)*, ADHD, and other neurological and immune disorders, as well as asthma, chronic allergies, and gluten intolerance. All this has created an open door for Big Pharma to introduce even more medications, necessary according to them, to give us *"better life through chemistry."* Would you believe I see patients on as many as 20 medications? And to top it off, the side effect of many of these medications is dementia *(loss of memory).* Anti-anxiety and depression medications, opioid analgesics, high blood pressure medications, and even cholesterol-lowering medications are stealing our memory and causing mental illness. [17] And when we don't have our memory, Big Pharma and the rest of the chemical industry profiting from our *"ill- health" (caused by their medications)* can get an even better stranglehold on our bodies without being noticed.

We are not living the healthy lives that we deserve *(nor the ones promised to us by DuPont's commercial).* And while we do have to take responsibility for our own choices, we cannot make good choices without good information, like the knowledge you will gain from reading this book. What's worse is that whatever unhealthy lifestyle choices we may make, or whatever chronic illnesses we may develop from bioaccumulation of the toxic chemicals that infest our bodies, these effects alter our genes and can be epigenetically passed down to future generations. *(I'll go into greater detail on this in Chapter 2).*

We need to seriously come to terms with the fact that we live in a toxic world and we should understand the implications of this fact on our health.

"Chemicals have replaced bacteria and viruses as the main threat to human health. . . . the diseases we're beginning to see as the major causes of death in the latter part of the 20th century and into the 21st century are diseases of 'chemical origin'," writes Rick Irvin, toxicologist Texas A&M University. [18]

The most likely causes of the chemical insults that we experience every day include exposure to pesticides sprayed on crops, synthetic chemicals in the processed foods that we consume, insecticides, air and water pollution, and personal care products [19] that we use every day. Organophosphate pesticides, medications, vaccines, and industrial chemicals in every sector of our lives including flame retardants, lead, mercury, phthalates, and other plastics such as Bisphenol A *(BPA)* that can be found in food, water, furniture, food wrap, cookware, cans, carpets, shower curtains, electronics and even shampoo are all harmful. They are everywhere around us, and we don't know what the synergistic impact of the chemicals may be. [20] This sentiment was reflected in a statement from 2004 by the editors of Environmental Science and Technology, and American chemical Society Journal: *"It is a virtual certainty that other (chemical synergy) effects are occurring in the field that we are presently overlooking in the lab. How can all biodiversity be protected from the myriad of chemicals they are now exposed to when, we do not even know what is there?"*

Why Can't The Environmental Protection Agency Put A Stop To This Madness?

Of the 80,000 plus chemicals currently approved for use in the marketplace, as of 2016, the Environmental Protection Agency *(EPA)* has only been able to ban nine. That's it!! Just nine. [21]

Thanks to a manipulated and broken piece of legislation called the Toxic Control Substance Act *(TCSA)*, regulators like the Environmental Protection Agency *(EPA)* had to *"prove"* a substance posed an *"unreasonable risk"* before the they could act. The EPA was given the responsibility to enforce the TSCA but didn't have the authority because of the restrictive language contained in the TSCA law. So, what started as an attempt to protect people from dangerous chemicals actually became a shield of armor for the chemical industry. In addition, *(only the government can manage this kind of corruption)* all of the 62,000 plus chemicals that were already on the market were grandfathered in and no toxicity testing was required. That is appalling!

The EPA's power was severely restricted by the TSCA's burden of proof requirement that a chemical is toxic and dangerous only after people have been knowingly harmed or killed. But that supposedly changed when the TSCA was overhauled in 2016. Now, it is not so much the TSCA that is the problem, but it is the EPA that is engaging in bureaucratic shenanigans to keep from enforcing the totality and intention of the revised TSCA. Curiously, they seem to make strange bedfellows as evidenced by the recent attempts by the EPA themselves, to *"down-regulate"* the 2016-approved, newly acquired TSCA power to regulate. Now, I know that sounds bizarre, but that is one more of the head-scratching and boneheaded decisions made by our government bureaucrats. Not convinced? There's more as you read on. Here are just some of the heavy hitter chemicals that many of us are exposed to on a daily basis.

Asbestos

A couple of examples might help bring the severity of the problem into better focus. Remember asbestos? Many people think it was banned - it wasn't. It was restricted but is still used in many products thanks to a Federal court's down-regulation of the originally passed ban. Due to the ruling, proving the toxicity of asbestos became so difficult that the Environmental Protection Agency couldn't ban it completely, even though it is a known carcinogen that still kills approximately 12,000 to 15,000 people in the United States each year. That number is most likely low, since tracking deaths related to asbestos is difficult. [22]

Phthalates and BPA

Another example is phthalate which is a plasticizer used to soften plastics and improve the flexibility and durability of products made from harmful chemicals like Bisphenol A *(BPA)*, Phthalates are commonly used in products that we use in almost every aspect of our daily lives from baby toys and household cleaners to food packaging to fragrance, cosmetics, and personal-care products. Approximately 900 billion tons of plastic products have been made since the 1950s and 260 million tons of plastics are made every year, and production is increasing. [23]

Phthalates and BPA plastics are used all over the world and studies are emerging that clearly implicate them as a big-time health hazard. There are over 200 published articles alone describing the health hazards associated with BPA plastic, commonly described as endocrine system hormone disruptors, or xeno-estrogens, since they mimic the actions of estrogen. These endocrine system disruptor chemicals imitate our natural hormones by affecting any or all of the glands that produce hormones. This can trigger or disrupt our natural hormone production. Estrogens associated with the reproductive system are especially vulnerable to disruptor chemicals sometimes called *"gender bender"* synthetics. BPA affects development *(especially in children),* memory, and learning. Therefore, BPA has been shown to play a role in the pathogenesis of several endocrine disorders including female and male infertility, precocious puberty, hormone dependent tumors such as breast and prostate cancer, and several metabolic disorders including polycystic ovary syndrome *(PCOS).* Our hormone receptors cannot distinguish these toxins from the natural estrogenic hormone estradiol. [24]

In addition, their industrial wastes from processing plants are present in the air and in our water systems including our streams, lakes, and oceans. DDT, PCBs, and other toxins are absorbed in the water with plastic polymers. Fish eat the plastic pellets, and we eat the fish. [23]

In the past few years, researchers have linked phthalates to asthma, attention-deficit hyperactivity disorder, breast cancer, obesity and type II diabetes, low IQ, neurodevelopmental issues, behavioral issues, autism spectrum disorders, altered reproductive development, asthma, deteriorating birth rates and male fertility issues including a 50% loss of male sperm count since the 1930s. Hermaphrodite fish with both male and female sex organs are also being found in many lakes and streams, mostly downstream from industries dumping chemicals into the local water systems. [24, 25]

For example, Hermaphrodite shellfish and other fish have been turning up all along the northeastern coast of Chesapeake Bay along the Potomac River in Maryland. At least 60% of fish examined by scientists in 2003 and 2004 had mutated into hermaphrodites - or from male to female - with the fish born male having eggs growing inside their testes. Numerous pharmaceutical drugs were detected in the river. *"We might just be seeing the tip of the iceberg in terms of cumulative impact of all this,"* commented Thomas Burke Ph.D., then Associate Chairman of Health Policy at the Johns Hopkins

Bloomberg School of Public Health in Baltimore. He is also the former Deputy Assistant Administrator of Environmental Protection Agency's *(EPA)* Office of Research and Development *(ORD)* as well as EPA's Science Advisor.[24]

These findings were particularly alarming because Washington DC and other cities along the Potomac River drink water from the river. Such reproductive mutations in fish have been showing up across the United States.

From another perspective, a group of 120 scientists from around the world met in Prague in May, 2005, and issued a warning and an appeal to all governments to acknowledge their *"serious concerns about the high prevalence of reproductive disorders in European boys and young men."* The health specialists identified endocrine disruptor chemicals as the prime suspect for the epidemic of reproductive abnormalities being seen worldwide.

Studies in pediatrics and other medical journals reveal that since the early 1960s there has been an estimated 40% increase in male infants born in Europe and United States with symptoms of feminization. At least 10% of all couples in the United States are unable to conceive a child and the number seems to be growing. Among eight-year-old girls in the United States Britain and Australia one out of every six has already entered puberty with breast growth, pubic hair, and even menstruation. Just a generation ago, only one out of every ten eight-year-old girls had entered puberty. [27]

Early puberty in girls as young as eight years old becomes easier to understand when we look at the research. There are many hormone- mimicking chemicals that we are all exposed to on a daily basis including the environmental contamination with BPA, an estrogen-mimicking hormone. Recombinant Bovine Growth Hormones *(RBGH)* is found in store bought dairy products and in the school system's lunch programs and can also contribute to early puberty. It gets worse; RBGH, which increases the production of milk in cows, is reportedly banned in 27 countries including Europe, Japan, New Zealand, and Canada. It artificially stimulates a cancer-causing hormone in cows called IGF 1, which is in the milk that humans drink and has been linked to cancers including breast, prostate, and others. Developed by Monsanto, the chemical giant has been successful in deterring any significant restrictions on the drug in the United States. It is also in American made cheeses and most any other dairy product that we consume. Phthalates, BPA, and RBGH should be better controlled in a supposedly responsible government like the United States. [28]

Exposure to toxic environmental chemicals during pregnancy and breast-feeding is ubiquitous and is a threat to healthy human reproduction. There are tens of thousands of chemicals in global commerce, and even small exposures to toxic chemicals during pregnancy can trigger adverse health consequences.

In a special communication written in the Journal of the Gynecology and Obstetrics in 2015, the multi-author article said this about the current chemical toxicity that envelops the globe:

"Widespread exposure to toxic environmental chemicals threatens healthy human reproduction. Industrial chemicals are used and discarded in every aspect of daily life and are ubiquitous in food, water, air, and consumer products. Exposure to environmental chemicals and metals permeates all parts of life across the globe. Toxic chemicals enter the environment through food and energy production, industrial emissions and accidents, waste, transportation, and the making, use, and disposal of consumer and personal care products..." [29]

Trichloroethylene - TCE

Our water supply is poisoned, chiefly by industrial pollution via smokestacks and waste water runoff, by livestock excrement loaded with agricultural chemicals, and artificial fertilizers *(which is often recycled toxic sewage sludge loaded with heavy metals that accumulate in our body),* by pesticide runoff as well as the human and animal elimination of medication, and by cleaning chemicals and even medications routinely and indiscriminately poured down the drain. I have regretfully taken part in this when my father-in-law passed away from cancer. After he passed, the attending nurse in our home said she needed to pour all of his medications down the drain since she could not take them with her. I agreed at the time, since I didn't know how harmful this was. Guess who is drinking the water that has those chemicals and many others in it? Just imagine how many people a day *"eliminate"* their bodily waste laced with toxic chemicals and medications into our drinking water. Those chemicals do not get removed through the local municipal filtration system. Many studies have shown how contaminated our drinking water is with pharmaceuticals and their metabolites and other unsavory chemicals. In a 2008 study, one of many such studies, fifty-six pharmaceutical drugs and their metabolites were found in Philadelphia's drinking water.

One of the deadlier industrial chemicals in our water supply is TCE *(trichloroethylene)*, a cancer-causing solvent that contaminates the water supply of an estimated 14 million Americans. It is a poison that was most notably brought to the public consciousness back in 1995 in the book and film, a Civil Action. The contamination was again verified most recently in a 2018 release by the EWG. Previous studies in 2013 and 2015 found that TCE is polluting our water supplies throughout the United States. *"People whose water contains TCE can be exposed not just by drinking it, but also by inhaling it while bathing, washing dishes, and doing other household activities,"* said Tasha Stoiber, Ph.D., a senior scientist at EWG. *"Communities across the country have water with potentially harmful levels of this toxic solvent, but many people don't know about the risk they face when they turn on the tap."*[30]

TCE was also detected in EPA-mandated tests by more than 300 public water systems in 36 states. Drinking TCE-contaminated water has been linked to liver and kidney damage, and to cancers like leukemia. It has also been linked to birth defects, but EPA documents raise concern that the agency will downplay important evidence that TCE exposure causes heart defects in developing fetuses. [31]

DDT

Many people growing up in the latter twentieth century remember the controversy about DDT. It was partially banned by the US decades ago because it is a blatant carcinogen and endocrine disrupter, but it also persists or stockpiles in the environment as well as in our bodies. It has even been implicated as a major contributing factor to the polio-like symptoms seen in the late 1940's and 50s that caused the original polio panic. There will be much more on this in the Vaccine chapter. The United States still makes it and sells it to other countries, many of them Third World, even though it was banned here in our own country. African nations have brought DDT back in full force as a weapon against malaria. Scientists have tracked DDT containing clouds in the region that eventually rain over the United States soils and waters. DDT has even been found in the tissue of penguins in the South Pole region and polar bears in the North Pole region, supposedly the few remaining places on earth thought to be free from industrial chemicals. Aside from the trade winds and water currents that bring it back to us, many of these countries supply our foods that are also laced with DDT. In essence, organochloride pesticides, even the most carcinogenic ones banned decades ago, are unavoidable in our environments. Unfortunately, they are also among the most potent causes of cancer, other chronic diseases, and organ malfunctions. The body is unable to completely metabolize, detoxify, and permanently get rid of many parts of these pesticides.[32, 33]

Commenting on the current state of affairs with toxic chemicals especially related to pesticides impacting human health, the Pesticide Action Network of North America declared:

"The human body is not designed to cope with synthetic pesticides. Yet we all carry within our bodies a cocktail of chemicals designed to kill insects, weeds, and other agricultural and household paths. Many of the pesticides we carry in our bodies can cause cancer, disruptor hormone systems, decrease fertility, cause birth defects, or weaken our immune systems. These are just some of the known detrimental effects of particular pesticides at very low levels of exposure.

Almost nothing is known about the long-term impact of multiple chemicals in the body over long periods from chemical trespass." [34]

Cosmetics

The cosmetic industry in the United States is saturated with toxic chemicals. There are more than 25,000 chemicals in cosmetics sold in United States, yet less than 4% of these ingredients have ever been tested for toxicity and safety. The European Union has banned over 1,300 chemicals found in cosmetics. The FDA has only banned eight and restricted three. The average woman puts 515 synthetic chemicals on her body every single day without even knowing it. And 60% of what we put onto our skin is absorbed into our bodies. [35] [36]

Fluoride

Fluoride is not the knight in shining armor for resolving tooth decay that so many people think it is. Nor is it safe to be consumed in drinking water or toothpaste or in any other way. It is in just about every store-bought toothpaste and the American Dental Association estimates that 72.5% of Americans live in areas with fluoridated drinking water. [37]

Up until the 1970s, scientists in Europe prescribed fluoride to reduce the basal metabolism rate in patients with an over-active thyroid gland. One published clinical study from this period reported that doses of just two to three milligrams of fluoride - a dose that many, if not most, Americans now receive on a regular basis - were sufficient to reduce thyroid activity in hyperthyroid patients. [38]

It's actually quite a toxic substance and was used as a rat poison and insecticide in the early to mid 1900s. It was first used in a municipal water supply in Grand Rapids, Michigan, in 1945, and estimates suggest that over 65% of the water supply in the United States is fluorinated. For more than fifty years, there has been much debate about the health risks associated with fluoride exposure and the necessity of it, given that fluoride is contained in toothpaste. There were deeply flawed studies initially supporting the use of fluoride for prevention of dental cavities. But subsequent recent analysis in the Cochran's Collaboration report reveals that countries that don't have fluoride in their drinking water have as low or lower incidence of dental cavities than countries that do have it. [39]

As of June 2018, a total of 60 studies have investigated the relationship between fluoride and human intelligence, and over 40 studies have investigated the relationship between fluoride and learning/memory in animals. Of these investigations, 53 studies have found that elevated fluoride exposure is associated with reduced IQ in humans, while 45 animal studies have found that fluoride exposure impairs the learning and/or memory capacity of animals. The human studies, which are based on IQ examinations of over 15,000 children, provide compelling evidence that fluoride exposure during the early years of life can damage a child's developing brain. [40]

After reviewing 27 of the human IQ studies, a team of Harvard scientists concluded that fluoride's effect on the young brain should now be a *"high research priority."* Other reviewers have reached similar conclusions, including the prestigious National Research Council *(NRC),* and scientists in the Neurotoxicology Division of the Environmental Protection Agency. [41]

Dr. Dean Burk, Chief Chemist Emeritus, US National Cancer Institute in the 1970s attributed over 70,000 deaths a year to fluoridation based on *"conclusive scientific and biological evidence"* that he has come across in his 50 years of cancer research. Dr. Burk has also gone on record to say that fluoride causes more human cancer, and causes it faster, than any other chemical.

He also stated that according to the Delany Clause in The Food Additives Amendment of 1958, an amendment to the United States' Food, Drugs, and Cosmetic Act of 1938, that if a substance were found to cause cancer in man or animal, then it could not be used as a food additive. Dr. Burk says conclusively that fluoride is a cancer-causing chemical and should not be used in water. [42]

"In point of fact, fluoride causes more human cancer death, and causes it faster, than any other chemical." Dr. Dean Burk

Here are some interesting facts about the fluoride toothpaste that the vast majority of consumers put into their mouth every day:

- Over 95% of toothpastes now contain fluoride.

- A single strip of toothpaste covering the length of a child's brush contains between 0.75 to 1.5 mg of fluoride. This exceeds the amount of fluoride in most prescription fluoride supplements *(0.25 to 1.0 mg)*.

- Many young children swallow over 50% of the paste added to their brush, particularly if they use candy-flavored varieties and if they are not supervised during brushing to ensure they spit and fully rinse. Research has shown that some children swallow more fluoride from toothpaste alone than is recommended from all sources combined.

- Although dentists now recommend that children only use *"a pea-sized amount"* of toothpaste, many children use more than this, particularly when the toothpaste has bubble gum and watermelon flavors.

- Ingesting toothpaste during childhood can also cause symptoms of acute fluoride toxicity *(e.g., stomach pain, etc.)*. Excessive fluoride also causes dental fluorosis - changes in tooth enamel that range from barely noticeable white spots to staining and pitting.

- The FDA now requires a poison warning on all fluoride toothpastes sold in the US.

- Fluoride can also become concentrated in bone - stimulating bone cell growth, altering the tissue's structure, and weakening the skeleton. [43, 44, 45]

Have you ever looked at the warning label on the back of a tube of toothpaste? Antibacterial toothpaste contains fluoride and may contain triclosan, which is known to be carcinogenic. Aside from the serious implications on the warning label to call a poison control center if more than a normal amount for brushing teeth is swallowed, both absorb directly in the blood stream when it comes in contact with the superficial blood vessels under the tongue. So, you are getting the cancer-causing chemicals regardless. Besides that, you may also have aspartame *(artificial sweetener and propylene glycol (antifreeze))* in your toothpaste!

Deodorant, shaving cream, toothpaste, trash cans, clothing, cutting boards, credit cards - these are just a few of the ways consumers can come into contact with triclosan. A growing body of evidence suggests that it can be harmful, but should you be concerned?

The FDA banned triclosan's use in antibacterial liquid soaps in 2016. It did the same last year for over-the-counter antiseptic products, such as hand washes and surgical scrubs, in hospitals, doctors' offices, and other healthcare settings. The agency banned it from antibacterial soaps because, it said, companies failed to prove triclosan was safe. And yet we put it in our mouth every time we brush our teeth.

The FDA's ban was limited, however, in part, because of the way products are regulated. Soaps that make antibacterial claims are considered over-the-counter drugs and subject to FDA approval. But the agency has different regulatory power over products considered cosmetics, such as shaving gels and lotions, in which triclosan may be used as a preservative. These products don't have to gain FDA approval before being sold.

"Because of its use in so many products, it enters the environment, and into the sewage system," says Ted Schettler, M.D., science director for the Science and Environment Health Network in Eugene, OR. Triclosan has been detected in fresh water streams and rivers all over the country. It's been measured in fish that we eat and in vegetables. It has been associated with cancer, human reproduction disorders, allergies, asthma, antimicrobial resistance,

and destruction of gut bacteria, which is critical to a properly functioning immune system. There are much better toothpaste alternatives, which I discuss in the New Beginnings Chapter." [46, 47]

Chlorine And Chloramine

Chlorine and chloramine *(chlorine and ammonia)* are used as water disinfectants. Their use is widespread. Chlorination as a drinking water disinfectant had its beginnings in the early 1900s. Because of its disinfecting properties, it was very helpful in containing the spread of diseases through contaminated water during the difficult early years of the Industrial Revolution when so many people were crowding into cities and contaminating the local water supplies. The first municipal chlorination of water took place in New Jersey in 1908, and many other municipalities followed soon after. [48]

While the benefits of chlorination at that time in history are well recognized, there are some unintended side effects of chlorination that have been observed over the years, including the creation of a family of chemicals known as trihalomethanes or *"disinfection by-products"* or plainly, toxic trash. Four members of this family are regulated by the EPA, including chloroform, which is a familiar term to many. These are classified as *"probable"* human carcinogens and some scientists suspect that trihalomethanes in drinking water may cause thousands of cases of bladder cancer every year. These chemicals have also been linked to colon and rectal cancer, birth defects, low birth weight, and miscarriages. [49]

There are more than 600 unwanted chemicals created by the interaction of water treatment and pollutants in source water and many more are suspected. Most have not been studied in any depth for their impact on health. [50]

In recent years, many water utilities have tried to reduce chlorine-induced contamination caused by water treatment by switching from free chlorine to chloramines, compounds made from chlorine and ammonia gases. Yet switching to chloramines has not solved the problem, but rather moved the problem - and may have complicated it. [51]

Chloramines are toxic to kidney dialysis patients and extremely toxic to fish *(EPA 2012b)* and can form dangerous compounds called nitrosamines which according to Federal Government sources are *"reasonably anticipated"* to be human carcinogens.

In a 2011 report called *"The Chlorine Dilemma,"* David Sedlak, a professor of civil and environmental engineering at the University of California, Berkeley, detailed the *"dark side"* of water treatment and the new and unanticipated hazards of water treatment plants' shift from chlorine to chloramine. *"Nitrosamines are the compounds that people warned you about when they told you shouldn't be eating those nitrite-cured hot dogs,"* Sedlak told National Public Radio in 2011. *"They're about a thousand times more carcinogenic than the disinfection by-products that we'd been worried about with regular old chlorine."* [52]

Perchlorate

A 2005 study of lactating women in 18 US states found the toxin, perchlorate, in practically every mother's milk. The source was food eaten by the mothers that had been tainted from water, which was polluted by perchlorate seeping from defense industry plants scattered around the nation. Perchlorate is known to adversely affect the thyroid and other glands of the body. It inhibits iodide uptake and may impair thyroid and neurodevelopment in infants.

In an article published in the journal, Environmental Science and Technology, the authors wrote: *"Recently, we unambiguously identified the presence of perchlorate in all seven brands of dairy milk randomly purchased from grocery stores in Lubbock, TX. How widespread is perchlorate in milk? Perchlorate in 47 dairy milk samples from 11 states and in 36 human milk samples from 18 states were measured. Perchlorate was detectable in 81 of 82 samples. Perchlorate is present in virtually all milk samples, the average concentration in breast milk is five times higher than in dairy milk."* [53]

Your Grocery Store Experience

There are approximately 3,000 chemicals in our food supply and when the liver is unable to process the overload on a daily basis, many of these are stored in our fat and liver cells. Also, when you read *"made with natural flavors"* on a food label, that doesn't necessarily mean that it is good for you because natural flavors and artificial flavors usually contain the same chemicals. *"Natural"* may have originated from ingredients in nature, but chemical processing and manipulation can create a whole different product that can be harmful to our health. Also, *"natural"* can mean that there are synthetic ingredients that have been injected with yeast, so a manufacturer can call it "natural." Many lawsuits have been adjudicated regarding the food industry's indiscriminate and deceptive use of the term *"natural"* in their food and beverage products. [54, 55, 56]

At least 70% of the processed foods in the grocery store contain at least one genetically engineered ingredient that has never been tested for its potential harm. Artificial sweeteners in soft drinks and other foods have been linked to brain tumors, Parkinson's disease, Alzheimer's disease, and other neurological diseases. Very few of the 3000 synthetic chemicals that are regularly added to US food products have been tested for their synergistic toxin-producing effect in the human body. Even soy products have been shown to be detrimental to health, but soy continues to be promoted as a healthy food choice. Soy here in the United States is heavy laden with pesticides and is a mostly genetically modified product. In addition, soy contains high levels of an estrogen equivalent that babies may receive in their milk formula.

Don't think that just because you see a beautiful package of spinach at the grocery store that it is healthy for you. Aside from the many chemicals laced throughout, it is most likely lacking in essential nutrients. Mass farming techniques may give us a bigger and prettier harvest, but the crops are severely lacking in the micronutrients necessary for optimal cell function.

Processing of food removes vital macro and micronutrients from our food sources. USDA nutrition information reveals nutrient levels in our food. Between 1973 and 1997 for every vegetable grown in the United States, every single nutrient that can be measured in each category of vegetable has undergone huge declines. For raw broccoli, average calcium levels dropped 53%, riboflavin declined 48%, thiamine nose-dived 35%, niacin 29%. Similar nutrient declines were found in cabbage, carrots, cauliflower, onions, and a long list of others.

When whole wheat is refined into white flour for white bread, the percentage and range of nutrients lost is extraordinary: fiber 95%, iron 84%, vitamin E 95%, manganese 82%, niacin 80%, and vitamin B 281%. Most foods are also irradiated to neutralize insects and microorganisms, but this process further destroys vitamins and other essential nutrients in the food and eliminates the soil organisms that produce natural antibiotic content. To compensate, the food processors have resorted to synthetic food additives. *"No functional food can ever replace the full range of nutrients and phytochemicals present in and fruits, vegetables, and whole grains,"* writes Marion Nestlé.

A scientific nail in the coffin of the quote, *"We get all the supplements we need in food,"* myth came in 2002 when the Journal of the American Medical Association published an article that reviewed 30 years of medical research about the relationship between vitamins and chronic diseases. The trend was clear, showing that most people get less than optimal intake of vitamins from food and that puts them at an increased risk for cardiovascular disease, cancer, and other ailments. *"All adults should take one multivitamin daily,"* the Harvard researchers concluded. [57]

The Environmental Working Group has put out its annual *"Dirty Dozen"* list of fruits and vegetables that have the greatest amounts of pesticide contamination - the 15th such list - and strawberries are once again top the rankings. The 2019 complete list shakes down like this: [58]

1. Strawberries

2. Spinach

3. Kale

4. Nectarines

5. Apples

6. Grapes

7. Peaches

8. Cherries

9. Pears

10. Tomatoes

11. Celery

12. Potatoes

Before you buy that grocery store steak, you might want to know what's at stake. In feedlots, the cattle are directly or indirectly given growth hormones, pesticides, antibiotics, herbicides, and genetically modified feed. One hundred percent of the cattle prepared for the general marketplace are fed five or more sex hormones including progesterone and testosterone to accelerate weight gain and these hormones are known to cause reproductive dysfunction and cancers in humans.

In the book, *The One Hundred Year Lie*, author Randall Fitzgerald notes that medical evidence is emerging that suggests artificial sweeteners and diet soft drinks may cause brain tumors and other neurological diseases such as Parkinson's and Alzheimer's, headaches, and addictions. The occurrence of these diseases has risen dramatically in proportion to the expanded use of those synthetic sweeteners.

Most vitamins and supplements sold in the United States that are advertised as natural are actually synthetic chemical concoctions that contain coal tar, preservatives, artificial coloring, and a vast range of other potentially harmful additives. For the most part, they are a waste of your money. Synthetic vitamins are arguably not processed by the body the same way as whole food vitamins, which are generally a *"complex"* of intimately, connected natural compounds that the body prefers. Synthetics also have a different *"optical activity"* or *"stereochemistry"* where the synthetic form may have the same chemical makeup, but the way it is organized is different. The body is smart and recognizes this difference and cannot use it in the same way as the form coming from nature. The science studies demonstrating the superiority of naturally occurring vitamins over synthetics have been published in such journals as the Annals of the New York Academy of Sciences, American Journal of Clinical Nutrition, and Britain's Royal Society of Chemistry. While we should be eating healthy foods to begin with, it is also a wise idea to cover our vitamin and mineral needs with a good whole food vitamin/mineral/ micronutrient complex. We can use the extra support living in a world of high stress and toxic overload. [59]

What other chemicals are found in the grocery store foods?

Flame Retardants: These have been linked to cancer (PBDEs, a bromine compound) and they contaminate grocery products such as fish, pork, turkey, cheese, butter, milk, cheese, chicken, and turkey. Tests have found these chemicals to be carcinogenic and damaging to the nervous system for motor functions and reproductive organs. [60]

Methyl Bromide: A highly toxic gas fumigant and pesticide used on tomatoes, strawberries, and other crops. Lungs can be severely injured even by short-term exposure and neurological damage can occur with longer exposures. . While short and long-term exposure is not likely for the average grocery store consumer, the residues may pose a threat.

Phthalates/BPA: Used in food packages and is known to leach into whatever it wraps or containers such as water bottles, baby bottles, meat wraps, plastic containers that get microwaved including such as those plastic spaghetti sauce storage containers, all leach this chemical into the foods.

Fruit and vegetable cans are lined with a plastic, Bisphenol A, *(BPA)* which also coats the receipts that you get at the checkout counter. If you handle receipts regularly, or your hands are sweaty, or you have on a hand lotion that absorbs into your skin, you will absorb BPA into your body. When used in thermal paper, BPA is present as *"free" (i.e., discrete, non-polymerized)* BPA, which is likely to be more available for exposure than BPA polymerized into a resin or plastic. When handling receipts, there is some concern that residues on hands could be ingested through incidental hand-to-mouth contact. [61]

Sweet Poison

Most everyone now is aware of the dangers of consuming too much sugar. Too much sugar can lead to diabetes, heart disease, obesity, cancer, and a whole host of other diseases. It is frequently referred to as *"sweet poison."* However, high fructose corn syrup (HFCS)is a much more deadly poison. The FDA only controls *"acute"* toxins. Because fructose's negative impact on health occurs over an extended time, it is conveniently considered a chronic poison so the FDA does not regulate it.

HFCS is particularly dangerous because it is hidden in so many products. For example, did you know that a typical carbonated soft drink could have 55 mg of salt? Why does that matter? It matters because the sodium makes you thirstier. The salty taste is then hidden by the sweetness of HFCS. Additionally, the caffeine that may be in coke type beverages acts as a diuretic, which causes you to lose water through urination. It's a vicious cycle of dependence, the more you drink, the more you urinate, the thirstier you become, the more you drink. The equation is simple: more thirsty = more coke = increased manufacturer profits - absolutely calculated. [62] I will cover HFCS in greater detail in the *Hunger Games chapter.*

Warnings about the toxicity of aspartame were issued in 1991 by the National Institutes of Health, and in 1994 by the United States Department of Health and Human Services, detailing 88 documented symptoms of aspartame toxicity. A partial list includes birth defects, depression, mental retardation, chronic fatigue syndrome, brain tumors, epilepsy, multiple sclerosis, Parkinson's and Alzheimer's. And yet, even though this is a toxic chemical, it remains widespread as an additive throughout the US food supply and that of many other nations. [63]

The best defense is a great offense in the grocery store. Look at labels before you put those groceries in your cart!

Chronic Diseases

Toxic chemicals that envelop every part of our lives inescapably lead to chronic diseases and premature death. Disorders such as heart disease, cancer, lower respiratory disease, Alzheimer's disease, asthma, allergies, diabetes, etc. reduce our quality of life and are the leading causes of death and disability. They affect over 133 million Americans. Roughly forty-five percent of the adult population has at least one chronic disease, and they are responsible for seven out of every ten deaths. [64]

Cardiovascular Disease has gone from rare up until the late 1800s, to the number two killer recently upstaged by cancer, now the number one cause of death in those less than eight-five years old. The incidence of cancer has risen dramatically with lung, breast, prostate, and colorectal cancer occupying the top four spots. Breast Cancer has gained national attention in recent years because of the increasing incidence. It is the most commonly diagnosed cancer and the leading cause of cancer death in women. The problem is that about 40% of people undergoing the rigors of cancer treatment who survive, will die of cancer or a reportedly unrelated disease within seven years. But, research does show connections between the cancer treatment and those diseases. [65]

In most cases of treated breast cancer, the cause of death is cardiovascular disease. Treatments such as chemotherapy and radiation used for breast cancer end up damaging muscle and nerve tissue. Cancer deaths have been declining since the 1990s, but the way these stats are calculated leaves out important information that makes the numbers look better, but in reality these *"unrelated"* deaths are directly or indirectly related to the cancer and/or treatment for the cancer. Women have been convinced that chemo, radiation, and surgery are the only way. And that is just not the case. There are other options that work even better and without the side effects.

Since 1950, the explosive growth of certain types of cancer has become mind-numbing. Skin melanoma cases are up 690%. Prostate Cancer up 286%. Thyroid cancer up 258%. Non-Hodgkin's lymphoma up 249%. Liver and intrahepatic cancer up 234%. Kidney and renal pelvis cancers up 182%, and the list goes on. During a speech in 1994, Dr. Samuel Epstein, an international expert in toxicology, laid the blame squarely on the synthetics in the chemical revolution. Dr. Epstein stated that in 1940, we produced about 1 billion pounds of new synthetic chemicals. By 1950, the figure had reached 50 trillion pounds, and by the late '80s it became 500 trillion pounds. Most of these chemicals have not been tested for toxic, carcinogenic, or environmental effects. Also, a report done by Columbia University School of Public Health estimated that 95% of cancer cases are caused by diet and environmental toxicity. [66, 67, 68, 69]

In 2018, an estimated 1,735,350 new cases of cancer will be diagnosed in the United States and 609,640 people will die from the disease. It is the leading cause of death among people ages 65-84. [70]

Diabetes has gone from .2% in the 1890s to over 9.4% with near epidemic levels in both adults AND children, accounting for over 30.3 million people and getting worse every year. There are an estimated 84.1 million people with pre-diabetes, which works out to 34% of American adults. By 2020, it is estimated that 50% of the population will have diabetes or pre-diabetes. [71]

Obesity in adults as well as in children is near epidemic levels. A probable low estimate is that 70% of Americans are overweight, with 40% that are obese affecting over 93,000,000 Americans. Compare this to 1960 when only about 10.5% of Americans were overweight. Obesity is projected to 50% by 2030. Childhood obesity is at 18.5%, triple the levels in the 1970s. Obesity-related conditions include heart disease, stroke, type 2 diabetes and certain types of cancer, some of the leading causes of preventable death. There are multiple causes of the obesity epidemic, which many researchers report can be traced back to Ancel Keyes and the low fat, high carb movement.[72]

Arthritis remains a serious health crisis in the United States - and it's a global epidemic as well. Recent estimates show that as many as 91 million Americans may have arthritis *(37%),* including a third of those aged 18-64, plus an estimated 300,000 children. Arthritis is very common, but not well understood. Actually, *"arthritis"* is not a single disease; it is an informal way of referring to joint pain or joint disease. There are more than 100 different types of arthritis and related conditions. People of all ages, genders, and races have arthritis, the leading cause of disability in the United States. We don't know the true number of people with arthritis because many people don't seek treatment until their symptoms become severe. Osteoarthritis is the most common form of arthritis. Gout, fibromyalgia, and rheumatoid arthritis are other common, arthritis-like conditions. [73, 74]

More than one million Americans have been diagnosed with rheumatoid arthritis *(RA),* and about 75% of those are women. Unlike osteoarthritis, which is a wear and tear degenerative joint disease, rheumatoid arthritis is where the immune system is triggered to eat its own joint flesh and other cells. It is crippling people, and the incidence is increasing, especially in females.

Between 1995 and 2007, there was a 20% rise in RA in women. It affects more than 2,000,000 Americans. Other autoimmune diseases such as lupus, celiac, and type 1 diabetes, continue to rise mostly from immune system reactions to environmental chemicals.

Leading Causes Of Death

If you search the available literature, there is some debate on the top causes of death, but most of that is because the trends are generally broken down into age categories *(which can get a little troublesome to interpret)* and, would you believe, an incomplete, inefficient, and sometimes manipulated reporting system.

The discrepancy becomes more important with the third leading cause of death, which is generally listed as chronic lower respiratory disease. But, it is little known or publicized that the actual third leading cause of death in the United States is medical errors after heart disease and cancer, causing at least 250,000 deaths every year.

"People don't just die from heart attacks and bacteria, they die from system-wide failings and poorly coordinated care," says the study's lead author, Dr. Martin Makary, a professor of surgery and health policy at Johns Hopkins University School of Medicine. *"It's medical care gone awry."* [75, 76]

Leading Causes of Death
Cancer
Heart Disease
MEDICAL ERRORS
ADVERSE DRUG REACTIONS
Accidents
Alzheimer's
Diabetes

"Throughout the world, medical error leading to patient death is an under-recognized epidemic," Makary and his co-author, Dr. Michael Daniel, also of Johns Hopkins, write in the British Medical Journal. They define medical errors as lapses in judgment, skill, or coordination of care, mistaken diagnoses, and system failures that lead to patient deaths or the failure to rescue dying patients, and preventable complications of care. The Hopkins team used evidence from four studies that analyzed medical death rate data from 2000 to 2008, including one by the US Department of Health and Human Services' Office of the Inspector General and the Agency for Healthcare Research and Quality. Using this data, they were able to calculate a mean death rate for medical errors in US hospitals. Applying this rate to the 35 million admissions in 2013, they calculated that 251,454 deaths resulted from medical mistakes.

And, to make matters of trust in our healthcare providers worse, the actual fourth leading cause of death in the United States, is again, not at all a chronic disease and not generally publicized. It is Adverse Drug reactions. ADRs represent over 100,000 deaths per year. Aren't drugs supposed to be safe? Add in reasonable estimates for ambulatory patients, death due to medication cross reaction, and nursing home patient ADRs deaths (*none of these are monitored*) and it turns out that our health care system may very well be the leading cause of death in the United States.

There have been so many adverse drug events that in some situations, the Federal Government has made it very difficult to sue drug companies for harming people. Take vaccines for example, the government set up a federal fund to compensate those harmed, but they have also made it very difficult for the injured party to actually receive compensation for their injuries, essentially immunizing drug companies from consumer lawsuits through government legislation. Getting a favorable verdict from the Feds is like passing an act of Congress. [77, 78, 79, 80]

Alzheimer's Disease

Alzheimer's Disease *(AD)* is an irreversible, progressive, and degenerative brain disorder that slowly destroys memory and thinking skills and, eventually, the ability to carry out the simplest tasks. It is the most common cause of dementia among older adults.

Although researchers still do not know exactly what causes AD, over the past three decades, there have been significant advances in our understanding of the emergence of symptoms and the course of the disease. Approximately 20 genes have now been associated with the risk of developing AD, but studies of identical twins show environmental rather than purely genetic causes for the changes in genes that lead to AD. [81, 82]

As a result, some researchers have shifted their attention from genes to the environment - especially to certain toxins that may affect the brain. Their studies of pesticides, heavy metals such as aluminum, mercury, and cadmium, food additives, air pollution, and other problematic compounds are opening a new front in the battle against this devastating malady. They are finding that exposure to numerous environmental stresses causes brain inflammation which can lead to AD and other neurodegenerative diseases. [83, 84, 85] There will be a more thorough discussion about AD on the Brain Drain chapter.

Vaccines

Are vaccines safe? That debate is longstanding and frequently characterized by heated arguments and slanderous accusations. Vaccines have proven most beneficial as an emergency medical treatment when epidemics rage out of control. For instance, in 1998, about 350,000 people, mostly in West Africa, lost their eyesight from River Blindness caused by a parasite carried by the black fly. The drug company, Merck, produced a drug called Ivermectin to cure this scourge, and distributed it through the World Health Organization to affected countries, virtually eliminating this contagion. But vaccines aren't always safe or effective. To be sure, the research demonstrates that vaccines are much more than harmless shots that protect us from disease. They have killed, maimed, or destroyed the lives of many innocent people, in some cases harming more than they have helped. The surprising and horrifying details will be covered in the Vaccine chapter. Just know the debate goes back a long way.

Government Corruption - It's As Real As Real Gets

Well, isn't there someone out there who can protect us from all this harm, like the Food and Drug Administration *(FDA)?* Most people don't know that the FDA is not a proactive watchdog group. By design, they only get involved when there is a problem, and by that time it is often too late as thousands have died and tens of thousands more have been harmed in various ways.

But many people still believe that the US FDA protects them from anything dangerous in our drug and food supplies. That is far from the truth. The fact is that when the FDA approves a new drug for public use for instance, it has not necessarily studied that drug's safety research. The agency relies on information from the drug manufacturers to make its approval decisions. I don't know about you, but that seems a little like the fox guarding the henhouse. Additionally, the FDA does not test the safety of ingredients in cosmetics, food, and personal care products either. They wait until enough people get injured, and then they may investigate.

Also, in the United States up to 99% of the ingredients in some products can be withheld from labels under the trade secrecy laws if they are categorized as *"inert."* Most inert ingredients are in bug sprays, insect repellents, and other pesticide products. Toxins expert, Doris J. Rapp, claims that at least 200 chemicals classified as inert are environmental pollutants hazardous to human health.

These laws have enabled the chemical industry to obscure its operations under a shroud of secrecy that has hampered efforts to protect public health. Due to these trade secrets, it is nearly impossible to get complete information about these chemicals even for physicians treating poisonings.

Also, consider the many pharmaceutical drugs over the years that have ended up killing or harming so many people before they were finally recalled from the worldwide marketplace - one hundred and seventy-five of them! Also contributing to the ADR *(Adverse Drug Reaction)* events is the fact that in 1992 the FDA established PDUFA *(Prescription Drug User Fee Act)*, which established an application and processing fee to be paid by the pharmaceutical drug companies applying for approval of a new medication. Drug companies could get approvals through the regulatory pipeline faster, and patients would get new drugs more quickly. Previously, the FDA was taking too long for the drug approval process because it was underfunded and understaffed, and the pharmaceutical industry and even some consumer advocacy groups *(supported by the pharmaceutical industry to the tune of $116 million per year)* were getting frustrated with the delays. That sounds like a good problem to solve; but there may be a dark side as well. PFUDA puts FDA squarely in the hands of the drug companies who, considering the exorbitant application fees, expect a quick approval for drugs that may not have even been tested properly. [86]

Since the FDA does not do drug safety or efficacy testing, they only require seeing and reviewing testing results from the drug companies themselves, or from outside research groups that support the claims. The standard application fee was $100,000 in 1993. In 2012, the fee for filing a new drug full application with clinical data was $1,841,500. [87]

In 2018, the FDA fee for a full application was $2,421,495 for applications requiring clinical data, about a 30% increase over 2012. In 2017, the FDA collected $837,500,000 in user fees for prescription drug approvals. This, in essence means that the drug companies are now *"funding"* about 75% of the FDA's drug review budget. There would certainly be an expectation by the drug companies to get the approvals. In 2008, the FDA rejected *"never-before-marketed drugs"* 66% of the time. By 2015, the rejection rate had dropped to 4%. Regulatory agencies should not need to depend on the industry that they regulate for their budget.

As patients or their insurers shell out millions of dollars for unproven drugs, manufacturers reaped the windfall. For them, expedited approval can mean not only sped-up sales, but also, if the drugs are intended to treat a rare disease or serve a neglected population, FDA incentives worth hundreds of millions of dollars can be thrown in. *"Instead of a regulator in a regulated industry, we now have a partnership,"* said Dr. Michael Corome, former US Department of Health and Human Services official. *"That relationship has tilted the agency away from a public health perspective to an industry friendly perspective."*

The FDA approved 46 new drugs where the chemical structure hadn't been previously approved in 2017, the most in at least fifteen years. In that same year, the FDA's Center for Drug Evaluation and Research denied 19.7% of all applications for new drugs, biologics, and efficacy supplements, down from a 2000 peak of 59.2% in 2010. In return for accelerated approval, drug companies commit to researching how well their drugs work after going to market. But these post-marketing strategies can take 10 years or longer to complete, leaving patients and doctors with lingering questions about their safety and benefit. *"Clearly accelerated approval has greater uncertainty,"* says Dr. Janet Woodcock head of FDA's Center for Drug Evaluation and Research.

The more the FDA relied on industry fees to pay for drug reviews, the more it showed an inclination towards approval, former employees say. *"You don't survive as a senior official at the FDA unless you're pro industry,"* said Dr. Thomas Marciniak, a former FDA medical team leader, and longtime outspoken critic of how drug companies handle clinical trials. *"Nobody gets congratulated for turning a drug down, but you do get seriously questioned if you do,"* said the former staffer. Higher-ups would also send congratulatory emails to medical review teams when a drug was approved. [88]

In his book Overdose, Dr. Jay Cohen quotes a study by three university professors in the Journal of American Medical Association that determined that at least 51% of all FDA approved drugs *"have serious adverse effects not detected prior to approval."* This revelation prompted Cohen to write, *"Think about this: more than half of our drugs, after being deemed safe by the FDA and then prescribed to millions of people, are subsequently detected to have previously unrecognized medically serious side effects."*

A Prescription For Disaster

A new study from Mayo Clinic researchers reveals how many Americans are on prescription drugs - and it's a lot of us. Research shows that nearly 70% of Americans take at least one prescription drug, and more than half take two. The most commonly prescribed drug is antibiotics - taken by 17% of Americans - followed by antidepressants and pain-killing opioids - each taken by 13% of Americans. Twenty percent of patients are on five or more prescription medications, according to the findings. Drugs to lower lipids, such as cholesterol came in fourth *(11%)* and vaccines were fifth *(11%)*.

As mentioned earlier, Adverse Drug Reactions *(ADR)* is the fourth leading cause of death in the United State. Think about that for a moment. The people that are supposed to care about our health are actually killing off a whole bunch of us. Let that sink in for a moment.

In addition, that does not consider the number of other *"serious"* ADRs in hospitalized patients, which are estimated to be 6.7%. If these estimates are correct, then there are more than 2,216,000 serious ADRs in hospitalized patients, causing over 106,000 deaths annually.

What's worse is that these statistics do not include the number of ADRs that occur in ambulatory *(non-hospital)* settings, which adds up to 4,300,000 per year according to a study done between 1995 and 2005. [89]

Also, it is estimated that over 350,000 ADRs occur in US nursing homes each year. The exact number of ADRs is not certain and is limited by methodological considerations. However, whatever the true number is, ADRs represent a significant public health problem that is, for the most part, preventable.

The statistics on medication usage among elderly patients in the US are eye-opening: more than one-third of prescriptions drugs used in the US are taken by elderly patients; the ambulatory elderly fill between 9-13 prescriptions a year *(including new prescriptions and refills)*; the average elderly patient takes more than five prescription medications; the average nursing home patient takes seven. [90]

Dr. Russell Blaylock, a well-known retired neurosurgeon, and now health and nutrition specialist, has this to say about the aging population in this country:

"Our nursing homes are filled with an alarming number of decrepit, sick, disoriented, demented, and crippled elderly. Most health experts have lamented that all of the degenerative diseases have been increasing in incidence, but even more alarming, they are occurring at a younger age. This is especially so with neurodegenerative diseases such as Alzheimer's dementia, Parkinson's disease and amyotrophic lateral sclerosis (also known as ALS and Lou Gehrig's disease). They are wracked with arthritis, cataracts, macular degeneration, detached retina's, arthritis, tendinitis, hypertension, diabetes, asthma, chronic lung disease, kidney failure, heart disease, poor circulation, vertigo, digestive problems, poor hearing, aching muscles, fatigue and poor immunity."

I would also add insomnia, depression, and anxiety - assuming of course that they would even have a presence of mind to think that there may be a problem. While the past two generations have grown up in a world where heart disease, diabetes, cancer, Alzheimer's, and the rest of body ravishing diseases in the now fifty and up population are all part of a day's walk in the park, these are not a normal state of affairs. Something is very wrong!

A Pandemic Of Behavioral Disorders

Neurodevelopmental disorders such as autism, attention deficit and hyperactivity disorder, depression, anxiety, and others can have a life-long devastating impact on individuals and their families and friends. But why is there such a dramatic increase in these behavioral disorders over the last fifty years? The reasons are now clear and will be explained in detail in chapters to come. Clearly, epigenetic mechanisms including environmental toxins, insufficiently tested and dangerous drugs marketed by an overzealous pharmaceutical industry, and cultural mores that accept the false premise that doctors know best and that there is a pill for every little ill play an important role in the development of these disorders. From the sources already mentioned to cholesterol-lowering medications, vaccines, and many other drugs, your brain is being damaged, which can lead to a variety of neurobehavioral disorders. That may sound a bit counterintuitive since it is understood that drugs are supposed to prevent, treat, or cure diseases and not cause them. But, they do! Add kickbacks from the pharmaceutical industry to mental health and other medical professionals for promoting mind-altering drugs and safety and efficacy cover-ups by the FDA and pharmaceutical industry and the picture that emerges is a pretty shocking indictment of the healthcare industry - worthy of prosecution? When mental health professionals start toying with the minds of innocent people, especially children, people become outraged when they do find out what is happening to harm them. So, get outraged.

Doctors, Take Them Off The Pedestal

As a practicing medical and surgical specialist for over thirty-five years, I can say this - stay as far away from the doctor's office as reasonably possible. Now, having said that, let me add some clarification. There are times when we really do need their help. However, overall, the general medical profession is not what many trusting people think it is. While, in my opinion, allopathic medicine *(Western medicine, evidence-based medicine or modern medicine)*, is great at trauma care, emergency care services, necessary surgeries, anesthesia, and diagnostics, we are the pits *(literally, near the last)* when it comes to keeping people healthy and out of the doctor's office. We don't belong on the pedestal on which we have been placed over the last one hundred or so years.

While most docs do not take swearing to any oath seriously, there are some very important tenants of integrity contained within the Hippocratic Oath. The words, *"I will use treatment to help the sick according to my ability and judgment, but never with a view to injury and wrong-doing. Neither will I administer a poison to anybody when asked to do so, nor will I suggest such a course. Similarly, I will not give to a woman a pessary to cause abortion. But I will keep pure and holy both my life and my art."* Sounds high and mighty, and certainly worthy of this high calling as a healer. This is not the whole document, which does contain some out of step tenants such as never using a knife for surgery, but, at its core, there are deep and morally sound maxims that can certainly provide guidance for the journey as a healthcare provider. Following such, however, is but a fantasy in today's medical community. Evidence of this may be clear by these statistics. According to a 1993 survey of 150 US and Canadian medical schools, for example, only 14% of modern oaths prohibit euthanasia, 11% hold covenant with a deity, 8% foreswear abortion, and a mere 3% forbid sexual contact with patients - all maxims held sacred in the classical version of the Hippocratic Oath. [91]

Does it seem like it is indeed a relic of the past? What we docs perhaps held dear in this oath not three generations ago, now to many is but a fading memory of nonsensical jabberwocky by idealistic morons. Hmmm. With the medical profession being responsible for the third and fourth leading causes of death in the United States, perhaps instead of viewing the document at best merely as a rite of passage and best wishes, docs might take to heart the depth of privilege and moral responsibility that the oath espouses.

What we are taught in medical school is sick care, not healthcare. We get paid for treating sick people, period. I wish it were different, I mean, how cool would it be if doctors were paid by insurers to actually get people healthy, off medication, away from the operating room, and out of the hospitals and extended care facilities. It would be a win/win for everyone; the patient premiums would *(should)* go down, doctors would *(should)* get paid more for reducing the insurer and patient's healthcare financial burdens. But no, that is just not on their radar screen - maybe a blip *(a passing thought)* from time to time. They are too locked into an antiquated and frankly harmful system of sick care for profit. Insurers also don't have as much of an incentive to change as one might think considering the escalating healthcare costs. They will still make their share of the profits regardless. They just hike insurance premiums and reduce payments to doctors and hospitals and other clinical facilities to cover any expected reduction in future profits. They control the remote, so to speak.

The pharmaceutical industry is also intimately tied to what is taught in medical school. It can go something like this: *"Dr. Reed, you have a patient with metabolic syndrome. He has diabetes, high blood pressure, high cholesterol/ triglycerides, and is obese. How do you want to treat him?"* Now, if I don't spew back the diagnostic tests and multiple medications that are needed, then I fail the test. It is that simple. So, we all get out of school as Big Pharma automatons - a *(human)* machine that performs a function according to a predetermined set of coded instructions, especially one capable of a range of programmed responses to different circumstances.

While docs may be personable, and their kids play on the same teams as yours, and they have all the other social behavior skills in place, when they get in the office, it's *"symptom = drug"* most of the time. We are a product of our education, so we are not generally able to think past what we were taught. I did that for the first twenty-five years of my practice. Then, after the death of my father-in-law from cancer, I wised up, turned rogue, and started to re-examine the whole medical education and healthcare system. What I found was not pretty, which I will share throughout this book. Of course, there are exceptions to the rule, but for the most part, this is the reality of modern medicine.

But, this inherent indictment of the medical profession is still not the complete picture. I don't think that we will ever get that. There is too much *(money)* at stake. However, let's add a few other variables to the equation. Add in the third leading cause of death in the United States - Medical Errors, and fourth leading cause of death - Adverse Drug Events, ADR, and the controversy about the unnecessary deaths that occur in nursing homes and other skilled nursing care facilities *(although conveniently those statistics do not seem to be kept in any known national registry)* from lack of professional care or overdosing and the picture becomes more clear and macabre. It appears that the actual leading cause of death is the medical profession.

Despite all the medical marvels to help keep us alive and make our lives better through chemistry, we ARE sicker than ever before, and the research overwhelmingly bears this out. And, we are not winning the war on any of the major disease fronts. Listen to what Randall Fitzgerald, an investigative reporter and author of The Hundred Year Lie has to say after his exhaustive investigation of toxins in our environment.

"Over the last one hundred years, our species has been engaged in a vast and complicated chemistry experiment. Each and every one of us, along with our children, our parents, and our grandparents have been a guinea pig in this experiment, which uses our bodies, our health, our wealth, and our goodwill to test the proposition that modern science can improve upon the foods and medicines of nature."

In every practical sense, it is my hope that this book will show you the ropes to take control of your health and even force some very necessary changes in the marketplace. We do have a choice about whether or not we will become a victim. We can view ourselves as savvy consumers that help drive the markets or we can allow our food, medicine, and product ingredient choices to be made for us by institutions that are little more than interchangeable parts of an economic engine driven by self-serving money-grabbing interests. If we fail to recognize what is at stake here and do not act to stop the madness, we negatively impact our own well-being, the well-being of those others who care about us and who depend on us for good judgments, as well as our future generations.

CHAPTER 2

Epigenetics
Unraveling The Mystery Of Who We Are

Epigenetics is one of the most important scientific discoveries of our time, and our understanding of epigenetics may very well be a huge leap for mankind in the fight to cure diseases worldwide.

So, what is the science of epigenetics? You may have heard of genetics, - the DNA from mom meets the DNA from dad, then *poof!* There you are!! Epigenetics takes it from there. It is the science of understanding how life's events can impact the expression of our genes to produce a response to those events. From the moment you are conceived until the moment you take your last breath, epigenetics is involved. The old belief was that our genetic profile is set in stone and does not change. But in recent years, molecular biology has shown that the human genome is far more fluid and responsive to the environment than previously supposed. Epigenetics describes changes in gene activity in response to the environment without changing the DNA sequence itself. It takes us from the victim status of the old belief because we didn't have a choice about our genetics, to life-giving mastery over our destiny.

In the early 1990s, the Human Genome Project set out to discover the sequence of our DNA. You know, that double helix of information that looks like a twisted ladder and makes you, YOU! After the project was completed, a new project emerged *(epigenetics)* that would take that human genome with all of its now organized and labeled DNA and attempt to understand how that DNA expresses itself through genes, which are groupings of DNA.

The epigenetic palette provides the colors for painting the portrait of the person you will become. Alterations in normal gene function caused by activating or deactivating genes to various degrees occur in response to environmental and emotional signals. These alterations can be good or bad. If the environment is healthy, then it supports normal gene function. If it is not healthy, then normal gene function does not happen to one degree or another and you struggle down the highway of life. It is like having bad gas in your car; it just doesn't run right, the car stutters and shakes, the carburetor gums up, and the car may up and *"die"* before you've completed the intended journey. Of course, your genes are a much more complicated system, but the basic concept works. Good lifestyle choices support and strengthen normal gene function. Bad lifestyle choices degrade normal gene function. Both can be passed down to future generations. Genes are generational instructions for what to do and where and when to do it.

Our Legacy To The Next Generation

Success in mapping the human genome and our ongoing research into the epigenome has also fostered the complimentary concept of the exposome, developed by Dr. Christopher Wilde, a cancer epidemiologist. The concept is based on toxic exposure from our environment, diet, lifestyle, etc. That exposure begins before birth and interacts with our own unique characteristics such as genetics, physiology, and epigenetics that can impact our health. The toxins that we are exposed to that enter our body may seem small and insignificant, but over time the accumulation of toxins will lead to an overflow. Our detoxification organs are not able to handle the toxic load passing through the body and the resulting overflow, along with the associated gene damage, then results in a variety of symptoms. [92]

Today, a wide variety of illnesses, behaviors, and other health indicators have some level of evidence linking them with faulty epigenetic mechanisms, including cancers of all types, cognitive dysfunction, and respiratory, cardiovascular, reproductive, autoimmune, and neurobehavioral illnesses.

Known or suspected drivers behind the negative epigenetic effects involve many agents, including heavy metals, pesticides, diesel exhaust, tobacco smoke, polycyclic aromatic hydrocarbons, hormones, radioactivity, viruses, bacteria, plastics and other synthetic products that permeate our lives. [93, 94]

Many people believe that poor lifestyle choices are affecting only them, but that is not true. Research shows that the negative health impact poor lifestyle choices have on us, including the chemicals that we put in and on ourselves, and other unhealthy lifestyle choices such as addictions, emotional toxins such as unforgiveness, anger, bitterness, and resentment, can pass down to the third and fourth generations. That is important to understand, especially when considering raising a family. Our choices are NOT just about us!

National Institute of Environmental Health Sciences

Trans-generational *(to third and fourth generation)* effects have now been reported for chemicals including:
• Permethrin - Insecticide
• DEET - Insect repellant
• Bisphenol A used in plastics
• Phthalates used to soften plastics
• Dioxin & PCBs
• Jet fuel mixtures
• Tributyltin - Paint on boats
• Nicotine -Tobacco
• Methoxychlor- Insecticide
• Vinclozin – Fungicide
• DDT - Insecticide

Dr. Jirtle, an American biologist noted for his pioneering research in epigenetics, explains the transgenerational effect very eloquently: *"Every time we look into a mirror or step on a scale, we know we are what we eat; however, we now know that we may also be what our mother ate (was exposed to) while we were in her womb."*[95]

We may even be what our grandparents and great grandparents were exposed to during their lives. Thus, recent epigenetic investigations have brought a unique biological perspective to the biblical warning that the sins of the fathers are visited upon the children down to the third or fourth generation *(Exodus 20:5).*

The good news is that unhealthy epigenetic alterations of genes, passed down or through unhealthy lifestyle choices, are not necessarily a destiny, and they can become normal again if conditions change for the better. For the most part, it doesn't matter what genes you inherit, but more importantly it matters how they are expressed. By choosing a healthy diet and lifestyle, we influence optimal genetic expression for ourselves and generations to come. [96]

Think of your DNA as the Introductory Chapter in your own personal storybook of life. The words describe who you are when you are conceived. Ideally, it is well written without typos, misplaced, mis-spaced, or deleted words. Soon after you are conceived, Chapter One begins to be written. It takes the instructions of the intro and further develops that storyline of your life. The way the story unfolds depends on many factors, primarily environmental exposure in the womb, and emotion signals received from mom and others. The story *(gene expression)* can be written very smoothly all the way through the chapter, or there can be text typos, etc. *(epigenetic changes in gene expression)* that may or may not change the original storyline written in the intro.

Chapter Two begins postnatally when you are born. It takes the story written in the intro, the prenatal developmental experiences, good or bad, in Chapter One, and writes a new chapter about you based on the previous information and the new information experienced every moment of every day. It is an ongoing, ever-changing story based on life's experiences, and hopefully the original narrative is still in place and does not change much. As life has it, the story of our lives will always be filled with ups and downs, dings and dents, and some crashes and burns. Ideally, we recover and heal, and make changes to avoid future similar events. Sometimes, though, we don't learn from those valuable life lessons, and we continue to harm ourselves in various ways. The masterpiece described so beautifully in your intro, the one that made your cells and your spirit smile and dance, can get changed into a horror story. What began well doesn't end well. Then that story can get passed down to future generations and can make their beginning intro a theme of struggle from the start. The good news is, while your children and future generations may have been dealt a bad hand to begin with, that doesn't have to be their destiny. They can exchange the bad experiences for good ones and write their own stories of change, health, and healing and then pass that on to their children.

Cellular Communication

The DNA genome is like a twisted ladder. It has two sides with the rung in the middle, which is made up of two nucleotide base pairs *(either Adenine with Thymine, or Cytosine with Guanine)* connected by hydrogen bonds. There are roughly three billion base pairs that make up a human's 23 chromosomes stored in the nucleus. The twisted ladder is very long. If the DNA in the nucleus of a cell is removed and stretched out, it would measure about six feet. How in the world does

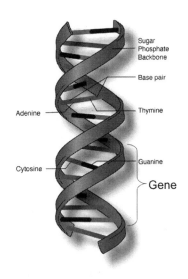

that compact into that tiny nucleus? I will get to that shortly. In the nucleus, the DNA is like jumbled spaghetti. When a cell decides to split in two, the DNA becomes more defined into the 23 pairs of chromosomes that you may have seen in pictures. Long segments of DNA base pairs make up the 30,000 genes. They are simply protein manufacturing centers responding to environmental signals. [97]

Cells talk to each other through a very sophisticated communication system. Some experts in the field of biological sciences believe that every one of our approximately fifty trillion cells in the body is aware of all chemical processes that take place in every other cell. It seems reasonable to consider since responses to stimuli are dependent on instantaneous recognition. It could be just cause and effect, but the field of Quantum Physics suggests that there may be more going on through the concept of *"entanglement"* of subatomic particles that established a relationship. All subsequent cells from the time of conception are inherently related, making entanglement a reasonable possibility.

There are many types of receptors on the outside of each cell awaiting chemical messenger signals to dock on a receptor landing pad and give an instruction that will pass through the cell membrane covering. The instruction will then be transported to the nucleus of the cell where a gene produces a protein. Cellular perception of the surrounding intracellular environment is what controls biological processes - not genes. [98]

The created protein is an instruction, which is then passed back outside of the cell to initiate an action, or be part of a larger composite of responses, like maintaining normal blood sugar or responding to a viral attack. These normal response instructions can be altered by unhealthy environmental and emotional conditions to give an unintended result. For instance, the genes that protect women from breast cancer can be turned off from environmental toxins leaving the normal immune response helpless to act against the chronic inflammation and subsequent abnormal cell growth. Very similar to the adjustment controls on a TV where the *"quality"* of the picture can be altered depending on how the controls - contrast, color, tint, and sharpness are set. Anything that causes a stress response in the body will start messing with the picture quality. If there is acute short-term stress, the picture can self-adjust. If the stress is chronic, the picture quality remains poor, and the self-adjust mechanism can freeze up and no longer be able to compensate until the picture adjustment mechanisms are re-calibrated and set to the way they were first designed. Our genes function much the same way. We can have control over the way our genes are expressed. We just may need to make some adjustments and recalibrate to take back our health.

Our genes are vulnerable to hijacking throughout our lives. Fetal development and the period from childhood through puberty are the most vulnerable stages of life. When alterations of normal gene function do occur, they can be passed from generation to generation and have an observable negative impact on the body, disorders such as diabetes, obesity, autism, other mental health disorders, and cancer can develop. But, again, that it is not necessarily the destiny of future generations.

These changes in gene function can be passed down through *"epigenetic tags"* which act as cellular memory. A cell's epigenetic profile includes the DNA as well as a collection of tags that tell genes whether to be on or off and is the summation of environmental signals received during a lifetime. Most tags are removed within a couple of days after fertilization. Some of them remain throughout life unless lifestyle changes are made for unhealthy tags.

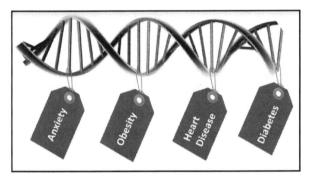

If epigenetic tags are passed down, it then comes down to a choice. Future progeny can return to normal gene expression by healthy lifestyle choices that are complementary to our nature, or they can choose to live in the past misery of the parents and grandparents' choices. I hear from patients way too many times in my office when someone comes in with diabetes, high blood pressure, heart disease, and most any other diseases that it runs in their family and their parents, and grandparents had it, and that is why they have it. It just doesn't have to work that way.

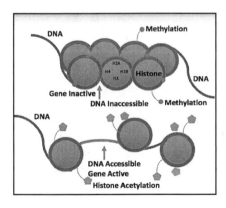

Unfortunately, that idea is also promoted within the medical community. It is not a destination unless one chooses to make it that way. There may be a *"tendency"* because genes have been *"conditioned"* but that is not destiny. Abnormal epigenetic gene expression can be normalized, and even some gene mutations can be overridden or corrected. But how do all these alterations in normal gene expression take place in the cell? Most of them come from gene activities called methylation and histone acetylation. Methylation mostly involves the *"silencing"* of a gene, so it won't express. It leaves a *"mark"* on the gene to be silent. Methylation is truly a multi-tasking marvel that allows us to be healthy and human. This highly intricate process occurs within each cell, and it is responsible for the most vital undertakings throughout the body chemistry.

Methylation determines who we are, what we look like, how we behave, and is central to our physical, emotional, and mental well-being. When first conceived, all dividing cells contain the same DNA. As they differentiate to become a muscle cell for example, the gene's capacity to become a bone cell is silenced through methylation. The differentiation continues and becomes even more sophisticated throughout life in response to environmental signals. Without methylation, we could not survive; hence, it is the perfect pathway to focus on for understanding the vast number of diseases that the world faces. Abnormal methylation patterns in a variety of genes can result in many poor physical and mental health outcomes, including cardiovascular and metabolic issues, immune system disorders, depression, psychiatric disorders and other mental health conditions, cancer, diabetes, and every life-sustaining process as well.

A gene *"activating"* mechanism is acetylation. It is like a dimmer switch that determines the degree to which genes are expressed. To pack the very long, six feet DNA inside the super small nucleus, it is wrapped around spools, like thread. There are about 30,000,000 spools of DNA in the nucleus. Acetylation unwinds the spool to access, activate, and copy a gene instruction to produce a protein to perform a function in the body. Both methylation and acetylation act in concert to produce a harmony of responses to internal, environmental, and emotional signals. It's epigenetics in action.

Evidence Of Epigenetics In Twins

Studies of changes in DNA over time in identical twins bring the power of epigenetics into perspective. Monozygotic twins are identical. They have the same DNA. The completion of the Human Genome Project and ongoing study of the Epigenome Project have created a unique opportunity to observe the similarities between twins through the lens of genes. This becomes especially significant with twins that were separated at birth and have different life experiences filtered through different personalities in most cases. From a macro viewpoint, they remain very much the same over a lifetime. An interesting example is the *"Jim twin"* story. In 1979, Jim Springer and Jim Lewis were reunited at age 39 after not knowing the other existed. As described in Nancy Segal's book on the identical Jim twins, Born Together- Reared Apart, both had been adopted and raised by different families in Ohio, just 40 miles apart from each other. Despite their separate upbringings, it turned out that both twins got terrible migraines, bit their nails, smoked Salem cigarettes, drove light blue Chevrolets, did poorly in spelling and math, and had worked at McDonald's and as part-time deputy sheriffs. But the weirdest part was that one of the Jim twins had named his first son James Alan. The other had named his first son James Allan. Both had named their pet dogs, *"Toy."* Both had also married women named Linda - then they got divorced, and both married women named Betty. Now, that's just weird. Their story is maybe not so unusual in that they both tested out having similar personalities, which may account for their parallel experiences.

From a DNA and gene expression standpoint, what researchers find in identical twins is quite different. While identical twins are virtually the same at birth, and maintain most external similarities over a lifetime, their gene patterns diverge to varying degrees depending on life's experiences. Also, personalities are for the most part very different in twins; their responses to life's experiences can be very different as well, creating epigenetic alterations, unlike the Jim Twins. [99]

Manel Esteller, a geneticist at the Spanish National Cancer Center in Madrid, and colleagues in Sweden, Denmark, Spain, England, and the United States studied 80 sets of identical twins, ranging in age from 3 to 74 years. Their aim was to explore what role epigenetics plays in generating phenotypic differences between genetically identical twins. Statistical analysis suggested that older twin pairs were more epigenetically different than younger twins. It also revealed that twins who reported having spent less time together during their lives, or who had different medical histories, had the greatest epigenetic differences. Gene expression analysis revealed that in the two twin pairs most epigenetically distinct from each other, the 3 and 50 year-olds, there were four times as many differentially expressed genes in the older pair than in the younger pair, confirming that the epigenetic differences the researchers saw *in twins could lead to increased differences in the way genes are expressed.* "*These findings help show how environmental factors can change one's gene expression and susceptibility to disease, by affecting epigenetics,*" Esteller told *The Scientist.* [100]

Environment seemed to play a critical role: Twins reared apart showed more epigenetic differences than those reared together. A serious illness in one twin seemed to correlate with greater differences between epigenetic profiles. "*Epigenetics may explain how DNA and the environment interact to give organisms their unique characteristics,*" says Esteller. The implications of this study and others are quite profound, helping to explain how dreaded diseases like cancer, Alzheimer's, and others develop. "*This study gives a remarkable demonstration of how environment affects our DNA "packaging,"*" says Stephen Baylin, a cancer biologist at John Hopkins School of Medicine in Baltimore, Maryland. [101, 102, 103]

Another study of identical twins was done with Scott and Mark Kelly. Scientists found that Scott Kelly, an astronaut who set the record for most consecutive days spent in orbit, underwent an "*unexpected*" genetic change. Post-flight, NASA investigators found "*hundreds of unique mutations.*" Some involved the circulation, others involved changes in the epigenome - the genetic control system that determines how genes are expressed. Still others involved a lengthening of telomeres, the caps on the ends of chromosomes that help regulate the aging process.

About 93% of the changes were temporary, with Kelly's genetic profile returning to normal comparatively quickly after his return to Earth; in the case of the telomeres, the lengthening vanished within 48 hours. But about 7% of the changes have remained two years since he returned to Earth. Those involved genes relate to Kelly's *"immune system, DNA repair, bone formation networks, hypoxia, and hypercapnia." "Mark and Scott Kelly are still identical twins,"* the agency said in a statement. Scott's DNA did not fundamentally change. What researchers did observe are changes in gene expression, which is how your body reacts to your environment. [104]

There are other studies as well supporting epigenetic changes due to environmental experiences. Historically, during the Dutch Famine of 1944- 45, food stocks in the cities in the western Netherlands rapidly ran out. The adult rations in cities such as Amsterdam dropped to below 1000 calories a day by the end of November 1944 and to 580 calories in the west by the end of February 1945. The Dutch Famine Birth Cohort Study, carried out by several departments of the Academic Medical Centre in Amsterdam, in collaboration with the MRC Environmental Epidemiology Unit of the University of Southampton in Britain, found that the children of pregnant women exposed to famine were more susceptible to diabetes, obesity, cardiovascular disease, and other health problems. Moreover, the children of the women who were pregnant during the famine were smaller, as expected, and significantly underweight. However, surprisingly, when these children grew up and had children, those children were thought to also be smaller than average but follow up studies on birth weight were not conclusive. These data suggested that the famine experienced by the mothers caused epigenetic changes that were passed down to the next generation. Subsequent academic research on the children who were affected in the second trimester of their mother's pregnancy also found an increased incidence of schizophrenia in these children. [105, 106]

In Overkalix, Sweden during the 1880s, children and grandchildren of Swedes who lived in famine actually lived longer than expected because genes adapted for survival. When food was plentiful, children died earlier.[107,108]

Women who smoke will have a greater chance of having offspring who will have asthma and other developmental disorders. Maternal cigarette smoking during pregnancy remains a relatively common but hazardous event for the developing fetus. Previous studies have associated prenatal smoke exposure with reduced birth weight, poor developmental and psychological outcomes, and increased risk for diseases and behavioral disorders later in life. Researchers are now learning that many of the mechanisms whereby maternal smoke exposure may affect key pathways crucial for proper fetal growth and development are epigenetic in nature. Studies have shown that there are more than 4,000 chemicals in cigarette smoke including benzo(a) pyrene, nicotine, and carbon monoxide, and more than 40 of these chemicals are known carcinogens and about 50,000 gene mutations take place in those who smoke for a two-year period. [109, 110, 111, 112]

A highly referenced study supporting the evidence of gene alteration due to environmental conditions puts a different spin on cause and the effect on epigenetic relationships. It shows how positive changes in environment can have positive and long-lasting consequences on the epigenome. In a landmark Duke University study published in the August 1, 2003 Issue of Molecular and Cellular Biology, Dr. Randy Jirtle and his colleague, Dr. Robert Waterland, found that a nutritionally enriched diet can even override genetic mutations in the Agouti Yellow mice. Members of this strain have an extra piece of DNA in the Agouti gene, making them obese, yellow, and predisposed to cardiovascular disease, diabetes, and cancer. When fed the vitamin B12, folic acid, choline, and betaine before, during, and after pregnancy, the animals gave birth to thin, brown pups. Control animals' offspring were fat and yellow. These methylated supplements and cofactors were chosen because a number of studies have shown that the methyl chemical group is involved with epigenetic modifications. When methyl groups are added to a particular gene, that gene is turned off or silenced, and no protein is produced from that gene. Silencing a gene can be good or bad depending on what the gene does when it is activated. Silencing a cancer-protective gene, for example, is not good when it's supposed to be active.

Dr. Jirtle, in an interview with ScienceWatch, explained the significance of these results: *"Our results provide compelling evidence that the specific composition of each individual's "epigenetic mosaic" is influenced by early nutrition. Methyl donors also counteract . . . Hypomethylation caused by Bisphenol A, an endocrine-disrupting agent used to make hard clear plastic and epoxy resins. Many other studies as well have found epigenetic mechanisms to be a factor in a variety of diseases including cancer, cardiovascular disease, diabetes, and others."* [113]

Autism Spectrum Disorders

Autism spectrum disorders *(ASD)* are complex and multifactorial, and the roles of genetic and environmental factors in its emergence have been well documented. The processes underlying this interaction are still poorly known, but there is evidence that epigenetic prenatal and postnatal modification from environmental toxins, vaccines, and nutritional deficiencies such as vitamins D and B9 folate could be involved. The changes in epigenetic marks following exposure to environmental factors known as *"autism risk factors"* are discussed in many reports and will be discussed further in the Brain Drain and Vaccine chapters.[114]

Bisphenol A - BPA

The poster-child molecule for framing the links between environment and epigenetic health is BPA. It was invented in 1891 by the Russian chemist A.P. Dianin and discovered in 1936 to cause responses similar to those of the natural hormone estrogen. That discovery took place during the rush of pharmaceutical research to find synthetic estrogens, and bisphenol A *(BPA)* lost out to its more powerful cousin diethylstilbestrol (*DES*) which went on to be used by millions of women to control difficult pregnancies before it was discovered to be a cancer-causing agent. Bisphenol A, a powerful estrogenic chemical, was put on the shelf until a polymer chemist discovered around 1950 that it could be combined in chains to make polycarbonate plastic and certain epoxy resins. Use since that discovery has skyrocketed, to the point that over six billion pounds are synthesized each year and the molecule is now included in countless consumer products.

Today almost all people sampled in the developed world have Bisphenol A in their body at trace levels *(in the low parts per billion),* including in amniotic fluid, umbilical cord blood, and placental tissue. A Centers for Disease Control study in 2005 detected low amounts of BPA in the urine of 95% of Americans sampled. Since 1997, well over 200 articles have been published in the peer-reviewed scientific literature showing that BPA has a biological impact on cells and animals at levels below the current federal standards, which were based on data gathered in the early 1980s. In cells, BPA has been shown to alter vital genetic signaling pathways at less than one part per trillion, equivalent to one droplet of BPA in an Olympic size swimming pool.

How does one molecule contribute to so much suffering? Research shows that BPA alters the behavior of over 200 genes, approximately one percent of all human genes. The genes affected aren't controlling minor traits like eye color. They are genes involved centrally in how cells multiply, how stem cells become more specialized, how metabolism is regulated, and how the brain gets wired as a fetus grows. It is not at all surprising, therefore, to see so many potential links to health problems.

Glyphosate

Glyphosate is a non-selective herbicide, which means that it will kill most plants. It is mostly applied to the leaves of plants to kill both broadleaf plants and grasses and is the active ingredient in many weedkillers. The sodium salt form of glyphosate is used to regulate plant growth and ripen fruit. Glyphosate was first registered for use in the US by Monsanto in 1974 and is now one of the most widely used herbicides in the United States. People apply it in agriculture and forestry, on lawns and gardens, and for weeds in industrial areas. But the science about its safety is far from conclusive.

In fact, Glyphosate has also been linked to high and low blood pressure, weight loss resistance, dizziness, inability to handle stress, exceptional malaise, brain fog, fatigue, headaches, hormone deregulation, insomnia depression/mood changes, muscle/joint aches and pains, cancer, and more. And in 2015, the International Agency for Research on Cancer, also concluded that glyphosate was *"probably carcinogenic to humans."* [115]

So, it was no surprise that in August 2018, a jury for the Superior Court of California ordered Monsanto, maker of the glyphosate, Roundup, to pay $289 million to a man, a former school district groundskeeper, because of Roundup's likely role in contributing to his cancer. Diagnosed with non-Hodgkin's lymphoma in 2014, his was the first lawsuit to go to trial alleging a glyphosate link to cancer. As a result, the number of glyphosate lawsuits against Monsanto has ballooned to more than 13,000 cases since that time. Three lawsuits have been prosecuted and won by plaintiffs, the latest one in May, 2019, where two billion dollars was awarded to a couple both of whom developed non-Hodgkin's lymphoma. [116, 117, 118]

Glyphosate is an endocrine system disruptor that impairs the CYP *(P450)* gene pathway in the liver. This gene creates enzymes to help break down and detoxify xenobiotics like chemicals, drugs, carcinogens, pesticides etc. Glyphosate inhibits the natural detoxification process, and in turn, it disrupts homeostasis, increases inflammation, and leads to a deconstruction of the cellular system. It is a major hormone disruptor and has been linked to the T47D and MCF7 breast cancer gene. An in-vivo study of Roundup administered to rats in drinking water diluted to 50ng/L glyphosate equivalence *(half of the level permitted in drinking water in the EU11 and 14,000 times lower than that permitted in drinking water in the USA,)* resulted in severe organ damage and a trend of increased incidence of mammary tumors in female animals over a two-year period of exposure. [119, 120, 121, 1222]

Glyphosate also has a severe effect on our micro-biome function. Studies have indicated that glyphosate disrupts the microbes in the intestine, causing a decrease in the ratio of beneficial to harmful bacteria. Thus, pathogenic bacteria are highly resistant to glyphosate but most beneficial bacteria were found to be moderately to highly susceptible. Current research indicates that disruption of the microbiome could cause diseases such as metabolic disorder, diabetes, depression, autism, cardiovascular disease, and autoimmune disease.

The Big C

Approximately 90% of chronic diseases are epigenetically induced and 10% are related to heredity - what is passed down to you from previous generations. For example, epigenetic gene modifications can have a considerable effect on cancer-related genes. *"The evidence for epigenetics being involved in cancer is very widespread. If you look at solid tumors and leukemia, there are tumor suppressor genes that we know are inactivated by epigenetic mechanisms in almost all of these tumors,"* said Adam Karpf, a cancer biologist and epigeneticist at the University of Nebraska Medical Center. Anything you consume can modify the epigenome of a cell.

Methylation was covered earlier in the chapter. Hypermethylation of what is called *"promoter"* regions in tumor suppressor genes can inactivate many tumor suppressor functions. Take BRCA1 and BRCA2 breast cancer gene mutations for example. Both are tumor suppressor genes. Reportedly, only about 5% or so are hereditary in origin. In these cases, breast cancer can run in the family. That means that nearly 95% of the gene mutations occur AFTER conception. About 70% of women with one of these mutations will get breast cancer before the age of eighty years old. Forty percent will get ovarian cancer. [123]

This has naturally created a lot of hysteria. These cancer suppressor genes have been turned off at some point by epigenetic experiences from the time of conception. The end result is that when there is chronic inflammation in the breast tissue from environmental toxins or even emotional trauma, these cancer-protective genes can mutate and be ineffective or just be turned off. The standard treatment for breast cancer usually involves chemotherapy, radiation, and surgery, none of which are pleasant or desirable. The physical and emotional trauma is beyond anything that someone should have to endure.

What if it were possible to just turn these cancer protective genes back on and have the cancer disappear! Wouldn't that be a game changer? No surgery, no radiation, no chemo? No nausea, vomiting, hair loss, chronic pain, welts in the mouth? No nerve damage, organ damage, or psychological damage from the pending doom? Just make some simple lifestyle changes, take some special formulations, and the immune system can turn back on and the cancer cells are attacked and destroyed. And what if this can happen in as little as a couple of weeks to a couple of months? Wouldn't that be a good thing? Is that possible? Yes! I have seen this happen with a number of people. In my opinion, it is more successful than anything else available. Not with everyone of course, because cancer can be complicated.

Benefits of Exercise

• Increases Weight Loss
• Reduces Oxidized Cholesterol
• **Reduces Breast Cancer by up to 60%**
• Increases Mental Clarity
• Reduces Incidence of Heart Attack
• Reduces High Blood pressure
• Improves Psychological Well-being
• Reduces Osteoporosis
• Reduces Risk of Diabetes
• Reduces Depression and Anxiety

Emotional trauma itself has been implicated in breast cancer, particularly when there has been a break in a relationship between two close females in a family or friendship. That is hard to qualify, but I have seen it in action and there are others out there in the trenches who deal with situations like this regularly. And not just breast cancer, but other types of cancers and chronic diseases as well. People around the world have successfully battled chronic diseases naturally for eons. It is just a matter providing the right tools and a wholesome and loving environment that the body needs to repair itself. And, supplementation with concentrated natural products is an absolute necessity in today's world where toxic chemicals are interfering with our body's ability to heal itself. There is so much stress coming from all sectors of our daily experiences that we cannot handle the overload without some help, physically, emotionally, and spiritually. Physical exercise has a major effect on epigenetic modifications that can be beneficial to health and cancer patients. Modifications in DNA methylation patterns as a result of physical exercise can increase the expression of genes involved in tumor suppression and decrease the expression levels of oncogenes - those can then transform a cell into a tumor cell.

The problem is that people who are chronically sick have been convinced that there is something wrong with them that only toxic drugs, mutilation of body parts, and organ destroying radiation therapy can fix. That is simply not true in most cases. But, the vast majority of the marketing efforts are designed to make you believe it is true. And, many of them that promote such therapies, will probably be really upset that I am making healing the body seem so easy. They are not necessarily at fault. They, like me years ago, are just a product of what they have been taught. When you invest so much time into a belief system, and the belief is not right, you still try to hold onto it for as long as you can. It doesn't make it right, it just is what it is, and they are not necessarily to blame. But when people are exposed to verifiable truth, and they choose to ignore it in favor of harming others, especially for profit, that is where I draw the line and say, now they are responsible.

The verifiable truth is now coming to light through the study of epigenetics. Unfortunately, you can count on this information being purposely suppressed by the profiteers in many sectors of the sick-care community who want to keep the money coming through maintaining the status quo of nonsensical and harmful treatments to the unsuspecting public. Others are so entrenched into a faulty belief system, that it is just too hard for them to get out of the pit.

Hippocrates asserted over two millennia ago that *"food is medicine!"* Sounds like wise advice! Of course, today we are dealing with contaminated food supplies, so we have to be even wiser about food quality choices. Eminent scientist and physician Dean Ornish also supports healing the body through health food and lifestyle options. He has found that by just changing diet and lifestyle for 90 days prostate cancer patients switched on the activity of over 500 genes. Many of the gene changes inhibited biological processes critical in the formation of their tumors. He further states, *"Changing your lifestyle changes your genes (by) turning on protective genes and turning off genes that promote inflammation, oxidative stress, and oncogenes that promote prostate cancer, breast cancer, and colon cancer... In addition, these lifestyle changes lengthen telomeres, the ends of our chromosomes that regulate aging, thereby beginning to reverse aging at a cellular level."* When we provide the natural nutrition that cells are asking for, the body says thank you by keeping us healthy.

There needs to be a life stimulus to kick off cancer, says Dr. Bruce Lipton. *"If you understand epigenetics, you don't need drugs. You can heal yourself... my research reveals conclusively that the environment in which the cells live determines genetic activity... it takes from 15-20 different genes that must be modified to get a cancer off the ground...the other genes...are genes that are activated in regard to our responses to life..."* [125]

There is another piece to this puzzle. Genetic testing is coming to the forefront as a dependable and preferred diagnostic tool. Many diagnostic tools tell us what is happening, but not why. Genetic screening has advanced our diagnostic capability and can get to the how - a gene is turned off so it cannot protect you against cancer, but the why can be elusive. Why is that cancer protective gene turned off? The typical causative factors are environmental toxins, viruses, emotional discord, etc. This is important to understand if you want to get to as much truth as possible to move into complete healing.

Here is a real-life experience of how that played out in my family. My wife, Angel, was plagued with chronic urinary tract infections *(UTI)* for the first thirty years of our marriage. She had been on probably one hundred or more rounds of antibiotics over the years. We just couldn't figure out what was going on. We took as many natural precautions as we could, but nothing seemed to work. The gynecologist would just culture for bacteria then prescribes some antibiotics. The symptoms would go away quickly, but not permanently. Any woman who has had a UTI knows that pain and will do anything to get rid of it. My wife was no exception.

The last time she had a UTI, I was already researching and teaching about epigenetics. At the same time, we had met a local PhD and natural health expert, Dr. Deborah Warner, who was performing DNA testing using very sophisticated equipment. We had lunch and talked about her research and her natural approaches to healing. When my wife had another UTI, we ordered a DNA test kit and sent in a swab from inside her mouth. What we found from that test was life changing. As it turned out, yes, she had a bacterial infection and the antibiotics were keeping it down. But that was not the cause of the chronic UTI. The cause was actually a third world microscopic blood parasite called schistosoma that she had somehow contracted. The larva form can enter through the feet and then travel to the bladder when it lives and thrives. She had gone on a mission trip before we got married, and we had been to some underdeveloped countries early in our marriage, but other than that, we couldn't figure out where it had come from. Curiously, because of mass global travel, the parasite is now more common in developed countries like the United States.

This parasitic infection can cause chronic inflammation, which also predisposes her to bacterial infections and bladder cancer. Her gynecologist of many years hadn't thought to test for this. It just wasn't on his radar screen. The DNA test that she received was different than others. It was able to test what abnormal conditions in the body are stressing the DNA. We were also told that she had some bladder cancer cells from the chronic inflammation of the bladder. We knew what to do at that point. She took some of our own essential oils to support the body's natural protective immune response to the parasites and cancer cells, some special natural preparations from the Doctor Warner, and, shortly thereafter, she was retested and was back to normal.

No cancer cells, no bladder parasites. As of 2019, three years later, she has not had any symptoms of a UTI. We both have seen some amazing similar results in others using this approach, both before and after her experience.

Big picture? Genetic testing is still in its infancy. While more and more DNA testing options are available, there are only a handful of people who have the best and most sophisticated testing equipment and who really know how to interpret DNA test results. The standard doc knows very little about genetic testing. People end up going to the online genetic testing sites, which can provide valuable, gene information, both good and bad, but they don't go beyond that. There are professionals who do genetic testing regularly and may be technically savvy at reading the results, but there are very few epigenetic artisans of interpretation. We just happen to know one.

Methylation And Vitamin B9 Folate Metabolism

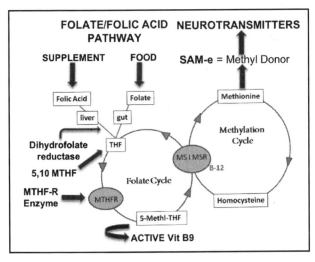

Since methylation plays such an important role in gene expression, mutations in genes within the methylation cycle can alter normal biological processes. One important gene in this cycle is for the production of the enzyme, methylenetetrahydrofolate reductase *(MTHFR)*. This gene is responsible for an important step in the conversion of non-bioactive folate *(vitamin B9)* from food sources to 5-MTHF, a bioactive form that the body uses for maintaining healthy brain chemistry. It is a precursor to the normal production of the neurotransmitters serotonin, melatonin, dopamine, epinephrine, and norepinephrine. These neurotransmitters are involved in a number of functions including short- term memory, concentration, sleep, motor control, hormone control, mood stability, motivation, and appetite control.

A variety of mutations in the MTHFR gene can interfere with this process. One normal gene *"address"* is C677C. The letters represent amino acids. The numbers represent the physical address on Chromosome 1. It is like a street address. A common variant of this gene includes the C677T or T677T single nucleotide polymorphisms *(snps)* where the normal amino acids are replaced causing the gene to function abnormally. Another less common variant is A1298C or C1298C. It lives down the street in the same town and neighborhood: Chromosome 1. In addition to neural tube defects and the brain functions mentioned above, polymorphisms *(changes)* in the MTHFR gene have been studied as possible risk factors for a variety of common conditions. These include heart disease, stroke, high blood pressure *(hypertension),* high blood pressure during pregnancy *(preeclampsia),* an eye disorder called glaucoma, and many types of cancer, autism, Alzheimer's disease, Parkinson's disease, diabetes, arthritis, and chronic fatigue.

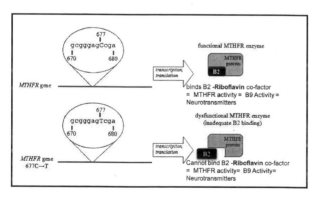

Studies show that variants are becoming common and that raises concerns since so many functions are dependent on the enzyme. One study shows the frequency in the general public of 677 C/T mutations to be 44%, and the 677 T/T to be 8% with total mutation frequency of 52%. Add to it the 8-12% frequency of the less studied 1298. In another study, Beth Ellen Diluglio, MS, RDN, CCN, LDN explains that individuals homozygous *(same variant from both mom and dad)* for C677T have at least a 50-60% reduction in MTHFR activity at body temperature *(98.6°F/37°C)*. Severe MTHFR deficiency with 0-20% enzyme activity can cause early developmental delay, neural tube defects, seizures, motor/gait dysfunction, and even schizophrenic disturbances. There does seem to be variation in the global studies, but regardless, they do present a bleak picture.[126]

Weighty Matters

Obesity is another major health risk, and few would argue that lifestyle and environmental factors have contributed to the epidemic. The World Health Organization estimates there will be more than 2 billion overweight and 700 million obese adults in the world by 2015, and by 2050, 90% of today's children will be overweight or obese. Just as important is the system-wide collateral damage that is associated with obesity such as type 2 diabetes mellitus, cardiovascular diseases, hypertension, and cancer. [127]

It is clear that lifestyle and environmental changes that have occurred over the past 50 years, including more high calorie and low nutrient food, appetite-stimulating chemicals in the food chain, higher stress levels, environmental toxins causing gene mutation, and decreased physical activity, underlie the obesity epidemic. What isn't so clear is why there is such a difference in the way that individuals respond to these lifestyle factors. Yes, genetics can play a part in gene mutations being passed down, but epigenetic influences from the point of conception are increasingly recognized as major contributing influences over the responses to obesity promoting factors. Research has revealed that SNPs such as the FTO gene on Chromosome 16 and others are associated with body mass index and obesity. [128]

The FTO gene SNP can be a lethal form of obesity gene and affects one in six of the population, making them 70% more likely to become obese. A study led by scientists at UCL, the Medical Research Council *(MRC)*, and King's College London Institute of Psychiatry shows that people with the obesity- risk FTO variant have higher circulating levels of the *'hunger hormone,'* ghrelin, in their blood. This means they start to feel hungry again soon after eating a meal. Real-time brain imaging reveals that the FTO gene variation also changes the way the brain responds to ghrelin, and to images of food, in the regions linked with the control of eating and reward. [129,130]

Increased exercise could counteract the effects of the FTO polymorphism. For example, the Amish have a high incidence of FTO - yet very few are obese. Why? Because each day, they labor on their farms for two or more hours. Hard physical labor keeps FTO from expressing obesity, making the Amish exemplify how an environmental trigger can modify gene expression. The good news is that you don't necessarily need two-four hours of hard physical labor. Many patients with this gene variant consistently exercise for 30 minutes, five days per week, and it can keep the gene turned off. Even better is the fact that the gene can be turned off with diet changes, healthy lifestyle choices, and genetic testing and gene normalization by a highly qualified epigenetic specialist. [131, 132]

Another gene affecting weight gain is the one that encodes for PPARG, a protein involved in fat metabolism. When activated, PPARG creates fat cells and helps with the uptake of dietary fats from your blood. Too much activation of PPARG can cause weight gain and increase the risk of heart disease, diabetes, and stroke. When individuals with PPARG polymorphism eat more unsaturated fats than saturated fats, they gain more fat tissue and have a higher BMI. By contrast, when they eat more saturated fats than unsaturated fats, the opposite is true - they are leaner. So here again we see how an environmental *(meaning non-genetic)* factor such as nutrition can trigger a gene and affect people's weight. [133]

There are many examples for correlation between epigenetic modifications and autoimmune diseases as well. For example, in patients with rheumatoid arthritis, both DNA hypomethylation *(under silencing)* and hyperacetylation *(over activation)* of histones *(the spool)* have been observed in synovial tissues. In addition, in patients with multiple sclerosis, the hypomethylation of DNA have been detected in central nervous system white matter in comparison to healthy individuals. In Systemic Lupus Erythematous *(SLE),* the main targets of autoantibodies are hypomethylated DNA and modified histones.

Vitamin D

Vitamin D is one of the most important vitamins for our overall health, but many people in the United States, as well as worldwide, are not getting enough of this vitamin. It is now clear that vitamin D plays an essential role in a variety of physiological processes. It facilitates the absorption of calcium and is critical for bone health. It helps to prevent bone fractures, osteoporosis, reduces the risk of cancer, especially colon cancer, prostate cancer, and breast cancer. It also reduces the risk of diabetes, protects against heart disease, high blood pressure, decreases the risk of multiple sclerosis, and improves mood and lung function. [134]

Vitamin D Binding Protein DBP is a taxicab for vitamin D. It is a multi-functional protein that transports vitamin D and its metabolites around the body. The bioactive form of vitamin D is 1,25-Dihydroxyvitamin D, a steroid hormone with many roles in the body including calcium and phosphorous metabolism, regulation of the immune system, and others. There are also vitamin D *(VDR)* receptors that bind with bioactive vitamin D in the cell nucleus. VDR can have mutations that interfere with vitamin D metabolism.[135]

Inefficient vitamin D metabolism has also been shown to be a factor in autism spectrum disorder *(ASD).* There are studies demonstrating that offspring of mothers with low vitamin D3 concentration were linked with an increased risk for development of autism. [136]

Similar results were presented by Humble et al., who showed below- normal *(31.5-40 nmol/L)* concentrations of vitamin D in the serum of patients with autism, schizophrenia, and ADHD. The relevance of epigenetic programming following dietary supplementation with vitamin D in the mother during pregnancy, which can induce a persistent functional positive vitamin D

epigenetic state in the newborn, thereby contributing to a decreased susceptibility to develop ASD despite its genetic risk, is hugely important. In recent
years, autism has grown to an *"epidemic"* with a 50-fold increase in prevalence during the last 25 years. It is important to search for new methods of
diagnosis and prevention. [137]

Emotional Health

Stress is an important environmental factor, and I think we all can attest to the
arguably unnecessary stresses we face almost on a daily basis. Of particular
epigenetic importance are the stresses during gestation, which have been
shown to be associated with neurodevelopmental and psychiatric disorders. Long-term studies on children exposed to stress in utero have shown
them to be predisposed to psychiatric disorders because of an increase in
the *"promoter"* activities of glucocorticoid receptors. Also, moving forward
in time, some studies have demonstrated that people with post-traumatic
stress disorder, who were abused during childhood, exhibit different levels
of DNA methylation and gene expressions in comparison to those who were
not abused. The way an individual's subconscious processes an experience
in life, especially during childhood, can vary greatly. Our lives are a printout
of our subconscious and patterns of behavior drawn from the subconscious
experiences will develop based on those stored experiences. Ninety percent
of our responses to life are said to come from the subconscious. While the
human mind is immensely complex, it is commonly understood that different
personality types as a group can process life's experiences in their own unique
way. Even identical twins mostly have their own unique personalities where
they each see the world through their own unique lens. So, the conscious
emotional response to a particular event is based on a very unique past
subconscious experience which can have profound epigenetic implications
since the normal healthy gene responses can be altered by that experience.

*"Along with behavior, mental health disorders may be affected by epigenetic
changes,"* says Arturas Petronis, head of the Krembil Family Epigenetics

Laboratory at the Centre for Addiction and Mental Health in Toronto. Numerous reports have pointed to the association of epigenetic DNA methylation with neurodegenerative diseases like dementia and other mental health disorders including autism, ADHD, schizophrenia, depression, and others. [138]

It is also now recognized that many dietary constituents may indirectly influence genomic pathways that methylate DNA, and there is evidence for biochemical links between nutritional quality and mental health. Deficiency of both macro and micronutrients has been associated with increased behavioral problems, and nutritional supplementation has proven efficacious in treatment of certain neuropsychiatric disorders. [139, 140]

Oxytocin is a powerful hormone that affects our mental health. It acts as a neurotransmitter in the brain, and regulates social interaction and sexual reproduction, playing a role in behaviors from maternal-infant bonding and milk release to empathy, generosity, and orgasm. It is even released while praying. Also, when we hug or kiss a loved one, oxytocin levels increase; hence, oxytocin is often called *"the love hormone."* In fact, the hormone plays a huge role in all pair bonding. The hormone circulates through the blood and is greatly stimulated during sex, birth, and breastfeeding. [141]

Oxytocin is also a hormone that, in some ways, is associated with trust, which is a very complicated social process. It is known to be an antidote to depressive feelings and to increase levels of feel-good hormones such as serotonin and dopamine, which may be why it has calming effects. If any of you see me at a conference, or on the street, feel free to come give me a hug, and just say that you want to hit me with some oxy and spread the love. We need more of that. [142]

It is evident that oxytocin plays a very important role in our lives. There are some epigenetically important gene mutations associated with the activation of oxytocin as well, like CD38, which can have some profound effects on social behavior and other systems. CD38 is a multifunctional enzyme. It regulates the release of oxytocin. The loss of CD38 function is associated with impaired immune responses, metabolic disturbances, and behavioral modifications including social amnesia possibly related to autism.

In today's world of autism awareness for example, the role of impairment in the gene that produces oxytocin becomes an important therapy consideration. In a review that examined autism spectrum disorder *(ASD)*, which is characterized by social and communication impairments, two single nucleotide polymorphisms *(snps)* in the human CD38 gene were found to be possible risk factors for ASD via inhibition of oxytocin function. [143, 144, 145]

There is some research on solutions to the social challenges experienced in autism. External nasal oxytocin therapy has been shown to improve social cognition in autistic individuals. Nasal oxytocin spray can modify social signals and the social feedback process in high-functioning autistic patients and can have symptomatic improvement with long-term treatment. [146, 147, 148]

The Effect Of Negative Emotions

Emotions, which again are based on our subconscious experiences, can also play a huge part in epigenetics and health. If they are healthy, then emotional grounding and self-control are epigenetically strengthened. If they are unhealthy, epigenetic changes can take place in DNA and cause a wide variety of temporary or even permanent changes. These tendencies can be passed down to future generations.

Anger, bitterness, unforgiveness, resentment, and depression can all have a negative impact on health, causing chronic diseases. In my opinion, all of these unhealthy emotional responses have unforgiveness at their core. Dr. Dean Ornish writes, *"Every time you feel unforgiveness, you are more likely to develop a health problem."* Forgiveness of others is crucial to our own health. It is unlocking the door to set someone free only to realize that you were the prisoner all along the way. Dr. Ornish continues, *"When I talk about forgiveness, I mean letting go, not excusing the other person or reconciling with them or condoning the behavior, just letting go of your own suffering... There have been over 1400 published studies on forgiveness and health."*

Having a chronic negative emotion towards someone gives that person power over your emotional health, and it can cause the same sort of chronic diseases and death as slowly drinking arsenic, DDT, or any of the other toxic chemicals mentioned throughout this book. And, depending on personality and subconscious processing of the longstanding experience, manifestation of the disease can occur in any number of organs through epigenetic changes in gene expression.

One story that demonstrates how emotional trauma may cause disease Another experience involved a phone call from the wife of a colleague who had recently been diagnosed with stage 4 breast cancer. I went through a litany of questions with her to try and pinpoint the cause. Everything was pretty normal. No meds or medical problems before this diagnosis. Angel *(my wife)* and I started to explore possible broken relationship contributions. Women, in general, are so much more relational than men. We knew that breast cancer can be caused from environmental chemical exposure, but that didn't seem to be the case here. We also knew that breast cancer can have emotional roots and be caused by a break in relationship between two females, either in the family or a close friend. So, we asked questions about her female family relationships. Nothing was unusual until I asked her if she'd had a break in a relationship with a close friend. She went silent, for an uncomfortably long time. When she spoke again, she said she'd had a falling out with her best friend in high school twenty some years before, and it was still a very painful emotional memory for her. We encouraged her, prayed for her, and helped her to understand how the cancer and that broken relationship could possibly be related. We encouraged her to seek out some counsel to cover that base, and we talked about forgiveness of herself for holding on to that old hurt, and forgiveness of her friend for whatever happened. She had already looked into medical intervention for her cancer and just wanted to look at some other possibilities.

Angel and I have seen on multiple occasions, in us, and in others, how devastating unforgiveness and other negative emotions can be on relationships and overall health. The progression of emotionally related diseases is stealth, and by the time the symptoms appear, recovery takes a lot of time and work, but it is worth every minute.

The Long-Term Impact Of Understanding Epigenetics

The importance of epigenetics in different human disorders has attracted much interest in the last decade, especially related to complicated disorders such as cancer, behavior disorders, memory, endocrine disorders such as diabetes, obesity, autoimmune disease, addiction, as well as psychological disorders and neurodegenerative disorders like Alzheimer's. It is becoming clearer why many therapeutic approaches have failed in the past. The only way to make future breakthroughs in disease causation is to involve experts in epigenetics as well as many other fields, including environmental epidemiology, genetic epidemiology, biostatistics, to name a few.

Poor nutrition and chemical intoxication, as a cause of epigenetic changes have been the focus of a great deal of research during the past 10 years. There is strong evidence that the degree to which certain genes are turned on or off has a greater effect on our risk for developing these chronic diseases than does the genetic code we inherited from our parents. Once it was demonstrated that genes could be regulated, we realized that our risk for disease could be directly tied to our lifestyle choices. At no time is this more important than during fetal development where toxic chemical exposure and nutrition will have the greatest impact on development. The risk of turning off *"good"* genes is highest during this time. If this happens, a person can be much more likely to develop chronic disease over their lifespan, but particularly as they age.

The good news is that growing evidence suggests that chronic diseases like diabetes, heart disease, obesity and others can be shut off in future generations, if we make sure everyone in this generation, especially infants, young children, and pregnant women, integrate healthy habits into their daily routines. Exercise alone, for example, will turn on hundreds of good genes and turn bad genes off. It is important to spread the word to everyone, especially women who may be thinking about becoming pregnant. Making changes to your diet and encouraging changes to the food culture and levels of toxic chemical exposure at your place of business or school and supporting public policies that encourage a healthy lifestyle for all, will help ensure that we are on the right track toward reversing the advancement of chronic diseases currently affecting the health of the US population now and for generations to come. [149]

CHAPTER 3

Brain Drain
Prelude To Orwellian Dystopia

Your brain HAS been hijacked. Those vying for your attention *(and your money)* wish to turn you into their own personal automatons, hitting you with a constant and daily barrage of information designed to *"make your life easier to manage."* Ethical marketing with the intent of selling goods is not necessarily a bad thing, at least not at face value. But there is a growing realization that many unscrupulous businesses and even the government want to take control of our lives by taking control of our minds. It reminds me what George Orwell warned about in his classic book, 1984. The term Orwellian dystopia describes a society in which language is manipulated to control our minds and actions, where harming people can actually be seen as love. Words are not used to convey meaning but to undermine it, and our brains are manipulated into a state of cognitive dissonance where we are stealthily convinced to disregard our own perceptions and replace them with officially dictated versions, which then become our reality. The result is that our privacy of thought is violated, controlled, and then stolen as we give over to the barrage of propaganda and mind control efforts. [150, 151, 152]

And, while humans have had control issues since the beginning of time, what is going on now is light years beyond anything we have seen in the past. It is covert in nature, with a bottom line that is always the same – control equals power and money. Experts in marketing strategies know that humans have three fundamental emotional needs: a need to feel safe, a need to belong to a group *(individuals are even willing to kill to be part of a gang who will accept them)*, and a need to do something that matters. This is why they no longer focus on what they are selling as much as they focus on *"why"* you need it. You need their product or service to make you feel good, to make you a stronger, more improved version of yourself. Whether they are advertising the newest app or a drug, the goal is to make you emotionally and physically dependent upon their product.

Large-scale strategies in mind-control techniques are troublesome, to say the least. In the social media world for example, there is high-level table talk among corporate execs and their tech teams about such strategies. According to Facebook, it is developing technology to read your brainwaves so that you don't have to look down at your phone to type emails, you can just think them. Facebook has assembled a team of 60 people, including machine learning and neural prosthetics experts, to study how to enable such a system. Its goal? To create a system capable of typing one hundred words per minute - five times faster than you can type on a smartphone - straight from your brain. Facebook plans to develop non-invasive sensors that can measure brain activity hundreds of times per second at high resolution to decode brain signals associated with language in real-time. *"No such technology exists today; we'll need to develop one,"* says Regina Dugan, the head of Facebook's innovation Skunkworks, Building 8. I wonder what suggestions will be put back into your brain secondary to what they measure and control coming out of your brain. [153]

Big Pharma is a major player in the marketing game and looking at their expanding sphere of worldwide influence and profits, no one should be surprised by their successful efforts. In 1983, they took to the streets with their first television ad. After some legal jousting on the ethics of advertising drugs to the public on television, the industry won the day. Instead of advertising just to the docs, the industry had full reign to go directly to the consumer. According to Kantar Media, a firm that tracks multimedia advertising, 771,368 such ads were shown in 2016, the last full year for which data is available, an increase of almost 65% over 2012. Global statistics depict the worldwide revenue of the pharmaceutical market from 2001 to 2016. In 2001, worldwide revenue was around 390.2 billion US dollars. Ten years later, in 2011, this figure stood at some 963 billion US dollars. In 2014, global pharmaceutical revenues for the first time increased to over one trillion US dollars. That's control! And for them, it is not about a better light bulb; it is about controlling your mind and the rest of your body for profit.

Mother's Little Helper

Perhaps the first to bring the dark side of pharmaceuticals to the public consciousness was the group, The Rolling Stones in the '60s! So many of the folk and pop groups of the time told stories of cultural shifts and struggles. We were first made aware of Big Pharma's large-scale efforts to control the minds of emotionally hurting people with their introduction of Valium in 1963. In the United States, it was the highest selling medication between 1968 and 1982, selling more than two billion tablets in 1978 alone. We were hooked, literally. The lyrics about Valium are quite telling:

Mother's Little Helper

What a drag it is getting old
"Kids are different today,"
I hear ev'ry mother say
Mother needs something today to calm her down
And though she's not really ill
There's a little yellow pill
She goes running for the shelter of a mother's
little helper And it helps her on her way,
gets her through her busy day

At the end of the song a warning is given to mothers:

"Life's just much too hard today,"
I hear ev'ry mother say

The pursuit of happiness just seems a bore
And if you take more of those, you will get an overdose
No more running for the shelter of a mother's
little helper They just helped you on your
way, through your busy dying day.

Fast-forward and we see that addiction to street drugs, while still a major problem, doesn't hold a candle to the drug pushers in the pharmaceutical world. The white-collar drug pushers have made their way into medical schools teaching docs that medications are the best and only way to keep someone alive. The docs get out and into practice and pass that message to their patients. It is a true and inescapable fact. I supported that mantra for years.

And, while you may casually accept paying for the recommended toxic medications and industrial chemicals that destroy the brain and the rest of your body, and you are hoodwinked into thinking that it is a good thing, the cold reality is that you have been hustled by chemical pimps that want you hooked - and they are winning, for now.

Physicians now face an ethical dilemma with prescribing medications that can also harm people. I would argue that most medications harm more than they help. Some are good for emergencies, but the ones to treat chronic diseases that *"help keep you alive,"* are generally more harmful than helpful, unless of course you have had organs removed or an organ has shut down, and then they may be necessary. Of particular concern are the mind-altering medications that can leave people prey to the Big Pharma profiteers. Dr. Ronald Hoffman, is recognized as one of America's foremost complementary medicine practitioners. He received his M.D. from Albert Einstein College of Medicine. He was trained in Internal Medicine and now specializes in complementary and alternative medicine. He writes, *"It recently came to light that a wide range of popular medications - used routinely by tens of millions of Americans - have a nasty tendency to accelerate cognitive decline and set the stage for Alzheimer's disease."* Anticholinergic medications (*they block the parasympathetic nervous system),* for instance, are associated with the development of memory disorders such as Alzheimer's. These medications block acetylcholine, a critical neurotransmitter in the brain. They include medications for bladder disorders, Parkinson's disease, depression, and are also found in many cold remedies used to dry up congestion. Other brain-stealers include anti-inflammatory meds, cholesterol-lowering medication, insomnia medication, and anti-anxiety medication.

Broadly speaking, there is no such thing as a *"clean"* side-effect-free drug. Medications are inherently *"dirty."* Vioxx for example, was the ideal non-steroidal anti-inflammatory drug embraced for years by the medical community before it was found to cause blood clots. Before it was yanked from the marketplace, it is estimated that the drug may have been responsible for tens of thousands of deaths due to premature heart attacks and strokes.

When doctors prescribe medications, many patients would say they feel compelled to do what is prescribed, partly because the constant drip, drip, drip of marketing by big Pharma has worn them down, and partly because they have been brainwashed into thinking that doctors belong on a pedestal, and their educated word is final. Shouldn't docs abide by some sort of bioethical precept such as *primum non nocere,* "first, to do no harm," which was embedded in the tenants of the Hippocratic oath? Or is that all passé now in a healthcare world of moral relativism driven by profit instead of compassion and common sense? Docs do their best with what they know, like I did for so many years. The problem with our knowledge base being so deeply engrained in pharmaceuticals is that what we have been taught is insufficient to protect the lives of the people placed in our care. Will that change anytime soon? I doubt it. So, you have to take control of your own health and well-being as much as possible and prepare your future generations to do the same. [154]

Increasingly, certain classes of medicines have been recognized as causing cognitive decline and impairment; these potentially preventable adverse events have risks that are a function of dose, duration, and individual susceptibility *(such as preexisting cognitive impairment or dementia or genetic makeup).* The impact of these medications on long-term cognitive function is an area of ongoing research. Pregnant moms especially need to be aware of the potential adverse effects on a fetus and breast-feeding baby as well as their own health and ability to effectively raise a family in a nurturing way.

Classes of Medications Causing Brain Impairment
1. Antianxiety drugs
2. Cholesterol drugs
3. Antiseizure drugs
4. Antidepressant drugs
5. Narcotic painkillers
6. Parkinson's drugs
7. Hypertension drugs
8. Sleeping aids
9. Incontinence drugs
10. Antihistamines

As we age, we are pretty much guaranteed that Big Pharma will directly market to us. And when I talk about aging, I am talking about 35-year olds and above. That is when hormone-related health challenges seem to emerge in today's toxic world. Guys, if you don't take care of your health, your gut will start to protrude, you will have less energy, less hair, be prone to diabetes, cardiovascular disease, and have less sexual prowess. You just start to feel less like a man and may look to other, not-so-healthy activities to take the edge off that stress. In the past, this may have started in one's late fifties and early sixties, but in today's world, environmental contaminants and poor nutrition will take you down to mush at a much earlier age. Ladies, you will experience heightened hormone disruption with emotional ups and downs, weight gain, a dysfunctional thyroid, loss of hair, early wrinkles, etc. Your PCP *(Primary Care Physician)* will then tell you that you are depressed, and you can guess what comes next - your brain is stolen from you because of the antidepressants and anti-anxiety medications that will be prescribed.

Your life, or lack thereof, will be determined by a seemingly soft but very cruel pharmaceutical taskmaster. Your life will not be lived out on your own terms. Then, you may also be subjected to suggestions of hysterectomies, brain implants, thyroidectomies, etc. all because you may be emotionally distraught through no fault of your own, but because of the chemical exposure that your body has tried to deal with for so many years. Your body systems finally start to shut down. You lose your autonomy, that special intimacy with your husband, your connection with your children, friends, and other loved ones. Just think about what it would be like for a child who is unnecessarily put on mind-altering medications at an early age. Their brains are essentially stolen from them. It may not seem so at the time, but it is true. Not that these scenarios will happen to everyone to the same degree, but you can bet that it will happen to some degree. There is no way around it. Do you really want to take that chance?

Older adults take an average of 14 prescription drugs per year, putting them at heightened risk for adverse drug reactions, drug-drug interactions, and drug-disease interactions. In 2015, the National Academy of Medicine published a report on cognitive aging. This report describes some groups of medications that may affect older adults' cognition. These groups include certain antihistamines, anti-anxiety and antidepressant medications, sleep aids, antipsychotics, muscle relaxants, antimuscarinics for urinary incontinence, and antispasmodics for relief of cramps or spasms of the stomach, intestines, and bladder. [155]

Health care professionals, particularly primary care providers, play a critical role in monitoring medications and avoiding inappropriate use by older adults, but too often they fail from lack of knowledge about the toxic chemicals they are recommending, or apathy, or both. Medicine is more of a business now than a healing art. Modern medicine as a whole no longer heals. It covers up and makes you think that you are okay when you are not. Yes, there are exceptions - necessary and corrective surgeries, trauma care, anesthesia, antibiotic intervention, emergency medicine, and some others. But, providing pharmaceuticals to take care of chronic health challenges like diabetes, hypertension, heart disease, etc. is unnecessary for most people. The risk of adverse reactions from medications far outweighs the benefit, as I mentioned in The Killing Fields chapter, with the third and fourth leading cause of death in the United States behind cancer and heart disease, being mistakes by doctors, and adverse drug reactions.

The Brain - A Masterpiece In Design And Function

The human brain has approximately 85- 100 billion neurons, each neuron connected to ten thousand other neurons. If it were a computer, it could process information at 38 thousand trillion operations per second. The world's most powerful supercomputer, the Summit, processes 200 trillion operations per second. Nerve impulses can travel up to 250 miles per hour, which translates to about 16-25 milliseconds from the time you think about moving your arm and then actually starting the process. That is incredibly fast. About a quarter of your body's metabolism goes toward operating and maintaining your brain. In order to process even basic information, billions of chemical signals are processed every second. [156]

Most of the brain is created in a matter of months. During the first few weeks of gestation, when your mother knew you only as morning sickness, and you were a layer of cells huddled in one corner of her uterus, those cells lined up, formed a groove, and then closed to form a tube. One end of that tube eventually became your tiny spinal cord. The rest expanded to form the beginnings of your brain. For a brain to develop properly, neurons must move to precise places in a precise sequence. They do so under the direction of hormones and chemical neurotransmitters like acetylcholine. The process is an intricate, fast-paced dance on a very tiny scale. At any point, that cell can be knocked off course. Many toxic chemicals like the ones already discussed have the potential to disrupt this journey, in a slight or serious fashion. [157]

By the third trimester, the surface of the brain begins folding itself into wrinkled peaks and valleys that make a brain look like a brain. Specific areas of that cortex learn to process specific aspects of sensation, movement, and thought, and that starts in the uterus. By age two, almost all of the billions of brain cells that you will ever have are in their places. Except in the hippo-campus and one or two other tiny regions, the brain does not grow new brain cells throughout your life. When brain cells die, they are gone. So, those initial months of formation, when the brain is most vulnerable, are critical. *"During these sensitive life stages, exposure can cause permanent brain injury at low levels that would have little or no adverse effect on an adult,"* write Grandjean and Landrigan.

From birth to about age 6, a child's brain develops more than at any other time in life. And early brain development has a lasting impact on a child's ability to learn. The quality of a child's experiences in the first few years of life - positive or negative - helps shape how their brain develops. From age 7-11, children become more aware of external events, as well as feelings about themselves and others. They become less egocentric and begin to understand that not everyone shares their own thoughts, beliefs, or feelings. From age 11 on, children are able to use logic to solve problems, view the world around them, and plan for the future.

In the adult, studies show that the very important prefrontal cortex will not fully develop until the mid-twenties, earlier for females, later for males. The prefrontal cortex coordinates higher-order cognitive processes and executive functioning. Executive functions are a set of supervisory cognitive skills needed for goal-directed behavior, including planning, response inhibition, working memory, and attention. These skills allow an individual to pause long enough to take stock of a situation, assess his or her options, plan a course of action, and execute it. Poor executive functioning leads to difficulty with planning, attention, using feedback, and mental inflexibility, all of which could undermine judgment and decision making. This brain region has also been implicated in personality expression, decision-making, and moderating social behavior. Any interference with this development, like that seen with medications *(and environmental chemicals)*, can alter brain function and have far-reaching and long-lasting effects. [158]

Antidepressant Medication

The US is in the midst of a mental health crisis. In 2017, 47,000 Americans died by suicide and 70,000 from drug overdoses, and 17.3 million adults suffered at least one major depressive episode. The answer so far? The rising denial of counseling treatment by insurance companies, doctors not taking insurance for those companies that do offer coverage because the reimbursements are so low, or blanket treatments with antidepressant medications dispensed by everyone from psychiatrists to quack shack docs. But why the rising denials for therapy care by insurance companies? Could it be that instead of paying out tens of millions for therapy that may be lifelong and ineffective, they would just rather sell drugs? [159]

Antidepressants are some of the most popular drugs in the United States, and their usage shows no signs of waning. Global revenue for antidepressants is projected to grow to nearly 17 billion dollars by 2020. Antidepressant use in the United States soared by 65% in 15 years. By 2014, about one in every eight Americans over the age of 12 reported recent antidepressant use, and women are twice as likely as men to be taking the medications.

It has been reported in the Journal of the American Medical Association's Jama, Internal Medicine, that 16.7% of 242 million US adults reported filling one or more prescriptions for psychiatric drugs in 2013." Most of those were for antidepressants. Most psychiatric drug use reported by adults was long term, with 84.3% having filled 3 or more prescriptions in 2013 or indicating that they had started taking the drug during 2011 or earlier.

In spite of a growing body of evidence that they are only nominally effective, their use is increasing with no end in sight. Antidepressants are also routinely prescribed for back pain, Post Traumatic Stress Disorder *(PTSD)*, Premenstrual Syndrome *(PMS)*, chronic pain, weight loss, muscle pain, obsessive compulsive disorder (OCD), smoking cessation, and sleep disturbance, just to name a few.

How Effective Are Antidepressants?

For people with mild to moderate depression, *"Nine out of ten studies showed that the new drugs were no more effective than placebos."* However, because of great marketing hype around the SSRIs, one of them, Prozac, now has the distinguished honor of having more adverse effects submitted to the FDA than any other drug in history.

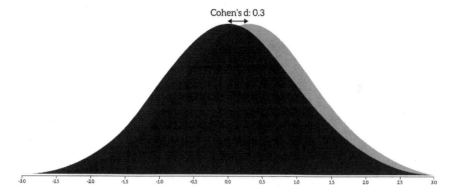

Irving Kirsch and his collaborators, in their meta-analysis of industry-funded random controlled studies, reported that the difference in symptom reduction between the medicated and placebo groups is insignificant in mild and moderate depression participants - less than two points on the Hamilton Rating Scale of Depression *(HAM-D)*.

Kirsch and others have calculated *"effect sizes"* of around .30 for antidepressants, but needed to be at least 3.0 on the scale to be significant. As is shown by the graph, this means that there is an 88% overlap in the distribution of outcomes for the drug-treated and placebo patients. Effectively, you need to treat eight people to produce one additional person who benefits from the treatment, as compared to the placebo. Thus, the risk-benefit equation from this symptom-reduction data can be summed up in this manner: 12% of patients will benefit from the treatment, while the remaining 88% will suffer the adverse effects of treatment without any additional therapeutic benefit beyond placebo. They concluded that there is a lack of evidence that antidepressants are effective in the majority of real-world patients, even over the short term. They *"work"* in only a minority of patients, and it may be that they don't provide any benefit over natural recovery rates at the end of six to twelve weeks. [160 - 165]

A Minnesota report on the real-world outcomes of 260,000 patients treated for depression from 2010 to 2013 found similarly low remission rates. At the end of each year, only about 5% of the patients were in remission. Another 10% or so were still considered responders to antidepressant treatment. The remaining 85% were categorized as chronically depressed. So, classic antidepressant medication does not work for the vast majority of people.

It is an indisputable, but well-hidden fact that not only are these drugs ineffective, *"the actual rate of death from suicide is higher in patients who take the new antidepressants then those who take older, tricyclic medication" (with major side effects)* or who received no treatment at all. In an article appearing in the Journal of Clinical Psychiatry in 1989, only two years after the release of Prozac, doctors were already starting to report drug induced neurological agitation. Similar results were being reported for Zoloft, Paxil, and Luvox, Effexor, Remeron, and Wellbutrin, all in the SSRI category and were also found to be *"no more effective than the older tricyclic antidepressants."* In fact, the newer drugs were not found to be even 10% more effective than placebos. The statistical results of all the published and unpublished data revealed, out of every 1,000 persons with depression that were treated with one of the newer drugs, 4.6 more committed suicide each year then would have if they had not received any treatment at all.

Keep in mind, in the studies that won SSRI initial FDA approval for seriously depressed patients, anyone suicidal, or with manic depression, children, and the elderly were typically excluded from the studies. Now, does that make any sense? These drugs are currently prescribed like candy to all of these other *"at risk"* groups even though they were not tested.

The Dangers Of Antidepressants

There are very legitimate and serious concerns about the overall safety of antidepressant medications and many studies and real-life observations about how dangerous they are. A Prozac clinical trial involving depressed adolescents was conducted by the University of South Carolina. The study was stopped abruptly because of the emergence of intense suicidal and or homicidal ideation in five patients.

In 1991, yet another group of researchers at the Yale University School of Medicine published a report on the *"emergence of self-destructive phenomena in children and adolescents during fluoxetine (Prozac) treatment."* In the report, the authors stated that self-injurious ideation or behavior appeared de novo, for the first time, or intensified in six of 47 patients being treated with Prozac for obsessive-compulsive disorder. Four of the cases required hospitalization and three required restraints seclusion or one-on-one nursing care. [166]

Peter Gotzsche, co-founder of the Cochrane Collaborative, the most respected source of information on medical standards, based on the most thorough meta-analyses of the scientific literature available - said at a European summit on depression: *"In relation to Zyprexa, and Eli Lilly's other blockbuster, Prozac, there were so many fundamental manipulations in the pivotal trials that they submitted for registration that in my view these drugs should never have seen the light of day. These are terrible drugs, both of them, but Eli Lilly made them blockbusters..."*

In human studies, prenatal SSRI exposure has been linked to increased rates of depression in early adolescence, lower birth weight, shorter gestational period, lower Apgar score *(a measure of the physical condition of the newborn infant and response to resuscitation),* and neonatal abstinence syndrome *(NAS).* NAS is often seen in newborns exposed to addictive opiates, alcohol, benzodiazepines, and results in withdrawal symptoms in the newborn. Overall, this study presents evidence that prenatal exposure to SSRI's can affect infant neurodevelopment and may be associated with increased susceptibility to anxiety disorders, hyperactivity, and maladaptive processing. [167]

Antidepressants are particularly dangerous because of the initial increase in availability of serotonin. Serotonin primarily affects mood, and this class of antidepressants increases availability of serotonin to the brain. However, while initially you may think you feel better, you won't feel like a butterfly like the ads suggest, nor will you float as you walk or smile from ear to ear. It is a dark world. You'll just be *"half there,"* in a sense because something else is controlling how you think and respond, but you just don't realize it. As each day passes, that sense becomes more of your reality, so you don't *"think"* anything is wrong. You live in that zone where the looking glass out into the world is not entirely clear.

The side effects reported with antidepressant use include mood swings, lack of emotion, dreams, altered personality, racing thoughts, restlessness, inability to sit still, unusual energy surges, inability to recognize reality, silly and giddy behavior, paranoia, blank staring, hyperactivity, aggression, self-destructive behavior, violence, suicidal thoughts and attempts, mania, and psychosis. It was the staggering increase in drug-related suicide that eventually resulted in the FDA's requirement for manufacturers to place a black box warning on all antidepressants regarding that increased risk in adolescents and young adults.

The British Medical Journal reported the following on SSRIs and suicide and violence:

"[. . .] we looked at 64,381 pages of clinical study reports (70 trials) we got from the European Medicines Agency. We showed for the first time that SSRIs in comparison with placebo increase aggression in children and adolescents... This is an important finding considering the many school shootings where the killers were on SSRIs...It can no longer be doubted that antidepressants are dangerous and can cause suicide and homicide at any age. It is absurd to use drugs for depression that increase the risk of suicide and homicide when we know that cognitive behavioral therapy can halve the risk of suicide in patients who have been admitted (even) after a suicide attempt..." I would go beyond that and state emphatically that DNA testing and therapy, lifestyle changes, good nutrition, essential oils, and a wholesome social support network are the major keys to successfully treating depression. While the mind is complex, simple lifestyle strategies have been shown to be very effective and DNA testing can identify some genes such as TAO, MTHFR, and COMT that may

be epigenetically altered. A sound approach to nutritional therapy can also help normalize gene function and alleviate symptoms. [168, 169]

In 2007, the FDA admitted that SSRIs can cause madness *(mental illness, insanity)* at all ages and that the drugs are very dangerous; otherwise daily monitoring wouldn't be needed and encouraged manufacturers to add this warning to product labels: *"Families and caregivers of patients should be advised to look for the emergence of such symptoms on a day-to-day basis, since changes may be abrupt. . . . All patients being treated with antidepressants for any indication should be monitored appropriately and observed closely for clinical worsening, suicidality, and unusual changes in behavior, especially during the initial few months of a course of drug therapy, or at times of dose changes, either increases or decreases. The following symptoms, anxiety, agitation, panic attacks, insomnia, irritability, hostility, aggressiveness, impulsivity, akathisia (psychomotor restlessness), hypomania, and mania, have been reported in adult and pediatric patients being treated with antidepressants...."*

I personally know of several cases that began with psychotropic meds for mild depression, anxiety, etc. that turned into nightmares. The studies clearly show that violent and suicide ideation are all part of the antidepressant package. My mom's suicide was one of those tragedies. But there are others that were well on their way off the cliff, and someone stepped into the gap for them and helped change their lives through simple caring and lifestyle changes, not medications, endless visits to the therapist's office, or electro-convulsive therapy.

There are many tragedies associated with the use of antidepressant medications. Most go unnoticed, and some are even removed in study models that try and support the use of medications to treat depression. But more notable are those that end up involving the murders and/or suicide of innocent people that hit the media outlets. Columbine mass-killer Eric Harris for example was taking Luvox - like Prozac, Paxil, Zoloft, Effexor and many others, a modern and widely prescribed type of antidepressant drug called selective serotonin reuptake inhibitors, or SSRIs." Along with fellow student Dylan Klebold, Harris shot 13 to death and wounded 24 in a headline-grabbing

1999 rampage. *"Luvox manufacturer Solvay Pharmaceuticals concedes that during short-term controlled clinical trials, 4% of children and youth taking Luvox - that's one in 25 - developed mania, a dangerous and violence-prone mental derangement characterized by extreme excitement and delusion."* That means out of 10,000 people taking this drug, 400 will develop a very serious mental derangement that may be a threat to other innocent people.

In November 2005, more than four years after Andrea Yates drowned her children in their own bathtub, Effexor manufacturer, Wyeth Pharmaceuticals, quietly added homicidal ideation to the drug's list of rare adverse events. The Medical Accountability Network, a private nonprofit focused on medical ethics issues, publicly criticized Wyeth, saying Effexor's homicidal ideation risk wasn't well-publicized, and that Wyeth failed to send letters to doctors or issue warning labels announcing the change. And what exactly does rare mean in the phrase rare adverse events? The FDA defines it as occurring in less than one in 1,000 people. But since that same year 19.2 million prescriptions for Effexor were filled in the US, statistically that means thousands of Americans might experience homicidal ideation - murderous thoughts - as a result of taking just this one brand of antidepressant drug.

In fact, as Channel 2, WCGH reported in 2009, *"One study shows a quarter of all children on drugs such as Paxil and Zoloft become dangerously violent and/or suicidal."* An investigation by a San Antonio television station in 2004 discovered that two out of every three foster children in Texas have been placed on psychotropic medications, many of them on two or more such drugs. One child was being forced to take 17 different prescription medications to alter or regulate behavior and sleep. At least 300 children under the age of seven were found to be on multiple mood and behavior medications. Today, with one out of six Americans on some psychiatric medication, we ought to perhaps bear in mind that just because a drug is on the right side of the law doesn't mean it won't bring you to the wrong side of sanity's line. [170, 171]

In Appendix B, I have listed the mass shootings that have been compiled and connected to psychotropic prescription medications. It is not just a few;

it is over 40. People can talk all around this issue but the facts pretty much speak for themselves. While there can also be extenuating circumstances, the balance of the evidence points to the medication that turned people to do unimaginable violent acts. As tragic as it was in all these cases, were the killers actually victims as well, and the real guilty party the manufacturer of the medications, since they knew could lead to such tragedies? Many psychiatrists and other mental health experts, as well as family and friends believe so, and the evidence seems to support that contention. Even the pharmaceutical manufacturers now have "violent and suicidal ideation" as a possible adverse drug reaction listed in the package inserts for psychotropic medications. [172]

Gwen Olsen is the author of Confessions of a Prescription Drug Pusher. As a high-level drug rep for fifteen years, she was very closely involved with the marketing of medications to physicians, hospitals, and med students. She was trained what to say, how to say it, and how to answer questions about medications efficacy and side effects. As a medical professional, I completely appreciate all that she shares in her shocking and very heart-moving book. She was no stranger to the side effects of antidepressants as she struggled with depression after a divorce. Gwen was placed on antidepressants and experienced a myriad of symptoms: *"I was 33 years old, and I had never taken antidepressants before. In just a few days I started having major side effects, including agitation, jitteriness, racing thoughts, and palpitations. I couldn't drive. I couldn't think. I certainly couldn't work and call on doctors."* Gwen's doctor doubled her dose and things got worse. *"My memory doesn't serve me as to what happened next but I fortunately kept a journal of my daily chemically-induced foray into madness. Apparently, after doubling the dose, I began experiencing psychotic delusions. . . . at one point I crawled up in a fetal position to hold myself while I shook uncontrollably. . . . at my insistence, he discontinued the Zoloft therapy. He prescribed Prozac next. The suicidal ideation came in intense and unrelenting urges. I played out every detail with obsessive-compulsive precision. My once sharp and brilliant mind was losing touch with reality, and I couldn't bear the mental pain."*

After her experience with antidepressants, she experienced a new awakening that transformed her life. She also realized that things were just not quite what they appeared to be in the pharmaceutical industry. The misrepresentations, marketing schemes, altered test results, and outright lies were all a part of their training to line the pockets of the Big Pharma profiteers. But it didn't really hit home how bad it was until her own niece committed suicide by setting herself on fire after being treated with a whole host of antipsychotics and other medications. [173]

To help give a heartfelt connection with this event, I am sharing this excerpt from Gwen's book as she came to the scene shortly after Meg's suicide:

I braced myself on my father's arm as we entered the house. The first thing I noticed was the melted, plastic venetian blinds next to the front door. Replaying the EMS report in my mind, I envisioned Meg struggling to open the door with her body engulfed in flames... my eyes next caught the exposed wires hanging from the living room ceiling where the fan used to be. She had first attempted to hang herself by fashioning a rope from her shoestrings and attaching them to the ceiling fan. The fan gave way to her body weight and she was unsuccessful. Feeling weak in the knees and nauseous, I can see my mother and sister, Meg's mom, moving about in the next room . . . a blood-soaked rag and bandanna found at the foot of her bed on a pile of clothes suggested she may have tended to a head wound caused by the ceiling fan. Next to her bedside were copies of "A Course in Miracles" and the "Living Bible." Her mother said she had spent a large portion of the night before on her knees as she prayed at the foot of her bed.

More melted blinds came to my attention as we proceeded to the center bedroom. This room belongs to Hayley, Meg's younger sister. In this room, Meg had poured oil from an angel shaped lantern over herself and ignited it. The intense heat of the fire had obviously risen to the ceiling and had melted the blinds into clumps of plastic at the very top on each side.

At some point, Meg had a change of heart and desired to live because she ran into the bathroom and tried extinguishing the fire in the bathtub. Apparently, she was unaware that this action would only strengthen the fire. Still struggling to survive, she had the presence of mind to call 911 and told them she had set herself on fire. The rescuers stated when they arrived at the scene, that she'd opened the door and fell backward onto the coffee table. She never spoke a word . . . she didn't die until they got to the hospital in Austin. [174]

Gwen writes that Meg was beautiful inside and out, but did experience emotional trauma from a turbulent childhood. Despite that, at 18 years old, Meg was an honor graduate and premed student at Indiana University. Following an automobile accident, Meg was given massive quantities of Vicodin and other anti-inflammatory drugs for pain. That began a downward spiral. Her performance at school began waning, and she became depressed. She was diagnosed as bipolar *(manic-depressive)* and was given a cocktail of chemicals that would lead to her ultimate demise. The partial list of drugs Meg took within a one-year frame clearly demonstrates how the lack of monitoring and coordination within he healthcare community can have devastating effects on a precious life: *Depakote ER, *Seroquel, *Vicodin, amoxicillin, penicillin, *Desyrel, *Zoloft, *Paxil, *Lamictal, *Flexeril, naproxen, Vioxx, *Trileptal, Voltaren, *Ultram, *Effexor XR, Phenazopyridine, Tinazidine, Septra DS, ibuprofen, *Darvocet N, XR, *Abilify, *Zyprexa, *Zanaflex, and Nabumetone. Those with the asterisk are very dangerous and mind-altering drugs.

Obviously, something was very wrong here. Shouldn't someone have been monitoring the number and kinds of medications being prescribed? Shouldn't her doctors have known about the side effects and drug interactions that even two medications would have caused? Shouldn't they have known that most of the medications she was prescribed would cause or exacerbate the spiraling out of control symptoms she was experiencing? There is no way that her liver or brain could have handled this type of abuse and poisoning. In the end, after some additional emotionally painful family circumstances, she couldn't take it anymore. She became a statistic and victim of an abusive system.

Corruption In The Healthcare And Pharmaceutical Industries

The cover-ups, misrepresentations of data, false advertising, and biased clinical research associated with SSRI *(Selective Serotonin Reuptake Inhibitors)* antidepressant drugs is staggering. There have been multiple reports of fraudulent clinical testing, forgery, bribery, racketeering, and endangering patients in the testing of psychiatric drugs.

American psychologist, Lisa Cosgrove, and others reveal the facts in their study *"Financial Ties between DSM-IV Panel Members and the Pharmaceutical Industry."* They found that *"of the 170 DSM panel members, 95 (56 %) had one or more financial associations with companies in the pharmaceutical industry. One hundred percent of the members of the panels on 'Mood Disorders' and 'Schizophrenia and Other Psychotic Disorders' had financial ties to drug companies."*

In a recent article by Citizens Commission on Human Rights International, CCHR, Shrink's for Sale: Psychiatry's Conflicted Alliance, the financial ties between psychiatrists and pharmaceutical companies were made abundantly clear. In March 2009, the American Psychiatric Association announced that it would phase out pharmaceutical funding of continuing medical education seminars and meals at its conventions. However, the decision came only after years of controversial exposure of its conflict of interest with the pharmaceutical industry, and after the US Senate Finance Committee requested in July, 2008, that the APA account for all of its pharmaceutical funding. Despite its announcement, within two months, the APA accepted more than $1.7 million in pharmaceutical company funds for its annual conference, held in San Francisco.

Also, within a month of the APA's announcement, its conflicts of interest came under criticism again with the release of a study that found that 18 of the 20 members overseeing the revision of clinical guidelines for treating just three *"mental disorders"* had financial ties to drug companies. Those three common diagnoses generate some $25 billion a year in pharmaceutical sales. With the United States prescribing anti-psychotics two children and adolescents six times greater than the United Kingdom and with 30 million Americans having taken antidepressants for a *"chemical imbalance"* that psychiatrists admit is a pharmaceutical marketing strategy, not a scientific fact, it is no wonder that the conflict of interest between psychiatry and Big Pharma in 2009, and is still on the radar screen today. [175, 176]

Depression And Nutrition

A growing body of research suggests that diet plays an important role in mental health/illness. It should be the first line of treatment and a priority future prevention. In addition, DNA testing for gene mutations involving the methylation process that produces neurotransmitters that keep you emotionally stable, and testing for glyphosate and other chemical toxicity should be employed. Why would nutrition have anything to do with depression? Over the last 60 years, we have seen a steady and significant decline in fruit and vegetable intake *(rich in folate)*, in fish intake *(rich in essential fats)* and an increase in sugar consumption, from two pounds a year in the 1940s to 150 lbs. a year in many of today's teenagers. Each of these is strongly linked to depression and could contribute to the increasing rates. Genes that are critical for nutrient metabolism are also being epigenetically altered because of the environmentally induced toxin overload that the body can't adequately process causing gene damage and eventual system-wide breakdown. In addition, the stressful conditions common to the 21st century lifestyle require more nutrients such as antioxidants, and essential vitamins and minerals which we do not receive in a processed food world. What are the common imbalances connected to nutrition that are known to worsen your mood and motivation? Excessive sugar intake, lack of chromium, selenium, zinc, amino acids, omega-3 essential fats, and B *(especially B9 folate and B12 cobalamin)*, vitamin D3, and TMG *(stands for tri-methyl-glycine)*. Great sources for TMG are quinoa and spinach and TMG is as important as folate in helping to produce neurotransmitters that prevent depression. [177]

Also, a good vitamin from whole food sources is very important. Recent research has demonstrated that persons who have experienced a first episode of psychosis *(FEP)* are likely to have significant nutritional deficiencies.

A study published in the Journal of Psychiatric Practice during 2005 found a direct link between typical depression and a deficiency of essential nutrients in the diet, carbohydrate cravings, and fatigue. A randomized, double-blind study of 113 people, 18 to 65 years old, with a typical depression found those exhibiting the most intense symptoms also tested positive for chromium deficiency. The patients in the eight-week study that were given a chromium supplement showed *"significantly great improvements"* in all symptoms related to their depression. Normally chromium is found in soil but the depletion of soil nutrients and food processing has taken most out it of our diets. John Daugherty, a professor of psychiatry at Cornell University, states, *"The use of antidepressants, mood stabilizers, and antipsychotics that are commonly prescribed to treat depression can often worsen carbohydrate cravings."* These findings strongly suggest that these synthetic drugs, which millions of people routinely take for depression, may be aggravating the underlying cause of their depression. In other words, your cure may be doing more harm than good while the real cure is the return of naturally occurring substances that have been depleted from your diet.

A major finding was a 50-fold greater rate of major depression among those women who had the lowest levels of seafood consumption. The substance in seafood that turned out to be responsible for providing protection against depression was omega-3 essential fatty acids. There seems to be a fairly clear connection between depression and a lack of essential nutrients. Processed foods, and a lack of education on the value of fresh organic whole foods in the diet are the most reasonable causes associated with these findings. St. John's Wort has been used for centuries as a natural treatment for depression. When buying St. John's Wort, look for tablets or capsules standardized to 0.3% hypericin. The usual dose is 300 milligrams three times a day. You may have to use it regularly for two months to get the full benefit of this treatment. [178]

Other natural remedies such as essential oils are very effective in supporting cognitive and emotional wellbeing. My family has used them for years and they are very effective, but you should be careful in choosing your essential oils company. Like supplements, not all essential oils are created equal, and there is a lot of junk out there that is a waste of your money. If you want the best possible outcome, be sure to purchase only the best essential oils. *(There will be more information in the New Beginnings chapter.)*

A new study also demonstrates an association between pro-inflammatory diets and depression in older adults. Researchers from across the US, Italy, and the UK used 8-year follow up data collected in North America and determined that participants with the highest pro-inflammatory diets had a 24% higher likelihood of developing depressive symptoms. Diets should be high in naturally occurring oils, like olive, coconut, palm, and other medium-chain triglyceride oils *(MCT)*, vegetables including raw, uncooked cruciferous vegetables, green beans, zucchini, cucumbers and leafy greens, as well as high quality/lower sugar fruits such as berries, avocados, kiwis, tomatoes. A diet with high natural/healthy fats, low simple carbs, and good quality proteins - all organic is also a great option. Processed foods with harmful food additives can contribute to depressive episodes, so avoid those like the plague. A healthy lifestyle can make a tremendous positive difference for those with depression. [179, 180]

Attention Deficit Hyperactivity Disorder - ADHD

ADHD, as we all have come to understand it, is the most commonly diagnosed neurobehavioral childhood disorder. It is characterized by three main symptom categories, inattention, hyperactivity, and impulsivity. Individuals with an ADHD diagnosis are also reported to have substantial functional impairment in academic, family, and social settings. [181]

How prevalent has an ADHD diagnosis become? A survey of 76,000 parents conducted by the Centers for Disease Control *(CDC)* every four years estimates that 1 in 11 children had been diagnosed with ADHD by a healthcare professional, an increase of 42% between 2003 and 2014. [182] The National Center for Health Statistics (NCHS), reported in the National Health Interview Study 9.5% or about 1 in 10.5 between 2011 and 2013. Looking at those teen years, diagnosis is now given to some 13.3% or one in 7.5 American children between 12 and 17, mostly boys, many of whom are placed on powerful drugs with lifelong consequences.

According to the Centers for Disease Control and prevention, of those diagnosed with ADHD, 18% between ages two and five, 69% between ages six and 11 come in 62% between ages 12 and 17 are treated with amphetamines. More alarmingly, more than 10,000 toddlers at ages two and three were found to be taking these drugs, far outside any established pediatric guidelines. Males are almost three times more likely to be diagnosed with ADHD than females. During their lifetimes, 13% of men and 4.2% of women will be diagnosed with ADHD. [183-186]

In 1961, the FDA approved Ritalin, the recognized prototype amphetamine for the treatment of ADHD, for use by children diagnosed with behavioral problems. More than 100,000 kids were taking the drug within the decade. By the mid-1980s, 1,000,000 children received the ADHD diagnosis and 67% were on meds. Current statistics show that 85% have only mild to moderate symptoms.

The term attention deficit disorder (ADD) was made of official in 1980, when it appeared in that year's edition of the Diagnostic and Statistical Manual (DSM). The diagnosis label was changed to ADHD seven years later. Subsequent editions steadily loosened the definition, and the diagnosis of ADHD skyrocketed accordingly. One in nine children, two-thirds of them boys, are being slapped with the ADHD label. Two-thirds of these children have been prescribed an addictive supplement that has been shown to more than likely cause negative lifetime alterations in brain function, even if the medication is discontinued. [187,188]

In addition, there are several other behavioral disorders that can get misdiagnosed as ADHD including depression, anxiety, autism, learning disabilities, parenting problems, medication side effects, hearing and visual problems, and heavy metal poisoning. Sleep deprivation in particular is becoming very common in the United States and Canada, as more and more boys stay up late playing video games, and more and more girls stay up late texting or interacting on social media. Sleep deprivation mimics ADHD almost perfectly. [189]

When the end result of a misdiagnosis turns into medicating innocent children, some as young as two years old, with amphetamines or other mind-altering drug cocktails that change their brains forever, and have shown multiple other adverse side effects, I think most would agree that something is very wrong, and the alarms are now sounding loud and clear. The sleeping giant of public outcry has awakened, demanding reforms and greater accountability for those responsible for the damage that is being done to our children. Not only is the over-diagnosing of ADHD a huge health problem, but also even its characterization as an actual disorder requiring treatment with medication is very controversial.

Is ADHD A Real Disease?

Many parents believe so, as they deal with out of control children. The vast majority of allopathically trained physicians and public health officials as well believe that it is real. Additionally, teachers, pastors, rabbis, scholars, politicians, and other leaders will all say the same thing. Of course, ADHD is real. It's a no-brainer! *(Pun intended!)*

But not so fast. There are more and more of those same people groups now saying the exact opposite, that ADHD is not real, and that the symptoms are the result of what is being done TO our children, not because there is something genetically wrong with them. What we believe is too often determined by what others try and make us believe, many with a self-serving agenda - money and power. What we end up believing may or may not end at the truth. We have seen this throughout history. In the world of healthcare, medical professionals and researchers are too frequently put up on the *"Hey, he is so smart, of course I will believe what he says,"* pedestal. After all, we trust and depend on others who spend their lives researching what we can't or won't take the time to do. So, we believe them to be honest as we are, and we drink the Kool-Aid. Are we too agreeable to follow the proverbial pied piper of supposedly honest and accurate medical researchers? Is this especially true when it involves telling us who we are, or what we are supposed to believe, and using medications to control and conform our minds because there is something wrong with us, or we just don't *"fit in?"*

There are many times over the centuries where the medical professional got it wrong. Medical experts over the centuries have had very different understandings of bacteria and viruses, and diseases like cancer, tuberculosis, HIV, and treatments such as bloodletting, morphine as a cough suppressant, and *"soothing syrup"* for unruly children, mercury for treatment for just about anything, and thalidomide for nausea in pregnant women producing children with missing extremities. We look at these past atrocities and may view them as appalling, but we are also thankful that, through some unfortunate and horrific lessons, we changed and grew from our ignorance. The tragedy is that many people are harmed in the process. Is unbridled collateral damage acceptable? I think we are facing similar challenges with ADHD as a real disease. We know what we are told, but is what we are told based on truth, or what others like the pharmaceutical profiteers and their sponsored research authors want us to believe?

So, do I believe that ADHD is real? No, not as the definition exists today. And there are more and more people who are standing up for the research confirming the fallacy of ADHD as an actual disease that never gets out to the public.

While various reports over the past 200 years have described a small subset of individuals with behavioral symptoms similar to ADHD, it is commonly understood that ADHD was essentially not even on the radar screen until the 1960s. People growing up then don't remember ever seeing anything like the classically described ADHD child. Sure, there was a very rare individual that was fidgety and those occasional dreamers that lacked focus - but, really, mostly, they were just bored boys looking for adventure. Not to exclude the girls, but I readily admit they were just more responsible than the boys. Some had more active imaginations than others. I did. *(I was a psychology major in college and my "active imagination" status was confirmed after some testing).* I had some of those distracting days in school as well. Hormones do that to boys, especially. Instead of sitting in a classroom listening to a teacher doing her best to teach me the ABCs, my mind would drift to playing baseball, or going out into the woods for an adventure. Spring, with the warmer weather and blooming flowers and fragrant smells, was especially distracting. If I were in school today, I probably would be put on Ritalin at the first sign of looking out the window.

Harvard psychologist, Jerome Kagan, one of the world's leading experts in child development, states: *"Let's go back 50 years. We have a seven-year-old child who is bored in school and disrupts classes. Back then he was called lazy. Today, he is said to suffer from ADHD (Attention Deficit Hyperactivity Disorder) . . . Every child who's not doing well in school is sent to see a pediatrician, and the pediatrician says: "It's ADHD; here's Ritalin."* In fact, 90% of these 5.4 million kids don't have an abnormal dopamine metabolism. The problem is, if a drug is available to doctors, they'll make the corresponding diagnosis. [190, 191]

The Evidence Is Compelling

So, what happened? Did genetics all of a sudden take a turn for the worse and create all these little monsters - most of them boys- that can only be controlled with medications? The evidence against ADHD as a disease is very compelling, and it also reveals another side to the controversy unknown by most. Dr. Leon Eisenberg, a prominent child and social psychiatrist who is considered by many as the scientific father of ADHD, made a jaw-dropping proclamation about seven months before his death. In a 2012 article in the German weekly publication, Der Spiegel, the author gives an account of an interview Eisenberg gave in 2009. It quotes him as saying, *"ADHD is a prime example of a fabricated disease. The genetic predisposition to ADHD is completely overrated."* Instead of prescribing a *'pill'*, Eisenberg said, *"Psychiatrists should determine whether there are psychosocial reasons that could lead to behavioral problems."* That statement about ADHD being a *"fabricated disease"* is so true, but it also pours salt into the wounds of those injured physically and emotionally by the diagnosis, stigma, and medications.

Many other researchers, doctors, and behavioral clinicians are coming to the same conclusion that there is no such thing as ADHD. There is nothing genetically wrong with the vast majority of these kids! Among them is Dr. Edward C. Hamlyn, a founding member of the Royal College of General Practitioners, who, as far back as 1998 stated: *"ADHD is a fraud intended to justify starting children on a life of drug addiction."* He's right!! Also Dr. Richard Saul, a behavioral neurologist and author of ADHD Does Not Exist, is convinced that ADHD is not a disease, but a set of symptoms. *"[. . .] after 50 years of practicing medicine and seeing thousands of patients demonstrating symptoms of ADHD, I have reached the conclusion there is no such thing as ADHD. Improving diet, exercising, and sleeping more can alleviate symptoms."* I agree and would add, be a student of your child's personality, strength, and weaknesses. The diagnosis of ADHD is mostly made in boys that are full of energy, they are adventurous, and are extremely smart.

Other researchers are now connecting the dots as well that ADHD has more to do with behaviors associated with environmental intoxication, and/or nutritional deficiency. Even a vitamin B folate gene mutation mentioned in the epigenetics chapter, now very common, can cause ADHD, depression, bipolar symptoms, and a whole host of other chronic disease symptoms. Give some methylated bioactive folate and poof, the symptoms can subside or completely resolve. Simple yes, but it generally involves additional nutritional supplementation.

Back in 2016, a 26-year-old man came into my office for evaluation. In the course taking his medical history, I found that he was on Ritalin for ADHD. I asked him how long he had been on medication, and he said since he was thirteen years old. He was married and had a young son. I asked him why he was still on medication. He said that he was told that he would be on this medication for the rest of his life because he had trouble focusing as a teen. I was shocked! I told him that, in my opinion, there was nothing wrong with him, and that he should consider working with his doctors to try and get off the medication. He actually started to cry and thanked me for my advice. You see, he was living in a jail that someone else created for him. He was told that something was wrong with him, and the only way to make him *"normal"* was to be on the medication for the rest of his life. To me, that is appalling. What I gave him was hope that he really WAS normal, and that there may be an end to his ADHD nightmare. For those who have had their brains rewired for years, it can take some work, but it can be done very effectively. I will go over some options in the New Beginnings chapter.

> *"ADHD itself is not an epidemic – ADHD misdiagnosis is an epidemic."*
>
> Alan Schwarz
> Investigative Journalist

Yes, there are individuals with symptoms of inattentiveness and hyperactive tendencies, but that is nothing new and has been mentioned in one report or another for hundreds of years with similar symptoms that have gone by many names. Yes, there is something going on, but it has very little to do with defining our children as abnormal or genetically deformed. As I mentioned in *The Killing Fields* chapter, there are many contributing factors to why someone may display symptoms of poor physical or mental health. Like so many other diseases of the 20th and 21st centuries such as diabetes, heart disease, cancer, Alzheimer's, and some others, the diagnosis of ADHD is occurring at epidemic levels. So, what's the deal? How can there be such a shift in human behavior in such a short period of time? If it has always been there, where is the historical evidence that parallels what we see today? Did all the teachers, parents, and physicians of 19th and 20th centuries miss it somehow? If it is genetic, then why haven't we seen it in past generations to the same levels as today? It was nowhere close to current levels in the past. ADHD does seem like a runaway train in today's world, but who or what is driving it?

> *"...after 50 years of practicing medicine and seeing thousands of patients demonstrating symptoms of ADHD, I have reached the conclusion there is no such thing as ADHD."*
>
> Dr. Richard Saul, Behavioral Neurologist

A growing number of medical professionals are trying to stop this train in its tracks before more children are harmed. After 50 years in practice, Dr. Richard Saul writes that there is no such thing as ADHD. Treating *"ADHD as a disease is a huge mistake,"* according to Saul. Instead improving your diet, exercising, and sleeping more can alleviate symptoms. *"The ADHD diagnosis and the stimulants have masked the real problem, as is so often the case."* Instead, he argues, this represents a cluster of symptoms stemming from 20 other conditions and disorders ranging from poor eyesight to bipolar disorder to giftedness.

Alan Schwarz, investigative journalist, writes that the epidemic is twofold. First, there are adults and adolescents who become addicted to stimulants, whether they first acquire them in clinical or recreational settings. Second, there is the enormous number of children who - it seems difficult to dispute - are being over-diagnosed with ADHD. Diagnosis rates, as Schwarz describes, are skyrocketing, whereas expert groups (*i.e. the American Psychiatric Association*) contend that ADHD is a mental illness affecting five percent of children. Numbers from the Centers for Disease Control indicate that today, some 15% of children in the United States will ultimately be diagnosed with the disorder by the end of their childhood.

The research and marketing of ADHD have been *"appallingly contaminated from its very genesis,"* writes Schwarz. *"Since that $5,000 check from CIBA in 1963 (to Dr. Leon Eisenberg/Dr. Keith Connors) "supporting" their research into ADD(ADHD), the pharmaceutical money has irrigated the channels running through every corner of the ADHD ecosystem, feeding researchers, patient advocacy groups, celebrity spokespeople, and advertisers."* Connors ultimately came to terms with the way that ADHD was hijacked by the pharmaceutical companies and has stated that ADHD misdiagnoses are a "national disaster of dangerous proportions." [192, 193]

> ADHD misdiagnoses is: *"a national disaster of dangerous proportions." "This is a concoction to justify the giving out of medication at unprecedented and unjustifiable levels."*
>
> Dr. Keith Connors,
> Child Psychologist and Scientific Father of ADHD

Psychiatry journals are teemed with more than a thousand studies on ADHD conducted by Pharma-sponsored scientists. Schwartz writes that "... *The Food and Drug Administration relied upon them when green-lighting medications as safe and effective. Their findings served as the backbone for the lectures that drug companies' key opinion leaders delivered on world tours. The whirlwind created a self-affirming circle of science, one that quashed all dissent."*

Schwartz goes on to say in an article written in Scientific American that there are additional considerations that never get brought out into the light of day. One is how medications to treat ADHD are being flippantly prescribed, then sold illegally under the radar to other children. None of the supposedly responsible medical professional organizations seem to care.

"When I looked deeper, it was obvious that our nationwide system of ADHD treatment was completely scattershot - basically, many doctors were merely prescribing with little thought into whether a kid really had ADHD or not, and then the pills would be bought and sold among students who had no idea what they were messing with. I asked the ADHD and child-psychiatry establishment about this, and they denied it was happening. They denied that there were many false diagnoses. They denied that teenagers were buying and selling pills. They denied that the national diagnosis rates reported by the C.D.C. - then 9.5% of children aged 4-17, now 11%and still growing - were valid. They basically denied that anything about their world was malfunctioning at all..."

What role has the pharmaceutical industry played? *"A completely predictable one..."* says Schwartz. He goes on to say, *"We are a very capitalistic country, particularly when it comes to medicine, and the pharmaceutical industry has massive financial incentive to produce drugs that address medical needs. The problem, in the ADHD world and others - particularly psychiatric - is that the companies hijacked the entire field. It corralled all the top researchers and doctors in the field and paid them five, six, even seven-figures apiece to conduct studies all written in the same key: That, ADHD is more widespread and dangerous than anyone knows, the drugs work wonderfully and with almost no side effects, and that if you don't diagnose and medicate a child, he or she will be doomed to academic and social failure, crash their car, get venereal disease and more."* [194]

Contributing Factors And ADHD

While essentially the whole of ADHD supporters would have you believe that ADHD is genetic, there are epigenetic factors that may more accurately describe the etiology. Risk factors that can be associated with the symptoms include premature birth, vaccines, maternal smoking and alcohol use, lead exposure, frequent maternal infections during pregnancy, personality, gender, and others. A 2009 German study found a significant link between having eczema, a rash caused by allergies, and developing ADHD symptoms, giving more credence to a controversial theory that at least some ADHD is the result of allergies or sensitivities to certain foods, food additives, or other environmental factors. Organophosphate pesticides - the kind used on most of the US food supply - were linked to an increased risk of ADHD in a 2010 Harvard School of Public Health study which found that higher concentrations of pesticides in a child's urine doubled the child's chances of being diagnosed with the disorder. In France, a study in 2004 found 84% of children diagnosed with ADHD were iron deficient, compared with 18% of 'non-ADHD' children. Yet time and time again, doctors miss the real problems - some serious, some easily correctable - by automatically reaching for the ADHD label. [195 - 197]

There are many other contributing factors to an incorrect diagnosis of ADHD, including personality, classroom structure, hyperstimulation from external sources, and even the proclivity of physicians to lean toward pharmaceutical intervention instead of doing the more difficult work of discovering the root cause of a child's inability to attend.

Many of those diagnosed with ADHD are already sensitive to overstimulation and certain personality types are particularly prone. Sanguine personalities *(one of the Four Humeral Personalities),* in particular boys, are *"wired"* for stimuli. There is nothing wrong with them; these personalities just react to the world with excitement, energy, and have a zest for life that other personality types don't have to that degree. They are always ready to go on an adventure with a big smile, are extremely intelligent, and they make the best salesman. They are the only ones that can get away with wearing a wild colored Hawaiian shirt without someone talking behind their back saying how weird they must be. Sanguines are always looking for the dopamine rush, an emotional high that creates a sense of pleasure and reward, but they can easily be over stimulated. From sugar to electronic video games till two a.m., stimulant food additives, endless social media opportunities, and other 'rush' opportunities, these all take their toll on this personality type, setting the stage for addiction. Parents should be students of their children and recognize their differences while they are young, and train them up, keeping strengths and weaknesses in mind. We all respond differently to the world around us based on genetics, personality, and epigenetic experiences and training. Sanguine personalities *(or 7 on the enneagram chart which you will see later)* have very busy minds and may need to be taught sitting, focusing, and concentrating skills at an early age, otherwise they may be unprepared to harness that energy during the school day, where the environment is so structured and unforgiving.

In today's hyper-stimulating digital world, with its vivid gaming and exciting social media platforms, and with the immediate gratification it offers, where practically any desire or fantasy can be realized in a blink of an eye, school can seem very boring, comparatively speaking. School would seem even more dull to a sanguine, novelty-seeking kid living in the early 21st century than in previous decades, and the boring school environment might accentuate students' inattentive behavior, making their teachers more likely to see it and drive up the number of diagnoses. Out of the box thinkers like Einstein and Edison, and high school dropouts like Richard Branson, Wolfgang Puck, Walt Disney, and others, may never have achieved their world-changing successes if they had been diagnosed with ADHD and their brains controlled by ADHD amphetamines.

Those prone to hyperstimulation from environmental causes like food and electronic stimulants, etc. have some commonalities that contribute to their responses. Non-ADHD brains are adequately aroused by the shifting internal and external stimulation of daily life. Regardless of fluctuations in stimulation, those brains can operate with reasonably sustained focus, fueled by the dependable coordination of neurotransmitters. They can self-regulate with relative confidence and exercise an adequate amount of control over their behavior.

Those with true ADHD-like symptoms have their own rules of engagement. They are motivated by their search for optimal stimulation, rather than by what others label as important. Their degree of arousal differs based on whether the request for attention comes from an internal desire or an external demand. The owners of these brains are not making conscious choices to ignore external demands, although it often appears that way. Instead, internal motivations are intrinsically more meaningful to their brains and, as a result, more dopamine becomes available. Concerns about time or consequences are dwarfed by the pursuit of pleasurable reinforcement, and they are more prone to addictive behaviors. Whether through sensation or hyperactivity, ADHD brains compel their owners to scan the environment for engaging stimulation. When mundane tasks can't be avoided, ADHD brains may be compromised in their ability to choose goal-oriented responses. [198]

So, the mantra in school seems to be let's just *force compliance* with medications. ADHD was created in response to heavy-handed restrictions that western cultures have naively allowed to be imposed. Ever know of a child that is on medication during the school year but not during the summer? Why is that? Is this customized ADHD?

Curiously, the prevalence of adult ADHD is only 4.4%, a fraction of the *"popular"* diagnosis of young people, at 9.5% with 15% being treated with ADHD medication. This suggests that a substantial number of people simply *"grow out of it."* How does that happen? Perhaps, one explanation is that unlike the closed in and structured school environment, adults have far more freedom to choose the environment in which they live and the kind of work they do so that it better matches their cognitive style and reward preferences. If you were a restless kid who couldn't sit still in school, you might choose to be an entrepreneur or carpenter, but you would be unlikely to become an accountant. Even at that, many teens growing into their adult years continue on medications because they are simply addicted or have been told that they will be on medications for the rest of their lives. When they do try and get off the medication after having their brains rewired for years, it can be a very similar experience to any other addiction withdrawal. Sometimes, when they try to separate themselves from the amphetamines, they find it very difficult, and, instead of realizing that they are going through withdrawals, they think that the difficulty is because they really do have ADHD, and they do need the medications to survive, so they give up and give into the addiction. No one ever told them about the addictive nature of amphetamines, nor that they can recover and live a healthy and free life. [199]

Another contributing factor can be age upon entry into the school system. Researchers in Taiwan looked at data from 378,881 children ages 4 to 17 and found that students born in August, the cut-off month for school entry in that country, were more likely to be given diagnoses of ADHD than students born in September. The children born in September would have missed the previous year's cut-off date for school entry, and thus had nearly a full extra year to mature before entering school. The findings were published in The Journal of Pediatrics. Other research has shown similar results. An earlier study in the United States, for example, found that roughly 8.4% of children born in the month before their state's cutoff date for kindergarten eligibility are given ADHD diagnoses, compared to 5.1% of children born in the month immediately afterward. [200]

Dr. Michael Manos, PhD, from Cleveland Clinic's Center for Pediatric Behavioral Health says, *"When you take people who are in a 15-minute pediatric primary care physician's office visit, and the mother describes hyperactivity and the physician automatically prescribes medication, that's a problem,"* Dr. Manos said. Many parents who describe concerns about children's behavior *"aren't describing developmentally inappropriate behavior,"* he said. *"They're describing behavior that does not meet certain expectations,"* and that can be the issue in classroom settings as well, where some students are older than others.

Teachers can perceive those younger children in the class as struggling with sitting, focusing, concentrating, and other behavioral issues, especially when compared to older children. When behavior struggles are identified at an early age especially, the path to an ADHD diagnosis can be paved. This is true, especially for live wire "sanguine" personality types entering the school system as one of the younger students in the class. They never have a chance.

My wife and I have seen this play out in families throughout many years of teaching parenting classes. We interact with parents who share their struggles raising their families, and what to do about the live wired kiddos, as well as the angry ones, the quiet, slower-paced ones, etc. They are just all different. While it is not always easy, our role as parents is to celebrate their differences and to be observant in training them how to cope with their extended environment and experiences, and to make emotionally and physically healthy adjustments for them as needed.

My birthday is in August. While my primary personality is more choleric *(doer, task driven, direct)*, I am secondarily sanguine *(fun-loving, lack of focus, impulsive)*. I was very immature compared to my classmates even through high school, and would have been better off starting school a year later or repeated a year, so I could be one of the older children which, by itself, instills confidence and a need to set a more responsible example for the rest of my classmates. According to today's loose diagnostic criteria for ADHD, I feel confident I would have been targeted, classified, and then drugged into compliance.

ADHD And Brain Size

There has been a lot of hype in the media and through research pundits that the brains are smaller in those diagnosed with ADHD. The research using brain MRIs completely contradicts that, but you have to know how to read the research in order to get there. What gets leaked to the media and brings accolades to the researchers is many times about money and self-promotion and does not always reflect the real truth. In a Mad In America *(MIA)* report by Michael Corrigan, Ed.D. and Robert Whitaker entitled Lancet Psychiatry Needs to Retract ADHD- Enigma Study, April 15, 2017, the authors clearly expose the truth of the study and challenge the authors' findings and frankly, their integrity. The Lancet publication, which is referenced so frequently by outside medical sources, is riddled with errors and important excluded data.

They write, "While the summary statement in the study and the Associated Press release tells of robust, definitive findings, leading to media headlines state that *'Study Finds Brains of ADHD Sufferers Are Smaller,'* a review of the reported *'effect sizes'* reveals that they found no such thing."

When the public reads that a study proved that children diagnosed with ADHD have smaller brain volumes, most people will naturally assume this is a characteristic found in all children so diagnosed. The assumption is that the researchers must have established a *"normal"* volume *(which would be the mean brain volume for a control group),* and then determined that most, if not all, of those diagnosed with ADHD have smaller brain volumes than the norm.

They continue by addressing the size of the nucleus accumbens *(NAc)* in the front part of the brain that has a high number of dopamine receptors, the pleasure/reward neurotransmitter that figures very prominently in ADHD research. The publication contains brain scan information suggesting that the accumbens is smaller in ADHD children. That is unsupported by their own data. That false information flew from coast to coast before truth could even get on its tennis shoes. The entirety of the publication was not available to the general public without an additional *"access fee."* That's right, you have to pay to get to the rest of the story that was not so complimentary to their conclusions. But here is the truth. The participants were 15 years old and younger. The younger participants in either group would naturally have smaller brain volumes, and yet that was never taken into consideration, nor included in the data results. Also, there were two groups - a control group was not on medication but the other group in the study was. Medication dosages were not included in the study, which they should have been. Previous studies have shown that amphetamines will reduce brain volume, which was not included in the publication. Also, without explanation, why did the authors exclude 545 patients *(1254 minus 719 accounted for in the results)* from the study without an explanation?

Curiously, and very important to the ultimate conclusion of the study, was the fact that 16 of the 20 sites that reported IQ statistics, found that the ADHD group actually had higher IQs on average than the control group. In the other four clinics, the ADHD and control groups had the same average IQ. Thus, at all 20 sites, the ADHD group had a mean IQ score that was equal to, or higher than the mean IQ score for the control group. If the participants with ADHD have smaller brains that are riddled with *"altered structures,"* then how come they are just as smart as, or even smarter than, the participants in the control group? But, again, in order to get that information in the publication, you have to pay *(about $31.50)*, then make a special request to receive the appendix. [201]

Is it possible that children diagnosed with ADHD are more intelligent than average? Maybe we are drugging millions of bright children because they are more easily prone to boredom and schools aren't providing them with stimulating learning environments. How much more could they contribute if they weren't drugged into submission, but instead were placed in a school environment more suited to their gifts and talents?

Medications For ADHD: An Epidemic Of Abuse

Stimulant medications on the market today, such as Adderall, Ritalin, Concerta, Metadate, Vyvanse, Focalin, Daytrana, are all variations on just two molecules, amphetamine and methylphenidate. They work very similar to cocaine by blocking the reuptake of dopamine and norepinephrine at the nerve-to-nerve connections, especially in dopamine rich receptors in the NAc and prefrontal cortex. This makes the neurotransmitters more available for acting on the reward/pleasure and focusing centers. There are also possible epigenetically induced gene mutations involved in some, where the reuptake mechanism is in overdrive and clears too much dopamine away from the nerve connections *(synapse),* requiring more to be made to compensate, or a mutation to occur that may reduce the actual number of receptors receiving the dopamine. The end result is the same - not enough dopamine is available and more is needed to make up for the deficiency. [202]

Dopamine is the brain's chemical messenger that is probably best known for its role in addiction to drugs, alcohol, sex, and even chocolate. But this chemical that carries information between nerve cells plays a far more

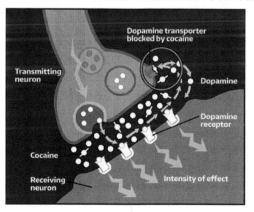

important function in human life than providing us pleasure from a cocaine or cupcake high. It uses reward - and the pleasurable feelings it supplies - to motivate us to pay attention, avoid distraction, or to pick out the most relevant information circulating in short-term memory when solving a problem or completing a task.

Many scholarly studies have now demonstrated that methylphenidate and amphetamine in animals can cause lasting changes to those areas of the developing brain where dopamine receptors are found. The disrupting effects appear to be centered on the NAc. This is not surprising, because the nucleus accumbens has a high density of dopamine receptors. While these studies are done on animals, they suggest the same effects will be experienced in humans and even short-term, low-dose exposure to amphetamine or to methylphenidate, particularly in the juvenile brain, may induce long-lasting changes both neurally and behaviorally. The risks could be very significant.

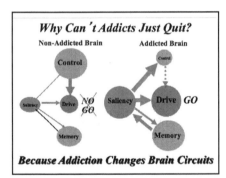

Why Can't Addicts Just Quit?

Because Addiction Changes Brain Circuits

Amphetamines, cocaine, nicotine, and morphine, all have similar actions, changing the structure of brain cells involved in incentive motivation and reward. Reorganization of neural conductivity alters their original function and can contribute to altered behavioral responses, including addictions. There is now substantial evidence that these medications may damage the nucleus accumbens *(NAc)*, an area of the brain crucial to motivation and drive. The NAc is not involved in cognitive functions like learning and memory. If the NAc is damaged, there will be no impairment of cognitive function. But the motivation to achieve will be diminished.

Dr. Leonard Sax, a family physician and research psychologist, author of in *Boys Adrift*, has seen many such people, mostly young men, in his practice. *"This boy was on Ritalin as a child and then Adderall as a teenager. Now he spends most of his time playing video games on his parents' 55-inch flat screen. He's 29 years old. He's guild master of his guild in World of Warcraft, but in the real world, he's nobody. His parents are frantic, but he is content.*

That may be the end result when the NAc is damaged. Medications are not solely to blame for this phenomenon - there are other factors in play - but the fact that this boy was on stimulant medications for many years is most likely a contributing factor." [202 - 205]

There can be changes and long-lasting hypersensitization to dopamine receptors upon stimulation after a long lapse without a stimulant as well. The memory of the high is embedded and when a stimulus comes and tells the brain, I'm BACK, there is an immediate recognition and intense pleasure high from the experience. There is also a stimulant-seeking phenomenon that takes place after discontinuation. The receptors send out long term signals that say, *"Feed me."* Over time, those urges may subside for the one stimulus, but the receptors will just encourage you to seek other stimuli to take its place.

But what is especially revealing is that even a single exposure to amphetamine is sufficient to induce some degree of changes at the behavioral, neurochemical, and neuroendocrine levels. [206 - 209] The good news is that the brain is changeable *(called neuroplasticity),* and you can discipline the brain to ignore or avoid certain unhealthy stimuli.

Side Effects Of Treating ADHD With Amphetamines

There are many dangerous and long-term side effects associated with the use of stimulants such as those for ADHD. The side effects include brain damage, addiction, loss of motivation, depression, reduced appetite *(dangerous for children who need a good diet),* sleep disturbance *(tiredness can exacerbate attention problems),* anxiety, irritability, depressed moods, and delayed puberty. And long-term use of stimulants makes people resistant to them, meaning they need higher and higher doses. The drugs can damage memory and concentration and have even been linked to reduced life expectancy and suicide. Yet stimulants are being prescribed more and more frequently, creating a health time bomb and neglecting the real causes of the problems.

Dr. Sax argues that there is a growing epidemic of unmotivated boys and underachieving young men. He describes social and environmental contributing factors including increased prescriptions of psychotropic medications that affect the motivational systems of the brain. [210]

"ADHD as a disorder is really taking a very substantial toll on our society," observed David Marks, a psychologist with the ADHD center at Mount Sinai Medical Center in New York. *"The adulthood individuals with ADHD miss more work, they're more likely to get fired, and they are more likely to receive negative work reviews. It does constitute a very substantial health burden."*

What is happening to an entire generation of children? For one thing, there is evidence that Ritalin use in the long term may actually be exacerbating a condition caused by other synthetic chemicals. A study published in the Journal of Biological Psychiatry found that high doses of vitamin B6 did a better job of reducing hyperactivity and children then Ritalin and for lower cost and with far fewer side effects. Yet physicians continue prescribing the drug to ever-greater numbers of kids by telling parents, *"Your child is abnormal, and this drug is replacement therapy."* As though the drug itself were a naturally occurring chemical in the brain.

"America's First Amphetamine Crisis," as the historian Nicolas Rasmussen describes it in a newspaper, *The American Journal of Public Health*, *"began soon after the drugs' discovery in 1929."* The drug firm Smith, Kline and French began marketing them first as a decongestant *(in inhaler form)*, he notes, and later as a treatment for depression and weight loss. During World War II, the US military provided amphetamines as a stimulant for soldiers, *"some of whom,"* Rasmussen describes, *"became addicted."* In the following decades, production skyrocketed, and addiction became a major public health problem. The addictive potential of amphetamines was well-known by the time ADHD pioneers and scientific fathers of ADHD, Eisenberg, and Conners, carried out their trials in the 1950s. They knew! [211]

Rasmussen gives a sense of the truly massive amphetamine use, addiction, and resultant suffering that followed. By 1962, he notes, 80,000 kg of amphetamine was being produced annually in the US, translating into some 8 billion typical 10 mg doses, or approximately 43 doses for every single person in the country each year. *"The original amphetamine epidemic,"* he asserts *"was generated by the pharmaceutical industry and medical profession as a by-product of routine commercial drug development and competition."* In other words, Big Pharma followed its usual approach to the mass-commercialization of a new prescription drug, and in so doing produced an epidemic of abuse. The pharmaceutical industry learned nothing from the first amphetamine epidemic it caused. And why would they? No one with any authority is challenging them on it.

> The pharmaceutical industry learned nothing from the first amphetamine epidemic it caused.

There is also a high unintentional and intentional abuse of ADHD medications affecting children of all ages. Whether it is engaging in sports, cramming for exams, or just looking for the excitement high, there are many abuses that too frequently end in tragedy. In addition to addiction, a 2009 report in Scientific American suggests that long-term Adderall use could change brain function enough to boost depression and anxiety. *(Young brains are particularly vulnerable, since they're not fully developed yet.)* In more rare cases, those abusing Adderall for an extended period of time may experience hallucinations, delusions, and full-blown psychosis. [212]

The side effects of Adderall have also resulted in multiple horrors. In 2011, class president and aspiring medical student, Richard Fee, hanged himself in his bedroom closet after struggling for years with an Adderall addiction enabled by careless doctors. More recently, in 2016, Scott Hahn caused a fatal crash on the New Jersey Turnpike after downing 10 Adderall pills. The crash took the lives of a local teacher and his five-year-old daughter.

Despite the very real warning signs - more than 116,000 people were admitted to rehab for an addiction to amphetamines like Adderall in 2012 - there's still not nearly enough research out there on exactly how extended Adderall use affects the brain. [213]

Why? These drugs have been available for over 60 years now, and there was already a major amphetamine epidemic! One reason, as lame as it may seem, is that millennials were the first generation to be *"routinely"* prescribed Adderall, and we've yet to see what happens to those who rely on the drug when they get old before determining if it is dangerous. *(Oh brother, you've got to be kidding! Here we go again!)* Let's create a reality program where they experiment on innocent children to find out how they may be harmed over a lifetime. Then what? Seventy plus years down the road, billions of dollars in profits, possibly hundreds of thousands permanently harmed, and then they may say, *"OOPS!"* But we've already seen the devastation of too many OOPS in the past. Do we really want to wait to see what happens with that grand experiment?

Autism

Autism Spectrum Disorder *(ASD)* is a complex behavioral condition with onset during early childhood and a lifelong course in the vast majority of cases. It is currently understood as a behaviorally defined syndrome manifested as impairment in social communication, repetitive routines, and restricted interests. Clinically, autism falls under a general category of developmental disorders, which also includes, Asperger's disorder, Rett's disorder, childhood disintegrative disorder, and other disorders not otherwise classified. Autism is the most studied of these developmental disorders.

Autism is also known as a *"spectrum"* disorder because there is wide variation in the type and severity of symptoms people experience. Autism spectrum disorders are characterized by behavioral symptoms including hyperactivity, stereotypic motor behaviors, sensory disturbances, language impairment, restricted interests, and self-injury. In some patients, it can also be associated with physical symptoms including seizure disorders, gastrointestinal disturbances, and autoimmune disorders. A dysfunctional folate pathway has also been identified in many individuals with autism. This pathway is crucial for DNA synthesis and methylation. As you may remember from previous chapters, the gene most recognized as responsible for abnormal methylation is C677T and A1298C on Chromosome 1. It is an enzyme producing gene that converts the folate and folic acid that we consume to a bioactive form and is critical to the formation of neurotransmitters and other cellular functions.

The incidence of autism increased from 1 in 5000 in 1978, to 1 in 36 in 2016, as reported in the NHIS *(National Health Information Survey).* These were mostly boys. That is an increase of epidemic proportions! This is the highest rate ever recorded in a national survey of children in the United States and was an increase from the rate of 1 in 45 children reported in the 2014 NHIS survey *(2).* The ASD information reported in these surveys includes children between the ages of three and 17 years of age and any diagnosis of an autism spectrum disorder, including Asperger's syndrome. The new report also described another record rate for ASD of 1 in 28 for boys born between 2014 and 2016. Clearly, these statistics are a major health concern. Over the last ten years, I have taught to large national and international audiences on health related topics including autism, and I hear too many tragic stories from moms about how their children were fine the day before vaccines and then a day or so after they received the combination of injections, they no longer have their child. The pain and fever from the vaccines taunted them throughout the night, then like a thief, stole their brains and the person they were. The alertness, smiles, joy, the innocent anticipation of learning moment by moment, every mother knows that look, now gone into the abyss of a blank stare.

> *"If the epidemic is truly an artifact of poor diagnosis, then where are all the 20 year-old autistics?"*
>
> Dr. Boyd Haley, a leading *authority on mercury toxicity*

So, what's going on here? Some professionals claim that we now have better diagnostic criteria. According to Mark

Blaxill, the increases cannot be explained by changes of diagnostic criteria to improve case evaluations. In a detailed analysis of 54 published reports on the incidence of autism, ASDs, and related disorders, published in 2004 in the Association of Schools Public Health, he concluded that *"...diagnostic criteria are unlikely to have had any meaningful effect on reported disease frequency."* Dr. Boyd Haley, one of the world's authorities on mercury toxicity also makes a simple observation when he asks the question, *"If the epidemic is truly an artifact of poor diagnosis, then where are all the 20-year-old autistics?"* And in the journal, Environmental Health, 2014, tracking trends suggests that ~75-80% of the tracked increase in autism since 1988, is due to an actual increase in the disorder rather than to changing diagnostic criteria. [214, 215]

University of California scientists also concluded that a sevenfold increase in autism cannot be explained by changes in doctors' diagnoses and most likely is due to environmental exposures. As reported in Scientific American in 2009, the scientists who authored the study noted a 700% increase between 1990 and 2001 in California *(and still increasing),* advocated a nationwide shift in autism research to focus on potential factors in the environment that babies and fetuses are exposed to, including pesticides, viruses, and chemicals in household products. Many researchers have theorized that a pregnant woman's exposure to chemical pollutants, particularly metals and pesticides, could be altering a developing baby's brain structure, triggering autism. Dozens of chemicals in the environment are neurodevelopmental toxins, which means they alter how the brain grows. Mercury, polychlorinated biphenyls, lead, brominated flame-retardants, and pesticides are examples. While thimerosal was taken out of most childhood vaccines starting in 1999, the problem persists in multi-dose flu vaccines, which even pregnant women and newborns are encouraged to receive. But, there are other heavy metal adjuvants *(additions that increase the immune response)* such as aluminum in vaccines, which are covered in more detail in the Vaccines chapter. And significantly higher levels of environmental toxins such as arsenic, cadmium, lead, and mercury are also clearly related to ASD symptoms and are reported in a meta-analysis of studies for both developed and developing countries. [216 - 218]

Aluminum has been implicated in a number of brain disorders including autism. There has been some controversy over its role in brain disorders, but current research by Dr. Christopher Exley has made a solid link. His findings will be explored more in the Vaccines chapter. [219]

Many vaccines also contain aborted human fetal cells and retroviruses, and studies show a very strong correlation between the introduction of these cells into vaccine development and a significant rise in autism. This was found in four separate countries. The study, *Impact of Environmental Factors on the Prevalence of Autistic Disorder after 1979* concluded that rising autistic disorder prevalence is directly related to vaccines manufactured utilizing human fetal cells. Increased paternal age and Diagnostic and Statistical Manual DSM revisions were not related to rising autistic disorder. These are used sometimes to help explain increases in the incidence of diseases. [220]

What is actually happening in the brain to cause ASD symptoms? First it may be helpful to understand some of the cell types in the brain. The neuron, for example, is the master of information processing and transfer. Another cell type, the astrocyte, provides nourishment and blood flow to the neurons and participates in the information transfer with its own system. Astrocytes also establish a protective structure for the neuron and are involved in immune functions. But it is the microglia that travels throughout the brain participating in surveillance, stimulation, cleanup, and maintenance tasks while communicating with all other cells. They are the immune cells that reside in the central nervous system. Like police officers, these cells constantly survey their environment for trouble and are often the first responders to injury or disease. On their surface is a tremendous diversity of receptors for various threats, including bacterial, viral, and fungal pathogens, and toxins, as well as noxious compounds released from dead or dying cells during traumatic brain injury, ischemia, and neurodegeneration. They have phagocytic (like Pac-Man) capacity, constitute 10% of the cells of the brain, and form a fairly regular three- dimensional network in which each microglia has a unique territory.

Microglial cells also make direct contact with nerve axons and dendrites, implying that microglia may be carefully listening in on nerve cell conversations that help them to respond more efficiently. If, for instance, a nerve is sending a signal to a neighbor saying that it is dying and can't send signals anymore, the microglial cells may respond by removing that nerve so that another one can take its place or redirect the signal through another nerve connection. Perhaps one way of explaining their function in removing foreign invaders is that microglial cells are somewhat like Pac-man. When there is an infection, or viral invasion, or some foreign substances like aluminum or thimerosal in the brain, the alarm sounds, and the immune system kicks in. As part of the immune cells of the central nervous system, microglial cells respond to eliminate the threat and perform cleanup. The problem is that when responding to the crisis, they end up eating brain tissue as well to try and remove the contaminants and reduce the chronic inflammation. [221]

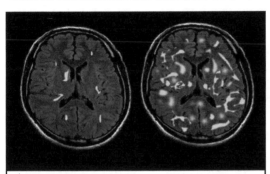

Created depiction of normal brain MRI on left and autistic brain MRI on right in young adult. Note white areas which represent inflammation of the brain.

Johns Hopkins University, in a collaborative effort with the University of Alabama at Birmingham, studied data from 72 autism and control brains. They found brain inflammation *(encephalitis)* as the *"hallmark of autism."* This was the largest study so far of gene expression in autistic brains. Previous studies had identified autism-associated abnormalities in cells that support neurons in the brain and spinal cord. This study was able to narrow in on microglial cells, which polices the brain for pathogens and other threats. In the autism brains, the microglia appeared to be perpetually activated, with their genes for inflammation responses turned on. *"This type of inflammation is not well understood, but it highlights the lack of current understanding about how innate immunity controls neural circuits,"* says Andrew West, Ph.D., an associate professor of neurology at the University of Alabama at Birmingham who was involved in the study. Mounting evidence indicates that microglial activation or dysfunction can profoundly affect neural development, resulting in neurodevelopmental disorders, including autism. [222-230] Other studies have also confirmed brain inflammation and activation of microglial cells with autism in both the neocortex *(front)* and cerebellum *(back)* parts of the brain. [231-233]

Postmortem studies have also unveiled neuroanatomical abnormalities in several parts of the brain that are suggestive of derangements occurring during the first/second trimester of pregnancy. Fetal sensitivity to a wide variety of environmental chemicals has been implicated as the cause. According to Andrey Rzhetsky, professor of genetic medicine and human genetics at the University of Chicago, *"Intellectual disability rates are linked with harmful environmental factors during congenital periods...there are certain sensitive periods (9-30 weeks gestation) where a fetus is very vulnerable to a range of small molecules-from things like plasticizers, RX drugs, environmental pesticides, and other things."* The strongest predictors of autism were associated with the environment. [234]

Gastrointestinal *(GI)* symptoms are commonly seen in patients with autism spectrum disorder. Wang et al., found more GI syndromes, including constipation *(20%)* and diarrhea *(19%)*, in children with ASD than in their unaffected siblings. Many studies have shown alterations in the composition of the fecal flora and metabolic products of the gut microbiome in patients with ASD. The gut microbes *(normal and necessary bacteria, etc.)* influence brain development and behaviors through the neuroendocrine, neuroimmune, and autonomic nervous systems. Patients with ASD who present GI symptoms might display significant behavioral manifestations, such as anxiety, self- injury, and aggression through what is called the gut-brain axis, regarded as a pathway of communication between the gut and the brain and a bidirectional communication system.

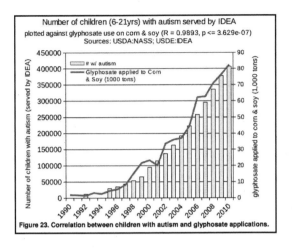

Figure 23. Correlation between children with autism and glyphosate applications.

Accumulating evidence demonstrates that the gut microbiota is directly or indirectly associated with ASD symptoms, in part by influencing the immune system and metabolism. A higher percentage of abnormal intestinal permeability was observed in 36.7% of patients with ASD and their relatives *(21.2%)* compared with control children at 4.8%. A fundamental factor underlying the relationships between ASD and the gut is the increased permeability of the intestinal tract of ASD individuals, referred to as a *"leaky gut."* [235]

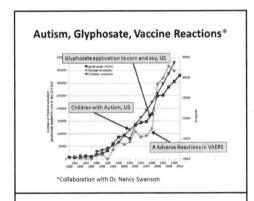

With permission: Stephanie Seneff Senior Research Scientist MIT Computer Science and Artificial Intelligence Laboratory

There has also been some new evidence for the role of glyphosate in creating brain and GI pathology. Dr. Zac Bush, a triple board- certified endocrinologist and cancer researcher has recently taught to thousands, including everyone from other doctors and healthcare professionals, to stay- at-home moms, that glyphosate *(Roundup),* an herbicide that was originally *"approved"* as an antibiotic, is the cause of many GI and brain disorders. The evidence is very convincing. Glyphosate not only destroys the microbiome in the gut, but it breaks the locks that hold together the cells lining the intestinal wall, causing chemicals like glyphosate *(and others)* as well as gluten, to pour through the opening creating the *"leaky gut"* syndrome. That floodgate opens the body to an onslaught of pro-inflammatory chemicals roaming the body and wreaking havoc, causing chronic diseases over time. Glyphosate can even cross the Blood Brain Barrier *(BBB)* causing microglial cell activation and brain cell destruction. Anything that may have glyphosate in it must be avoided. Also, just adding a probiotic/ prebiotic regimen can significantly improve GI symptoms. One of the best resources for actually healing ASD is Jodi Meschuk's book, *Speak UP, Buttercup, How I Brought My Son Back from Autism.*

Vitamin D3 plays a crucial role in the immune response, and in the development and function of the brain, and has been implicated in neuropsychiatric disorders, such as autism spectrum disorder. By interaction with the specific Vitamin D Receptor *(VDR),* the developmental and functional role of vitamin D in the nervous system can be modulated. It was shown that patients with mutations in their VDR receptor gene might have reduced activity of the gene.

A deregulated immune response may be contributing to the etiology of ASD. The active metabolite of vitamin D3 has an immunoregulatory role mediated by binding to the vitamin D receptor *(VDR)* in monocyte, macrophages, and lymphocytes., all important cells of the immune system. The effects of vitamin D and interaction with the VDR may be influenced by polymorphisms (SNPS-mutations) in the VDR gene. One precaution though, is that while the gene mutation may be correlated with the development of ASD symptoms by influencing functionality of vitamin D3, the blood serum levels may not be abnormal. It is just the receptor that is not receiving the signal. [236]

There is also some compelling evidence that drugs used during the labor and delivery process can possibly contribute to autism. Results of a published study showed that children in the drug-exposed condition, such as Pitocin, during labor were 2.77 times more likely to exhibit an autism phenotype. While the SARRC dataset only contained labor induction information, it was observed that mothers who received Pitocin to induce labor and analgesics during the birthing process were 2.32 times more likely to have a child diagnosed with autism later in life. [237]

Alzheimer's Disease

Alzheimer's *(AD)* is a chronic neurodegenerative disease that usually starts slowly and worsens overtime. It is the cause of approximately 70% of all cases of dementia. Every three seconds, someone is diagnosed with Alzheimer's or dementia. In 2015, there were approximately 29.8 million people world-wide with AD. Over a 16-year period, between 1999, and 2014, death rates from Alzheimer's disease increased almost 55%, according to findings in the US Centers for Disease Control and Prevention's Morbidity and Mortality Weekly Report. The most common early symptom is difficulty in remembering recent events *(short-term memory loss)*. As the disease advances, symptoms can include problems with language, disorientation *(including easily getting lost),* mood swings, loss of motivation, and behavioral issues. As a person's condition declines, they often withdraw from family and society. Gradually, bodily functions are lost, ultimately leading to death.

In 2015, a study published in the journal, Surgical Neurology International, highlighted a growing trend in the onset of dementia among people less than 65 years of age. The study, authored by Colin Pritchard and Emily Rosenorn-Lanng of Bournemouth University in England, found that dementia and other neurological diseases among people in 21 Western countries between the ages of 55 and 74 had dramatically increased during 1989-2010. By 2010, the average age of people developing dementia was 10 years younger than in 1989.

Dementia is increasingly being diagnosed in people in their 30s, 40s, and 50s. This phenomenon, known as *"early-onset" (or "younger-onset")* dementia, has been referred to as a growing *"silent epidemic"* affecting younger people - so much so that the media has begun to notice and report on individual cases. If growth trends in early-onset Alzheimer's continue, however, we could have more than a million young to middle-aged Americans with this disease within two generations. Clearly something is amiss.

There appear to be several contributing causes, including aluminum and mercury from several sources including vaccines, as well as industrial chemicals and the herbicide glyphosate. Activated microglia and neuroinflammation are hallmarks of Alzheimer's disease *(AD)* and other neurodegenerative diseases, including Parkinson's disease *(PD)*, amyotrophic lateral sclerosis *(ALS)*, and frontal temporal dementia. Another recently described hallmark event in neurodegenerative diseases *(NDs)* is the misfolding, aggregation, and accumulation of proteins, leading to cellular dysfunction, loss of nerve connections, and brain damage. Despite the involvement of distinct proteins in different NDs, the process of protein misfolding and aggregation is remarkably similar. A recent breakthrough in the field was the discovery that misfolded protein aggregates can self-propagate through seeding and spread the pathological abnormalities between cells and tissues. Dr. Zac Bush has made a very convincing connection between glyphosate, leaky gut syndrome, and the alteration of the amino acid glycine *(similar to glyphosate)* in proteins in the brain producing the typical prion conformation.

Dr. Russel Blaylock, retired neurosurgeon, and now natural health advocate writes extensively about AD. He practiced neurosurgery for 24 years before retiring and has spent the past 20 plus years studying the pathophysiology of neurodegenerative disorders including AD and how they can be prevented and treated. He has written 30 papers for peer review journals and has written four books and several chapters in medical textbooks on clinical neuroscience subjects. He states that amyloid plague is not the primary cause of Alzheimer's disease, and that even people who live up into their hundreds have amyloid deposit density in their brains equal to any Alzheimer's patient.

He continues, *"It may be an aggravating factor, but certainly not the cause. Researchers found that people with Alzheimer's had rather high mercury levels in certain areas of their brain. And the same thing was discovered true of aluminum. All of the proposed factors involved with Alzheimer's produce inflammation in the brain. And anything that produces inflammation will produce amyloid deposit and this would suppress the mitochondria. Inflammation also activates microglia cells. Microglial cells respond to inflammation and create an inflammatory process of their own while attacking damaged cells and cleaning up the debris."*

Dr. Blaylock is also concerned about mercury dental filings, which evaporate *(throughout the course of daily trauma)*, and turn into a mercury vapor. This vapor then enters the nasal cavities and travels along the olfactory nerve, which goes to the first part of the brain where we first see changes from Alzheimer's disease. Mercury and aluminum are high on the list as triggers for brain inflammation. Once it is absorbed into the bloodstream or by vaccination into the lymphatic system, it enters the brain and is stored. They act together as a toxin, making it even worse. Aluminum can come from several sources, and vaccines are one of the worst. A study by Pritchard and Rosenorn-Lanng suggests *"environmental factors"* is the cause. Neuropharmacologist, Richard Deth, Ph.D., and author of a major study on AD concluded, *"Mercury is clearly contributing to neurological problems, whose rate is increasing in parallel with rising levels of mercury. It seems that the two are tied together."*

Other Contributing Factors

The government says that every baby over the age of six months should have vaccines, and they know these vaccines contain a dose of mercury that is toxic to the brain. They also know the studies have shown that the flu vaccine has zero, - zero - effectiveness in children under five. *"Here's the bottom line,"* says Dr. Blaylock, *"The vast number of people who get the flu vaccine isn't going to get any benefit, but they get all of the risks and complications. Flu vaccines contain mercury in the form of thimerosal (ethyl mercury), a brain toxin, which accumulates in the brain and other organs. It's incorporated into the brain for a lifetime. After 5 or 10 years of flu shots, enough mercury accumulates in the brain that every single study agrees it's neurotoxic. Mercury is*

extremely toxic to the brain, even in very small concentrations, and there are
thousands of studies that prove it."

Pesticides and herbicides are also stored in the fat tissue in the brain over long periods of time, like mercury and aluminum. Herbicides, fungicides, and even *H. pylori* that are associated with stomach ulcers can store in the brain as well and contribute to chronic inflammation. We know that some chemicals, when they're in combination, produce much worse damage than when used alone. Everyone is exposed to aluminum, mercury, cadmium, lead, pesticides, and herbicides. All these accumulate over a lifetime and the bioburden increases as we age. Fluoride, plus aluminum, can form floroaluminum, which is infinitely more brain toxic than either alone. Almost all drinking water in the USA has floroaluminum in it. [238]

Another more recently reported and intriguing cause of AD is Tuberculosis *(TB)*, an historically devastating disease, which according to the World Health Organization currently affects one-third of the world's population. In his publication in the Journal of MPE Molecular Pathological Epidemiology, *Are the Infectious Roots of Alzheimer's Buried Deep in the Past,* Dr. John Broxmeyer presents a very convincing case for the inclusion of Tuberculosis *(TB)* as a cause of Alzheimer's disease. He has shown the TB organism can enter and infect brain microglial cells and alter their metabolism.

"A distinctive characteristic of infection with M. tuberculosis, a disease that
according to WHO (the World Health Organization) affects a third of the
world, is its capacity to enter and replicate within macrophages in the blood.
Within the brain, microglial cells are the resident macrophages. As such, human
microglial cells are productively infected with M. tuberculosis and are, in fact,
its principal target in the CNS" [239]

He goes on to say that the TB mycobacterium directs a frontal attack on the microglial cells and inhibits their ability to initiate an important immune response to microbes. The TB organisms can cause inflammation, interfere with vascular nutrition, and invade neurons causing degeneration of the brain and produce amyloid plaque.

Gluten And The Brain

Gluten can also cause brain disorders. Gluten, in patients with celiac disease, is strongly associated with risk for dementia, as was described in the Proceedings of the Mayo Clinic; it was a treatable cause of dementia.

People with gluten sensitivity can experience symptoms such as *"foggy mind,"* ADHD-like behavior, abdominal pain, bloating, diarrhea, constipation, headaches, bone or joint pain, and chronic fatigue when they have gluten in their diet. Gluten sensitivity has also been associated with autism, schizophrenia, and depression, as well as a newly identified condition called gluten psychosis. [240]

While symptoms of gluten sensitivity are common symptoms of celiac disease, these individuals do not test positive for celiac disease or for a wheat allergy. Having celiac disease is often confused with having a wheat or gluten allergy. People with a wheat allergy who consume any of the four classes of wheat protein, including gluten, can trigger an immune system response that causes an allergic reaction, with symptoms that span from itching, swelling and difficulty breathing to anaphylaxis. Individuals who have been diagnosed with gluten sensitivity do not experience the small intestine damage or develop the tissue transglutaminase antibodies found in celiac disease. [241]

Another disorder, called gluten ataxia, is an autoimmune response to gluten in which the antibodies attack the cerebellum in the brain. It can be related to non-celiac gluten sensitivity as well as celiac disease where there may be leaky gut syndrome. The intestinal cell wall lining is compromised and proteins and other chemicals can enter the blood stream as previously described by Dr. Zach Bush. Dr. Hadjivassiliou has conducted extensive research into gluten ataxia, having first described the condition in the 1990s after seeing a number of patients with unexplained balance and coordination problems curiously about the same time he began systematically testing these patients for gluten sensitivity and found a very high prevalence of antibodies in patients with ataxia, suggestive of a heightened immune response to gluten but not necessarily to a diagnosis of celiac disease. He described gluten ataxia as an immune-mediated disease triggered by the ingestion of gluten. Typical symptoms include difficulty walking or walking with a wide gait, frequent falls, difficulty judging distances or position, visual disturbances and tremor. Gluten ataxia can affect fingers, hands, arms, legs, speech, and even eye movements. Basically, the back of the brain gets eaten away by microglial cells. [242]

Carbohydrates

Insulin resistance as seen in diabetes and obesity can also drive brain disorders such as dementia. Dr. Robert Lustig, a pediatric endocrinologist, insists, *"There is no doubt in my mind that insulin resistance drives dementia. We have causative data in animals, and we have causative medical inference data in humans."* Neurologist, David Perlmutter says the number of people diagnosed with diabetes in the US has nearly tripled in the last twenty years, according to the CDC. *"That doubles your risk for Alzheimer's disease. We were told to eat more whole grain goodness. Eat more of what the US Department of Agriculture is producing for you, and that will be good for you. Nothing could be further from the truth. Diets that are high in fat actually lower cardiovascular risk factors and are absolutely associated with a reduced risk for dementia. This was published in The Journal of Alzheimer's Disease in January of 2012, research from the prestigious Mayo Clinic. People on a high-fat diet had a 44% risk reduction for developing dementia. Those on a high carb diet, which the government continues to recommend, had an 89% increased risk."* Perlmutter says that carbohydrates, even the whole-grain carbs that many of us think of as the good ones, are the cause of almost every modern neurologic malady. That includes dementia, decreased libido, depression, chronic headaches, anxiety, epilepsy, and ADHD. Over the last 40 years, people have become addicted to gluten. Perlmutter claims, *"In combination with carbs, gluten's influence on our diets explains why we get dementia - and every other common neurologic problem. Inflammation is the cornerstone of Alzheimer's disease and Parkinson's, multiple sclerosis - all of the neurodegenerative diseases are really predicated on inflammation."* [243]

Caffeine

I know I may get some nasty comments on this one but save your breath. It won't bother me, and I'll just end up owning some emotional real estate in your brain when you can't let it go. I am just the messenger who cares about you. Caffeine is the most commonly used psychoactive drug in the world, mostly because of its widespread acceptance, diffusion in many products, and addictive nature. It has been shown to enhance some physical activities and short-term memory and alertness, which is why most people use it. There may also be some benefit in some neurodegenerative diseases, but there is a tradeoff because of the negative side effects. A cup of caffeinated coffee now and then is not going to be a problem, but as a routine, it can be harmful to many systems and provokes psychological and physiological dependence, abuse, and addiction similar to other drugs like cocaine and amphetamines. Caffeine can cause electrical and blood flow disturbances in the heart, brain damage, and tooth and enamel erosion. And if that's not enough, it yellows your teeth, and makes your breath smell horrible. If you throw the book down now, you'll know for sure that you are addicted. But I appeal for you to hear me out, and then decide about your caffeine habits, and of course, read the rest of the book.

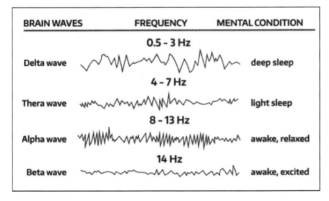

Caffeine has stimulant effects, and the more you consume, the more it reinforces future use, dependency, and addiction. Numerous controlled

laboratory investigations show that caffeine produces behavioral and physiological effects similar to other drugs of dependence. Caffeine's mechanism
of action is somewhat different from that of cocaine and the substituted
amphetamines, in that caffeine blocks adenosine receptors. Caffeine blocks
adenosine A1 that controls blood flow to the brain and relaxes the brain to
ready it for sleep. It can suppress Theta and Alpha brain waves that are calming, and promote Beta waves leading to increased stress and anxiety. [244, 245]

Caffeine also stimulates the adrenals to produce acetylcholine *(epinephrine)*
that puts body in fight or flight producing oxidative stress. An important
finding is that in most regular coffee drinkers, about half of the A1 adenosine receptors may be occupied by caffeine. It is likely that this blockage of a
substantial amount of cerebral A1 adenosine receptors will result in adaptive
changes and lead to chronic alterations of receptor expression and availability.
Adenosine is a by-product of cellular activity, and stimulation of adenosine
receptors produces feelings of tiredness and the need to sleep. Caffeine's
ability to block these receptors means the levels of the body's natural stimulants, dopamine and norepinephrine, continue at higher levels. Tolerance to
caffeine occurs when the physiological, behavioral, and/or subjective effects
of caffeine decrease after repeated exposure to the drug, such that the same
dose of caffeine no longer produces equivalent effects, and a higher dose is
needed to produce similar effects.

Caffeinated coffee inhibits the absorption of iron and circulating B6, a key
mineral involved with the synthesis of serotonin and dopamine, increases
stress hormones including cortisol and epinephrine, inflammation, and
insulin while decreasing insulin sensitivity to cellular uptake of glucose
thereby increasing blood sugar which leads to arterial deterioration and
cardiovascular disease - the perfect storm. It also steals oxygen from your
brain. Dr. Paul Laurienti, a radiologist at Wake Forest Baptist Medical Center
in a video broadcast on the Healthcare Channel, showed MRI images of the
brain before and after one cup of caffeinated coffee consumed by the news
station's interviewer. The results on screen showed a 40% drop in oxygen to
the brain after the MRI. Dr. Laurienti said during the interview, *"One cup*

a day will change your brain." Decreased blood flow to the brain was also noted in the journal Human Brain Mapping. [246]

John's Hopkins' School of Medicine published a study on caffeinated coffee and concluded that, because of the addictive potential of caffeine, routinely consuming 100 mg a day of caffeine can put an individual in a dependent or addicted category. Other studies have demonstrated similar results with physical dependence that would trigger withdrawal symptoms that include headaches, muscle pain and stiffness, lethargy, nausea, vomiting, depressed mood, and marked irritability. Of course, there are variations in response, but under a typical distribution curve, this holds up to be probable. The average cup of coffee contains 95 mg of caffeine. You can be sure to fly out of Starbuck's like a rocket ship if you suck down two cups of their Grande creations at 660 mg. [247 - 249]

In a general population survey conducted in the United States, 14% of caffeine consumers preferred to continue use, despite the harm that was explained to them. Many participants from this study reported that a physician or counselor had advised them to stop or reduce caffeine consumption within the last year. Medical and psychological problems that participants attributed to caffeine, included heart, stomach, and urinary problems, and complaints of anxiety, depression, insomnia, irritability, and difficulty thinking. In addition, two-thirds of those surveyed experienced at least one symptom associated with the clinical disorder, caffeine intoxication. [250]

We are not just talking about caffeinated coffee. There is an aggressive marketing of energy drinks with caffeine and other stimulants. While marketing efforts are spread across the age spectrum, they are targeted primarily at young individuals, for physical performance-enhancing and psychostimulatory effects. Furthermore, several studies suggest that energy drinks may serve as a gateway to other forms of substance dependence. Additionally, caffeine, like alcohol and tobacco, is legally used, but, unlike the last two, its sale in the form of high concentration drinks or tablets is not adequately controlled or restricted.

Caffeine in tea is generally much lower and has different effects. As was shared by one inspired person, *"The effect provided by tea is like being gently encouraged to do something by a loving grandmother, while coffee is like being kicked in the butt by a military officer."*

Caffeine, theobromine, and theophylline are active components of both coffee and tea. However, another component in tea called L-theanine has unique properties. In humans, L-theanine increases the formation of brain waves called alpha waves, which are associated with alertness, creativity, and relaxation making your brain sharper. This is perhaps the main reason for the different, milder buzz that tea generates. L-theanine may affect neurotransmitters in the brain, such as GABA. Additionally, L-Theanine has been found to help increase dopamine levels in humans. Dopamine is a naturally occurring chemical in the brain that is released during pleasurable activities and helps produce a sense of well-being. Some studies have suggested that L-theanine, especially when combined with caffeine, can improve attention and brain function. [251-254]

Tea is also rich in polyphenols. Especially abundant in green tea, epigallocatechin 3-gallate *(EGCG or EGC3G)* is found to be the most potent tea polyphenols for antioxidative, antimutagenic, and antipathogenic effects. Scientists isolating this substance from green tea for experiments discovered that it is often bonded with caffeine to form larger particles. Some found that the two substances *(caffeine and EGCG)* working together would be much more effective in the said preventive functions, particularly in burning more calories and preventing cancer. The many bioactive compounds in tea appear to impact virtually every cell in the body to help improve health outcomes.

So, caffeinated beverages can be good or bad, depending on context and source. Caffeinated coffee and *"energy drinks"* are generally not the best option for the reasons stated above. Organic caffeinated tea is a great option because of the lower caffeinated content and the L-theanine and polyphenol components that has significant brain function benefits. Because of the socially and chemically generated high addictive potential, focused restraint should be considered. If you like the taste and morning routine, just use decaf organic coffee. Teeccino is another option. It is an herb that smells and tastes very much like coffee. If you want the buzz, tea is a good option. I am a very active *"doer"* and need to stay at my physical and mental best. I sometimes drink organic white and green tea blends. These and other solutions are listed in the New Beginnings chapter.

Brain Drain And Our Children

And what of our children? What health legacy will we leave them? Most of us really do care, but we may not appreciate how important it is to get all the knowledge that we can about the things impacting our children's health. The damage can start at conception. The average pregnant woman will be exposed to a variety of toxins that can interfere with brain development. Studies have shown that over 200 toxic chemicals are in umbilical cords of the average woman, post-delivery. That does not include chemicals and medications that weren't measured or those that have already passed into the developing fetus over nine months but may have been eliminated, but not before the damage is done at the cellular level. Even when a pregnant mom gets vaccinated for whatever reason, more commonly with the flu vaccine, a 2.2-pound fetus at about 28-week gestation will get the equivalent of over 250x the EPA safety limit of thimerosal (mercury). But, the medical community at large is recommending that every pregnant woman get a flu vaccine shot. Dr. Russell Blaylock, has this to say about vaccinations: *"I cannot think of anything more insane than vaccinating a pregnant woman."* Prescription and over the counter meds, air, and water pollution, food additives, fertilizers, pesticides, weed killers, vaccines, heavy metals, radiation, stimulants like caffeine and antihistamines, fluoride, and many others all can impact brain development. It is very important that we parents be vigilant in this regard.

The number of industrial chemicals known to cause neurodevelopmental disabilities among children - such as autism, attention-deficit hyperactivity disorder *(ADHD),* and other neurobehavioral disorders, has doubled from 6 to 12 over the past seven years, according to a new study published in the journal Lancet, Neurology. The study also found that the list of recognized human neurotoxicants - chemicals known to injure the adult human brain but have not yet been linked definitively to neurodevelopmental disabilities in children - increased from 202 to 214 over that same seven-year period. These are chemicals that are widely used throughout the world and can be found in our food and air as well as in everyday products we use in our homes and gardens, including clothing, furniture, and toys.

But those numbers represent only the tip of the iceberg. As pointed out by the study's authors, Dr. Phillippe Grandjean, an environmental epidemiologist currently teaching at the Harvard School of Public Health, and Dr. Philip Landrigan, a pediatrician at the Icahn School of Medicine at Mount Sinai Hospital in New York City, *"Very few of the more than 80,000 pesticides, solvents and other industrial chemicals in widespread use in the United States and elsewhere have ever been tested for their toxic effects on the developing brain (or on the adult brain, for that matter)."* [255 - 257]

As a result, they say that we are in the midst of a *"global, silent pandemic of neurodevelopmental toxicity."* It usually takes decades to recognize the severe danger that an industrial chemical can wreak on the developing brain. Such was the case with lead and methylmercury. *"Early warnings of the neurotoxicity of those chemicals were often ignored or even dismissed,"* write Grandjean and Landrigan, primarily because the effects - such as population drops in IQ - were not immediately evident at the clinical level.

The developing human brain is incredibly vulnerable to chemical exposures, both in utero and in early childhood, and, during these sensitive growth stages, exposure to toxins of all sorts can cause permanent brain damage. Some of those industrial chemicals include lead, arsenic, methylmercury, PCB, Fluoride, toluene, BPA, and phthalates. [258, 259]

Perhaps the bottom line to this chapter is that each of us needs to consider how much of our autonomy and brain health we are willing to give away. We are being seduced from all sectors to give it up in some way, shape, or form. The first thing they are after is our brain; the last thing they can have is our brain - we have to voluntarily give it up. Even when medications are highly *"encouraged"* by our doctor, it is still our choice, but we should be diligent and search out the side effects of any medication that is recommended. The doctor will not necessarily tell you that. Yes, even with all of the toxic environmental chemicals mentioned that are harming our brains, it is still our choice whether or not to allow that to happen. That final decision becomes especially significant when we have been given critical tools in the decision-making process - knowledge.

Knowledge is power. You now have it, and the road you travel from here is your own. Choose wisely. There is too much at stake for you and your future generations.

CHAPTER 4

Vaccines
Blowing The Lid Off The Deception

To vaccinate or not to vaccinate, that is the question at the center of a very hotly debated topic these days, especially given the new research published on vaccine safety and efficacy concerns. If you would have asked me twelve years ago about vaccines, I would have said, *"Of course you should vaccinate. There is no reason not to because they are safe and effective!"* After twenty-five years of training as a medical and surgical specialist, I was sure of that. Like most everyone else in the medical profession, I marched to the tune of training I received, which, at the time, I thought was the best in the world. My heart was in the right place, but I was naive, and I contributed through blind trust and arrogance to the illusion that the medical profession, as we have come to experience it, is some sort of a Superhero. There was so much misinformation taught in medical school and residencies by well-meaning professors, and after that by drug reps, the CDC, FDA, NIH, and major research and teaching institutions funded by pharmaceutical companies. But now I better understand the depth of deception, even when it comes to vaccines.

As you read through this chapter, you will find some very disturbing compromises in the safety and efficacy of vaccine research and implementation that have been directly responsible for death and other damage to the health of the trusting *(albeit manipulated)* public. Essentially none of the standard scientific method protocols have been followed by the CDC or pharmaceutical industry. This is especially disturbing because the pharmaceutical companies have unbridled freedom to create whatever concoction they may want to try because, according to the National Childhood Vaccine Injury Act *(NCVIA)* of 1986, they can no longer be held responsible for the damage a vaccine may cause. The same is not true of other pharmaceuticals, even though that sector of the pharmaceutical industry is also riddled with corruption. But clearly, the vaccine industry is much worse. I am not necessarily anti-vaccine; so I won't say don't vaccinate, that is your choice, as it should be. But understand there is much more to the story. Personally, I am in favor of choice, and safe and effective treatment options recommended in a timely manner, based on long- term safety and efficacy studies. That is presently not the case, and I don't think it will be in our lifetime.

A fair argument may be made for crisis intervention use of certain vaccines in developing countries where adequate nutrition is lacking, hygiene is poor, and infectious diseases are out of control. Antibiotics, vaccines, and other practical sanitation and lifestyle changes may help end the crisis, but those situations are few these days. And when a crisis does emerge, the World Health Organization and many private organizations are quick to gear up and respond. Most responses involve antibiotics, antivirals, vaccines, improvement of personal hygiene, creating clean water sources, healthy nutrition, and healthy lifestyle education.

Historically, poor hygiene and contaminated water supplies in crowded areas are the main culprits for disease transmission. Even through the Dark Ages, many Europeans resisted bathing because they believed it actually caused diseases. This practice persisted even in their settling of the Americas, well into the 1800s, when the crowding of cities in Europe and America was brought on by the Industrial Revolution. The crowded city streets in London, New York, Boston, and Chicago especially were contaminated due to dead animal carcasses, and human and animal feces, which flowed into the drinking water. There was no real clean water infrastructure to speak of, which was the cause of many diseases. This total lack of sanitation in urban areas filled with rats and other vermin provided the perfect environment to spread disease.

Cholera spread easily through contaminated water and food and killed very quickly, often proving fatal within hours of the first symptoms of vomiting or diarrhea. The Infant mortality rate was between 25% and 70% in London during this era. Dr. John Snow, who later went on to become known as the Father of Epidemiology, traced the infection back to a well pump in London where one woman was cleaning dirty diapers.

Many similar stories occur around the world, and when the environmental and nutritional causes are addressed, the diseases go away. Typhoid Fever, Dysentery, Diphtheria, all respond to improved lifestyle conditions. Even the Smallpox epidemic subsided to very few cases after healthy sanitation and clean water plumbing practices were put in place. This occurred before the vaccinations became available, which did very little to eradicate the disease and caused statistically significant fatalities itself. Reports were as high as 1 in 200. But, the credit for stopping the epidemic was inappropriately given to the vaccines instead of the change in healthy sanitation and clean water practices.

We now have a better understanding of what causes diseases, resulting in more sophisticated preventative measures. Presently, it is estimated that 75% of infectious diseases are of animal origin. Infected fleas, rats, birds, pigs, and mosquitos, overcrowding, farm animal feces, poor nutrition and personal hygiene, and contact with infected wildlife are among the most common causes of the mass spread of bacterial and viral infections. And, while there can be a lot of collateral damage from the vaccines that have been developed for some of these epidemics, and their use and effectiveness may be questionable depending on the crisis, the benefit of intervention in a very serious situation may outweigh the risk. [260]

Compared to the 75-200 million deaths of the Black Death plague of the 14th century and other rare pandemics recorded over the last 2500 years, what the world faces today pales in comparison to the epidemics and pandemics of the past. Most of those were also isolated to specific geographical areas. Today, cholera and influenza account for most of the deaths and occur in the hundreds to thousands, not 100 million or more, and some are worldwide statistics, not just isolated to regions like those pandemics seen in past centuries.

Perhaps the worst human pandemic of recent times was from the Spanish Flu of 1918. More recent investigations, based mainly on original medical reports from the period of the pandemic, found that the viral infection itself was not more aggressive than any previous influenza, but that the special circumstances of the pandemic during the World War 1 era set the stage for the perfect storm. Malnourishment, overcrowded medical camps and hospitals, poor hygiene, mass movement of troops and civilians, and lack of knowledge about viruses promoted the spread of the virus in three separate waves, and caused bacterial *(mostly respiratory)* superinfections that killed most of the victims, largely between 20 and 40 who did not have natural immunity like the previous generations.

Unfortunately, this rare pandemic is frequently referenced to incite fear to convince people to be vaccinated with the flu vaccine. But let's take a look at the reality of a typical flu season. From a purely statistical standpoint, there are about 325 million people in the United States. There is a grossly inaccurate report of 60,000 people dying in the US from the flu virus each year. The reason I say inaccurate is because the CDC includes secondary causes of death, and not so many people actually die from the flu itself. But even leaving it at that number, the chances of dying from the flu are 1 in 5800 or .017%. Yet, there are global efforts to vaccinate for an extremely low risk and generally minor symptom disease with a vaccine that has been shown to be minimally effective at best with no long-term safety or efficacy studies. The flu vaccine has been shown to have extremely toxic ingredients that can cause devastating damage to developing brains and contribute to other brain and immune system disorders. Innocents are being harmed for no reason. Now, does that make much sense?

Despite this type of pro-vaccination propaganda and blatant verifiable lies by the pharmaceutical industry and FDA, the reality of vaccine injury and death is making the news, and objections to proposed forced vaccinations are mounting. But this is not a new phenomenon. It was controversial as well when the first vaccines were forced on British citizens almost 200 years ago and almost 150 years since the first compulsory vaccination laws were passed in the United States. This time the rising anti-vaccination sentiment has scientific research backup for the objections. The stakes are much higher today with the multitude of injected vaccines forced upon children whose parents are threatened to have their children taken away if they refuse. There is good reason to be concerned on many levels. One that is not discussed much is that the human immune system is not fully understood - in fact, man understands only the fringes of this complex system. More commonly discussed is that vaccines, with a concoction of harmful ingredients injected directly into the circulatory system, force immune responses that have never been studied for long-term effects. In addition to foreign microbial proteins, vaccines often contain toxins like aluminum, mercury, polysorbate 80, herbicides, live viruses, and even aborted fetal tissues.

But how would you like to find out that you have harmful viruses in your body causing symptoms from a vaccine that you never received! Is that possible? Yes, it is!! The dangerous SV40 virus from the polio vaccine used in the 1950s and early '60s in the United States, and elsewhere for decades after, contained SV40, a cancer-causing virus that is passed down to future generations. As you will see, there is no doubt that the vaccine manufacturers, the Federal Government's CDC, FDA, and other healthcare entities know about the dangers of vaccines, but their stated mission is to quell any fears about the effectiveness or safety, even if it means manipulating research results and using fear-based marketing tactics, so mass vaccinations will be accomplished.

Any discussion of the effectiveness or safety of a drug must be accompanied by published research and clinical observations. In the case of vaccines, it would seem unconscionable to proceed with injections into anyone without first demonstrating concrete evidence of safety and effectiveness testing. Gary Null, who holds a Ph.D. in human nutrition and public health sciences, elaborates on the gold standard of scientific method that should be used in vaccine research. There are some basic questions about vaccines that should always be answered before injecting someone with chemicals and potentially deadly microscopic life forms:

Are vaccines effective based on long accepted scientific standards? If so, where is the proof? If they are not effective, where is the proof?

Are vaccines safe? If so, where is the proof? If vaccines are not safe, where is the proof?

Are there long-term individual and multi-vaccine combination studies and double-blind placebo control studies? If not, why not? If performed, did these studies compare fully vaccinated groups of individuals against groups that were non-vaccinated? Have there been trials that compared one group vaccinated and another put on a lifestyle modification program?

I would also ask, is the public health information about the disease threats and the need for vaccines true and accurate? If not, why not? [261]

Vaccines - Are They Effective?

Vaccines are suspensions of infectious agents used to artificially induce immunity against specific diseases. The aim of vaccination is to mimic the process of naturally occurring infection through artificial means. Theoretically, vaccines produce a mild to moderate episode of infection in the body with only temporary and slight side effects. But, in reality, they may be causing diseases rather than preventing them. As mentioned in the beginning of this chapter, some vaccines have shown themselves to be effective in certain circumstances, especially in third world countries, collateral damage notwithstanding. But that does not reflect the reality of all vaccines. According to Jamie Murphy, an investigative journalist on vaccines and author of What Every Parent Should Know About Childhood Vaccination, *"Vaccines produce disease or infection in an otherwise healthy person... And so, in order to allegedly produce something good, one has to do something bad to the human body, that is, induce an infection or a disease in an otherwise healthy person that may or may not have ever happened."* When children contract a disease such as measles or mumps, they generally develop a permanent protection against that disease. Such is not necessarily the case with vaccines. As Murphy observes, *"The medical profession does not know how long vaccine immunity lasts because it is artificial immunity. If you get measles naturally, in the vast majority of cases you have life-long immunity . . . However, if you get a measles vaccine or a DTaP vaccine, it does not guarantee 100% immunity, or that the vaccine will prevent you from getting the disease. The problem is that the medical profession and science do not know, and have never known, what the infecting dose of an infection really is. It's not something that can be measured. So they're really guessing at the amount of antigen and other supplementary chemicals that they put into the measles and mumps vaccines."*

Dr. Richard Moskowitz, past president of the National Institute of Homeopathy, and a cum laude graduate of Harvard and New York Medical School has stated, *"Vaccines trick the body so that it will no longer initiate a generalized inflammatory response. They thereby accomplish what the entire immune system seems to have evolved to prevent. They place the virus directly into the blood and give it access to the major immune organs and tissues without any obvious way of getting rid of it. These attenuated viruses and virus elements persist in the blood for a long time, perhaps permanently. This, in turn, implies a systematic weakening of the ability to mount an effective response, not only to childhood diseases but to other acute infections as well."*

John Anthony Morris, M.D., was a virologist at NIH from the 1940s to 1976 when he was fired for blowing the whistle on the ineffectiveness and hazards of the Swine Flu vaccine. As the former Bacteriologist, Division of Biologics Standards, and Research Virologist, FDA, he stated, *"There is no evidence that any influenza vaccine thus far developed is effective in preventing or mitigating any attack of influenza. The producers of these vaccines know they are worthless but go on making them anyway."* Yet, we continue the injections that are laced with mercury.

Furthermore, Jamie Murphy insists that introducing antigens directly into the bloodstream can prove dangerous. *"When a child gets a naturally occurring infection, like measles, which is not a serious disease, the body reacts to that in a very set way. The germs go in a certain part of the body through the throat and into the different immune organs, and the body combats the disease in its own natural way. There are all sorts of immune reactions that occur. When you inject a vaccine into the body, you're actually performing an unnatural act because you are injecting directly into the blood system. That is not the natural port of entry for that virus. In fact, the whole immune system in our body is geared to prevent that from happening. What we're doing is giving the virus or the bacteria carte blanche entry into our bloodstream, which is the last place you want it to be. This increases the chance for disease because viral material from the vaccine stays in the cells and is not completely defeated by the body's own defenses."* [262]

> *"When you inject a vaccine into the body, you're actually performing an unnatural act because you are injecting directly into the blood system..."*
>
> Jamie Murphy, Investigative Journalist

Vaccine-induced protection is temporary unlike real immunity gained from contracting the actual disease. A recent study confirmed that measles could be spread from fully vaccinated people to other fully vaccinated people. Recent outbreaks of measles occurred in both fully vaccinated and unvaccinated people. In some measles outbreaks, a majority of the cases occur in fully vaccinated people. Thus, vaccine-induced protection is unreliable, but outbreaks in vaccinated people are blamed on the unvaccinated. How can that be? If vaccines are effective in preventing disease, how can the fully- vaccinated become infected?

One of the reasons that vaccines fail, as recent evidence seems to indicate, is because the wild virus may need to be in greater local and global circulation to boost vaccine-induced immunity. Protective antibodies wane more quickly when they are not periodically re-challenged by the freely circulating virus. This happened with the varicella *(chickenpox)* vaccine. Studies show that a reduction in the circulation of the natural varicella virus due to high vaccination rates caused an epidemic of herpes zoster *(shingles)*. The elderly, especially, relied on these periodic exogenous boosts to their immune systems *(when they went out in public)* to keep shingles from occurring. The chickenpox vaccine reduced cases of chickenpox, but the circulating cases actually provided a valuable function.

Vaccines - Are They Safe?

Are vaccines safe? Isn't that the question we all want to know? As with most things, it depends on whom you ask and how one defines *"safe."* The front lines of the vaccine battles are very definitive with their feelings about vaccine safety - it is either yes or no with very little in between. Many times, when people passionately disagree about something, it is commonly said that the river of truth flows in the middle where there is truth to be appreciated on both sides, maybe leaning one way or the other. But in this case, I would say, there is no middle ground; there are no SAFE vaccines. There may be some with a certain level of effectiveness, but none are proven safe because there have never been any studies showing that vaccines are safe. But the opposite IS true, that vaccines have been shown to be harmful. They have notable side effects and are therefore not *"safe"* for anyone for a variety of reasons. Not that everyone will experience noticeable and immediate side effects, but unless proven otherwise with long-term prospective double-blind safety studies including DNA and gene studies, vaccine proponents cannot rationally promote them as safe. What does a *"safe"* vaccine mean anyway to the vaccine proponents? As Inigo Montoya said to Vizzini in The Princess Bride on his constant use of the word *"inconceivable,"* *"You keep using that word. I do not think it means what you think it means."*

Many on the front lines of the vaccine controversy make emotional appeals for their position without being privy to scientific validity. More often than not, consumers know little or nothing about the vaccine safety testing process and assume that vaccine manufacturers and regulatory institutions have exercised due diligence in ensuring that vaccines are as safe as possible. But what IS true is that according to a recent study, the anti-vaccine crowd tends to be significantly more informed about the science *(or lack of science)* involved. I believe they have done their homework because they generally have experienced harm, in some way, that vaccines have caused a friend or family member. There are several parts to this puzzle, which constitute the big picture of vaccine safety. Some pieces are bigger and more important than others, but they all come together to help give definition to the question of safety.

At this point I hope you can appreciate that vaccine effectiveness is questionable as a preventative measure. But safety is where the rubber meets the road with most people on the front lines. So, what's in vaccines that may add to the safety question? We have heard about thimerosal used as a preservative, and aluminum used as an adjuvant to increase the effectiveness of an ineffective microbial antigen, but how about cells from monkey kidneys, chick embryo, beef blood and heart, caterpillar, pig stomach, cocker spaniel cells, retroviruses, and aborted human fetal cells. Yes, you read that right. Since the 1960s we have used aborted human fetal cells. Dr. Theresa Deisher, Ph.D. is world renowned in stem cell research. She writes that vaccines manufactured in human fetal cell lines contain unacceptably high levels of fetal DNA fragment contaminants and rising autistic disorder prevalence is directly related to vaccines manufactured utilizing human fetal cells. In addition, there are known adverse effects from vaccine additives such as formaldehyde, phenooxyethanol, glutaraldehyde, sodium, sodium acetate, monosodium glutamate *(MSG)*, hydrochloric acid, hydrogen peroxide, lactose, yeast protein, bovine and human serum albumin. [263 - 266]

More On Safety And Efficacy

The US childhood immunization schedule requires 26 vaccine doses for infants aged less than one year, at the moment, the most in the world. It is reasonable to assume that the purpose of infant injections is to reduce mortality and disease. The infant mortality rate *(IMR)* is one of the most important indicators of the socio-economic well-being and public health conditions of a country. Is it surprising to you, then, that the United States is #1 in infant mortality deaths? While there are some minor fluctuations in rankings, there are 33 developed nations with better infant mortality statistics - about 5.8 deaths /1000 live births, and we rank in the bottom one third for life expectancy. What does this say about the people and government agencies that are *"forcing"* supposedly safe, researched, and effective vaccine protocols upon the general public? [267]

The published conclusion to these findings demonstrates a counter-intuitive relationship: *nations that require more vaccine doses tend to have higher infant mortality rates.*

Most vaccines are shown to have only short-term effects requiring more frequent injections with harmful added ingredients. These vaccines may have been tested individually for immediate, observable laboratory effects, but not in combination, and none have been tested for long-term effects. No studies anywhere in the world were ever conducted for safety or to provide scientific evidence that infants or anyone else are not subjected to synergistic toxicity from the simultaneous administration of eight drugs. In fact, there is much evidence to the contrary. As babies receive more vaccines concurrently, they are more likely to be hospitalized and die. [268, 269]

Another variable to consider with regard to vaccine safety is the *"one size fits all"* approach to vaccinating children, which has been a dismal failure. There is essentially no pre-screening for genetic sensitivities, family history, etc. to determine those *"at risk."* When these morally and ethically responsible procedures ARE incorporated, then parents should then make their decisions on vaccinations based on known risks determined by safety studies. But that is not done and cannot be done any time in the near future. Why? Because there have been no prospective studies on safety or effectiveness done. One cannot determine risk when risk assessment studies have not been done.

In a study on Autism, *Family History of Immune Conditions and Autism Spectrum and Developmental Disorders...* published in 2019, the authors show a significant correlation between those moms and primary relatives who have autoimmune *(inflammatory)* disorders. An increased number of autoimmune disorders suggest that in some families with autism, immune dysfunction could interact with various environmental factors to play a role in autism pathogenesis. Now, adding to that picture is that the lives of the average person in developed countries are significantly impacted on a daily basis by *"pro-inflammatory"* environmental conditions. These conditions cause the immune system to always be on alert and over-reactive. The immune system microglial cells in the brain react very aggressively to chemicals crossing the blood brain barrier, and when they do, they eat brain tissue while trying to react to chemicals like thimerosal, aluminum, and other chemicals in vaccines.

Aluminum

Aluminum is used as an adjuvant in some inactivated vaccines. Adjuvants hyper-stimulate a stronger immune response to the vaccine in an effort to produce more antibodies that confer protection. According to the John Hopkins Bloomberg School of Public Health, 27 vaccines licensed in the US contain aluminum in varying amounts, including anthrax, DT/Td, DTaP/Tdap, hepatitis A, hepatitis B, Hib, HPV, meningococcal and pneumococcal vaccines. As a general rule of thumb, live vaccines will not contain aluminum. Only vaccines made with killed/inactivated viruses and so-called *"toxoid"* vaccines may have it, and this goes for both childhood and adult vaccines. When you orally ingest aluminum, your body will absorb between 0.2 to 1.5% of it. When aluminum is injected into muscle, your body absorbs 100%, which is why aluminum-containing vaccines are likely far more dangerous than eating aluminum. Since aluminum is used as an adjuvant in so many vaccines, it seems reasonable to assume that extensive tests have been done to ascertain its safety.

Reasonable or not, such an assumption would be false. There is in fact no real evidence at all to support the idea that injecting aluminum-containing vaccines is safe. Studies on human infants show that no aluminum is excreted short term at all. Two-month-old infants were given a total of 1,200 mcg of aluminum in the form of three intramuscular vaccines, as per the standard vaccination schedule. Blood and urine levels of aluminum were measured over the following 12 hours. The authors were *"reassured"* to find there was no rise in blood levels of aluminum following vaccination. But no aluminum came out through the urine either. So where did it all go? When Dr. Humphries M.D. and nephrologist asked the authors what happened to the aluminum, Dr. Tammy Movsas, wrote back saying: *"So... we don't really know what happens to the aluminum at this point in time. As you said, more research is needed in this area."* And yet, it's okay to give known toxin to infants? And, when finally tested, the results aren't as expected, those with the power to implement change, just shrug their shoulders, and allow it to continue without demanding a stop to the madness? Excretion of aluminum is not as efficient in infants and young children, yet this fact is almost never taken into consideration. That which is not excreted ends up accumulating in various organs, including the child's brain, kidneys, and bones!

There is no known biologic need or use for aluminum in the human body but aluminum can enter the body through the gastrointestinal tract *(such as by using aluminum cooking utensils and drinking beverages in aluminum cans),* via injected aluminum-containing vaccines or kidney dialysis products, and intra-dermally from use of antiperspirants. If an individual cannot efficiently excrete the aluminum through body fluids *(urine, feces, perspiration),* it is deposited in various tissues, bone, brain, liver, heart, spleen, and muscle.

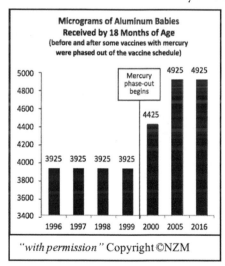

Micrograms of Aluminum Babies Received by 18 Months of Age
(before and after some vaccines with mercury were phased out of the vaccine schedule)

"with permission" Copyright©NZM

Aluminum is a known neurotoxin and scientific evidence shows that it can play a significant role in neurological diseases, including dementia, autism, and Parkinson's disease. While mercury preservative has been mostly removed from vaccines because of its known neurotoxicity, the levels of adjuvant aluminum have virtually no upper limit in the vaccine program, and the number of aluminum-containing vaccines American children receive has quadrupled over the past 30 years. In the 1970s, American children got only four aluminum-containing vaccines within the first 18 months of life. Now, they typically receive 17. In the US, babies end up getting up to 4,925 micrograms *(mcg)* of aluminum within the first 18 months of life, and an additional 170 to 625 mcg by the age of six. In all, American children end up getting about 6,150 mcg of aluminum if they get all of the recommended vaccines on the childhood vaccine schedule.

The administration of aluminum into vaccines is most commonly justified by the fact that a person usually accumulates more aluminum in their body each day simply by eating, but what people fail to take into account is that your body has a different method of flushing it out of your system. The body is very good at doing this but when you inject aluminum as a vaccine adjuvant, it does not come into the same mechanism of excretion as it would, say, from the aluminum you accumulate in your body as a result of wearing deodorant.

Injected aluminum does not enter the body or leave the body in the same way as environmental aluminum and that's the whole point of adjuvants - they are meant to stick around and allow that antigen to be presented over and over again. It can't be excreted because it must provide that prolonged exposure of the antigen to your immune system. Intramuscular injection of alum-containing vaccine was associated with the appearance of aluminum deposits in distant organs, such as spleen and brain in microglia and other neuronal cells where they were still detected one year after injection.

With its wide organ distribution, aluminum has been linked to several neuro-degenerative disorders and diseases, including Alzheimer's, Parkinson's, multiple sclerosis, amyotrophic lateral sclerosis *(ALS)*, autism, and epilepsy, and systemic lupus erythematous, chronic fatigue syndrome, Gulf War syndrome, macrophagic myofasciitis, arthritis, and autoimmune/ inflammatory syndrome induced by adjuvants and cognitive manifestations.

Dr. Christopher Exley is a professor in Bioinorganic Chemistry and an honorary professor at the UHI Millennium Institute. He is arguably the world's leading expert on aluminum toxicity. According to Dr. Exley, many of the adverse effects that you see in people who have suffered following vaccination are very similar to the known effects of aluminum intoxication and that aluminum adjuvants in vaccines have not undergone adequate toxicity testing. *"There are no clinically-approved aluminum adjuvants only clinically approved vaccines which use aluminum adjuvants."* [270 - 272]

He also published a definitive position on the relationship between aluminum and autism stating, *"We have made the first measurements of aluminum in brain tissue in ASD, and we have shown that the brain aluminum content is extraordinarily high. We have identified aluminum in brain tissue as both extracellular and intracellular with the latter involving both neurons and non-neuronal cells. The presence of aluminum in inflammatory cells in the meninges, vasculature, grey and white matter is a standout observation and could implicate aluminum in the etiology of ASD"* [273, 274]

In 2017, researchers, including Exley, published an article in the Journal Toxicology that investigated the toxicity of a commonly used aluminum adjuvant in vaccines. Study authors said, *"Concerns about its safety emerged following recognition of its unexpectedly long-lasting bio-persistence within immune cells in some individuals, and reports of chronic fatigue syndrome, cognitive dysfunction, myalgia, dysautonomia, and autoimmune-inflammatory features temporarily linked to multiple Al-containing vaccine administrations."*

On one hand, public health agencies acknowledge that further scientific investigation is needed to study the possible link between antiperspirants *(with aluminum)* and breast cancer. On the other hand, they actively promote and endorse vaccines containing aluminum as safe despite the fact that aluminum is neurotoxic and aluminum adjuvants have not been thoroughly tested for safety. Standard toxicity tests technically only assess acute, short-term toxicity of a substance. Although chronic studies examine adverse effects over a slightly longer period of time than sub-chronic and acute studies, a maximum observation period of twelve months is not adequate to be considered a long- term study given that children in the United States are repeatedly exposed to ingredients in vaccines during the first six years of life, starting on the day of birth *(The CDC recommends that infants and children receive 50 doses of 14 vaccines by the age of six).*

In addition to the limitations of toxicity testing for individual vaccine ingredients, there is also a lack of basic scientific research on the synergistic negative effects on the human body when vaccine ingredients interact with each other. In toxicology, synergism refers to the effect caused when exposure to two or more chemicals at a time leads to detrimental health effects that are greater than the sum of the effects of the individual chemicals. When chemicals are synergistic, the potential hazards of the chemicals should be re-evaluated, taking their synergistic properties into consideration.

Before the pharmaceutical industry and regulating agencies can even begin to claim that vaccines are safe, the synergistic relationship between all ingredients used in vaccines must be studied thoroughly.

Polio - A Contaminated Vaccine For An Epidemic That Didn't Exist

Vaccines are also noted to be contaminated with other known harmful ingredients. The most famous case of the contamination of vaccines was when rhesus monkey kidney cell tissue was used in the production of polio vaccines by Salk and Sabin in the 1950s. These monkey cells were infected with a monkey virus *(SV40)* that contaminated both the inactivated and live virus polio vaccines and both Salk and Sabin knew it. Since they never stopped to test the safety of a virus in the vaccine, they did not know that it actually was a very deadly virus. It was discovered by Dr. Bernice Eddy,

NIH virologist and epidemiologist, that the SV40 virus caused aggressive cancer in lab animals. Today, SV40 DNA has been identified in human brain, bone, lung cancers, breast, lymphomas, and others. An analysis of cancer risk published in Anticancer Research in 1999, indicated increased rates of ependymomas *(37%)*, osteogenic sarcomas *(26%)*, other bone tumors *(34%)* and mesothelioma *(90%)* among the over 98 million exposed to the virus through the polio vaccine. In 2002, the journal Lancet published compelling evidence that contaminated polio vaccine was responsible for up to half of the 55,000 non-Hodgkin's lymphoma cases that were occurring each year. This is serious folks. If there is a concern in your life about cancer, it is best to include testing for SV40 through DNA analysis. [275, 276]

The SV40 virus has also been shown to pass down to future generations. Dr. Deborah Warner mentioned previously has found evidence of SV40 even today in 40% of DNA samples she has tested. This finding parallels other studies. In 1996, Tognon and his collaborators reported that they had also found the virus in 45% of the sperm samples. [277]

While the last doses of that monkey cell culture were given out in the United States in 1963 *(even AFTER the virus was found to be cancer-causing),* the same cultures were used throughout the world. Italy was said to be the last country to stop using the kidney cell culture in 1999. [278, 279]

So there is a very real probability that billions of people are infected with the SV40 virus and those infected can pass it to others through sexual intercourse and from mothers to babies in the womb. And, all it takes is a significant breakdown in the immune system to activate the virus, and it will most likely be fatal for the infected person. Dr. Carbone M.D., Ph.D. and expert on mesothelioma *(a type of lung cancer),* has said that because of its unique viral structure, SV40 is *"the perfect little war machine."* Since 1994, Carbone has written more than twenty studies and reviews investigating SV40's link to human cancer. *"There is no doubt that SV40 is a human carcinogen,"* he says. *"SV40 is definitely something you don't want in your body."* There is also evidence in the book Dr. Mary's Monkey, that, after it was found to cause aggressive cancer, SV40 was being tested as a bioweapon to kill Fidel Castro, president of Cuba at the time. The relationships and storylines are intriguing and well documented. [280]

Was it all worth it? I mean, isn't polio a devastating disease, and don't we need to be vaccinated - granted without the monkey virus thing? Actually, an infection with the poliovirus itself does not mean that someone will get paralytic polio or die. Like many other viral infections, the symptoms are mild in most cases as long as the immune system is functioning properly, and the body is receiving adequate nutrition. Also, in case you didn't know, there are more bacteria in our body than human cells. And, to make things even more head scratching, we have an estimated 10 times more viruses in our body than bacteria, an estimated 380 trillion. It is all a balancing act that keeps us healthy. There are viruses that attack bad bacteria on our behalf. There are viruses that take up residence in us, held in check by our own immune systems, and some viruses that enter and try to take over our cells and wreak havoc if we are not able to mount a quick response. Of course, there are always those unusual cases where we can't explain why someone gets stricken with a life- changing infection when they are otherwise healthy. We are in the infancy of understanding how the immune system works. [281]

An infection with the poliovirus is generally mild, if even noticed. Ninety-five percent of those exposed to the poliovirus won't experience any symptoms. Nearly five percent will experience mild symptoms. Only one in 1000 children will experience muscle paralysis, but even that is generally temporary with a rare exception that paralysis is permanent. Adults will experience a higher incidence of paralysis with an infection. Generally other contributing factors allow the wild virus to cause permanent paralysis and death. Polio is transferred by contact with contaminated feces - while changing an infected baby's diapers for example, and through airborne saliva droplets, in food, or in water. It travels to the intestines and bloodstream where the body's immune system is quite efficient at stopping the progression of the infection. When this occurs, the individual should have permanent immunity against the disease.

Several studies also show that paralytic polio symptoms can occur as a result of other vaccine *(such as DTP single or combo)* and antibiotic injections during a period of active local polio infection or after vaccination with live oral attenuated polio vaccine. This is called provocation poliomyelitis. In 1995, the New England Journal of Medicine published a study showing that children who received a single injection within one month after receiving a polio vaccine were eight times more likely to contract polio than children who received no injections. The risk jumped 27-fold when children received up to nine injections within one month after receiving the polio vaccine. And with 10 or more injections, the likelihood of developing polio was 182 times greater than expected. A similar study of provocation poliomyelitis was published in the 1940s. [282 - 284]

Paralytic polio has also been misdiagnosed and confused with other neuro-muscular diseases such as Guillain Barre' Syndrome *(GBS)* that have similar symptoms. Historical research into the medical records of President Franklin Roosevelt for example, shows a high probability that he had GBS instead of poliomyelitis as was reported in the media. His diagnosis in 1921 was a major contributing factor for the worldwide efforts to eradicate polio. There was not enough medical knowledge at the time to distinguish paralytic poliomyelitis from GBS, which was not on the radar screen since it was newly discovered in 1916. The symptoms are similar, but there are distinguishing features that separate the two. In 1912 and 1915, Roosevelt had a bacterial food poison infection, which can be a major causative agent of GBS. He was reportedly also physically compromised for a couple of days before the initial symptoms, which very well could have made him more susceptible. [285]

Major polio epidemics were almost unknown before the 20th century. While self-limiting, infections ending in paralysis and deaths started to cluster in developed countries in the late 1800s, around the time of the Industrial Revolution, when sanitation was poor, sewage disposal systems were not effectively in place, and clean water sources were not available in the major cities. While there is something to be said for natural immunity by immersion *(into some dirt)*, deplorable living conditions and poor nutrition can overwhelm the body's ability to respond to infections. One United States epidemic in 1916 was short-lived. There is a theory based on research that suggests the cases clustered around a poliovirus testing facility in New York City which did not have adequate safety protocols and the infection spread from there. Over a thirty-year span between 1923-1953 before the Salk vaccine was introduced, the death rate from polio had already declined by 47% in the United States and 55% in England, several years before the introduction of the polio vaccine. But there was a major hiccup with the introduction of the Salk vaccine that caused polio in tens of thousands. In what became known as the Cutter incident, some lots of the polio vaccine produced by Cutter Laboratories - despite passing required safety tests - contained live poliovirus in what was supposed to be an inactivated-virus vaccine.

The Cutter incident was one of the worst pharmaceutical disasters in US history, and exposed several thousand children to live poliovirus on vaccination. All five pharmaceutical companies producing the vaccine had trouble completely inactivating the poliovirus. The mistake by Cutter at least produced 200,000 doses of polio vaccine that contained live poliovirus. Of children who received the vaccine, 40,000 developed abortive poliomyelitis *(a form of the disease that does not involve the central nervous system),* 200 developed varying forms paralytic poliomyelitis - and of these, ten children died from polio. The vaccination program was temporarily put on hold, and then resumed after safety concerns were addressed. [286, 287]

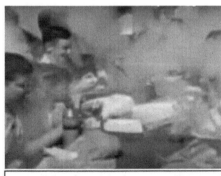

Classroom of children being sprayed with DDT circa 1947.

There are other contributing factors that may help explain the increase in polio-like symptoms in the 1940s and early 1950s. There is compelling evidence that symptoms of neurotoxicity from chemical poisons introduced at the same time when the polio epidemic peaked in the late 1940s and early

1950s. A significant rise in poliomyelitis began in the 1940s, at the same time DDT was recognized as a potent insecticide and was being produced during WW2. It was released for public use in 1945 and was sprayed over cities and in crowded swimming pools and school lunchrooms in an effort to eradicate polio and other diseases thought to be carried by insects. The symptoms mimic many of the polio symptoms including paralysis - that is how they work on insects. DDT *(pesticide),* BHC, lead, and arsenic are representative of the major pesticides in use during the last major polio epidemics. They persist in the environment as neurotoxins that cause polio-like symptoms, polio-like physiology, and were dumped onto and into human food and water supplies at dosage levels far above that approved by the FDA - drinking milk from cows eating grain laced with DDT for example. They directly correlate with the incidence of various neurological disorders, including polio and could have been co-factors in the epidemic. The chemicals were utilized, according to Dr. Morton Biskind, in the *"most intensive campaign of mass acidic poisoning in known human history."* He and Dr. Ralph Scobey both presented their concerns to the United States House of Representatives. When DDT and other similar pesticides were introduced to the public, they were produced in mass amounts, and the incidence of paralytic polio-like symptoms went up in concert with production and distribution. When the neurotoxicity became obvious *(shouldn't that have been determined BEFORE being released of public use?),* it was removed from such easy access and the incidence of paralytic polio-like symptoms decreased. This all occurred before the polio vaccine was developed and distributed. This is not to take away from the effectiveness of the polio eradication campaign, only to supplement cause and effect observations. [288, 289]

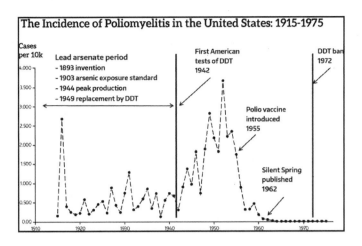

In addition, during the same period in the mid-1950s, criteria for determining a poliomyelitis infection was changed. Some symptoms that would ordinarily identify classified as characteristic of polio were removed and reclassified into other categories. The impact of doing that was an artificial *"reduction"* in the number of polio cases. Polio was redefined. The credit however was inappropriately given to the *"effectiveness"* of the polio vaccine rather than a major change in diagnostic criteria.

Yes, the polio vaccine appears to have been very helpful in reducing the *"wild"* poliovirus worldwide. But remember, 99.5% of wild virus polio infections go unnoticed or there are mild symptoms. Immune deficiency and malnutrition are the two most important factors in contracting polio. The Inactivated Poliovirus Vaccine *(IPV)* is the only one used here in the United States because of the adverse side effects such as contracting polio itself. The Live Poliovirus *(LPV)* is used in third world countries because it is easier to administer and less costly but certainly more dangerous and can be spread by various mechanisms but mostly fecal shedding or secondarily by saliva contact. There have been 21 countries reporting outbreaks of polio flaccid paralysis from circulating Vaccine Derived Poliovirus *(VDPV)* injections using the LPV vaccine. As a result, more deadly mutations are developing. Have we opened Pandora's Box? [290 - 292]

The truth is, while vaccines are promoted with a cure-all image, in actuality they have not been proven *"safe"* for anyone, they clearly do not work for everyone long-term, and implications of introducing active and inactive vaccine components into the body have never been studied. Even when they do work, you oftentimes end up with more virulent and hardy viruses, which is a very dangerous game to play. Such information is never discussed when the anticipated success of a vaccine program is announced, yet it is a health outcome of the vaccine that should be taken into account, not hidden. [293-296]

Challengers, Whistle-Blowers, And Researchers

There are many health professionals who challenge the safety and effectiveness of vaccines. A list of over one hundred professionals with their comments will be listed in Appendix A and a few are included below.

Robert Mendelsohn, M.D., renowned pediatrician, prolific author, TV and radio personality, was an early outspoken critic of mass vaccinations during his career spanning thirty years until his death in 1988. He was an early critic of medical paternalism, and he denounced unnecessary and radical surgical procedures and dangerous medications, reminding his readers of public health failures such as the 1976 swine flu vaccine fiasco.

Mendelsohn wrote a syndicated newspaper column called The People's Doctor, and also produced a newsletter with the same name. He published five books, including *Confessions of a Medical Heretic, Mal(e) Practice: How Doctors Manipulate Women, and How to Raise a Healthy Child, In Spite of Your Doctor.* And, he appeared on over 500 television and radio talk shows. He has commented, *"The greatest threat of childhood diseases lies in the dangerous and ineffectual efforts made to prevent them through mass immunization... There is no convincing scientific evidence that mass inoculations can be credited with eliminating any childhood disease and . . . there are significant risks associated with every immunization and numerous contraindications that may make it dangerous for the shots to be given to your child..."*

Furthermore, *"There is growing suspicion that immunization against relatively harmless childhood diseases may be responsible for the dramatic increase in autoimmune diseases since mass inoculations were introduced. These are fearful diseases such as cancer, leukemia, rheumatoid arthritis, multiple sclerosis, Lou Gehrig's disease, lupus erythematous, and the Guillain-Barre syndrome."* And current research adds autism, ADHD, and Alzheimer's disease to that list.

Toni Barks, M.D., a nationally recognized natural health advocate comments, *"The kids that come to me from other practices and are fully vaccinated, often are the kid,... well, they are the kids in my practice with asthma, panic disorders, OCD, pandas, autism, and Asperger's. The kids who have never vaccinated in my practice, I don't see those issues. I don't have one child who is not vaccinated who also has asthma or food allergies or Asperger's or autism or Crohn's or ulcerative colitis."* Dr. Paul Thomas, M.D., and a pediatrician with over 13,000 children in his practice in Portland, Oregon, has also noticed that the children who are the most vaccinated in his practice are also the least healthy. *"As unpopular as this observation might be, my unvaccinated children are by far the healthiest."*

Suzanne Humphries, M.D. spent 14 years as a nephrologist. She found that too many times within 24 hours of a vaccination, kidney function went down, and people showed up at the emergency room. She researched vaccines, especially related to the effects on the kidney, and found a disturbing correlation between vaccines and kidney damage. She left that job to become a vaccine and natural health researcher. In her research, Dr. Humphries found that 56% of Focal Segmental Glomerulosclerosis *(FSGS)* kidney disease patients were positive for SV40, the cancer-causing monkey virus that contaminated the first-generation polio vaccines that still haunt much of the world's population. She also states that physicians are not taught about the details of vaccines in medical school. I can testify to that as well. [297]

Deborah Warner, Ph.D., a researcher who heads up one of the most sophisticated DNA testing facilities in the world, Clinic Solutions-Houston, says that when she tests the DNA of Type 1 diabetics, she finds pertussis bacteria antigens 100% of the time. She writes that these come from the pertussis component of the combination vaccine including diphtheria and tetanus, and there is a causal relationship between the pertussis antigens and Type 1 diabetes. She agrees with an earlier concern of a causal relationship between Type 1 Diabetes and the pertussis vaccine, shared by Dr. Mendelsohn who suggested further research into the connection.

Other studies provide evidence of scientific malfeasance with regard to some well-publicized studies purporting to show no link between vaccines and severe safety hazards. Brian Hooker, et al, noted in his 2014 publication, *Methodological Issues and Evidence of Malfeasance in Research Purporting to Show Thimerosal in Vaccines Is Safe,* noted "[...] *the studies upon which the CDC relies and over which it exerted some level of control report that there is no increased risk of autism from exposure to organic Hg in vaccines, and some of these studies even reported that exposure to thimerosal appeared to decrease the risk of autism.*"

These studies are in sharp contrast to research conducted by independent researchers over the past 75+ years who have consistently found thimerosal to be harmful and associated with neurodevelopmental disorders. Several studies, for example, including three of the six studies covered in this review, have found thimerosal to be a risk factor for tics. In addition, thimerosal has been found to be a risk factor in speech delay, language delay, attention deficit disorder, and autism bringing into question the validity of the methodology used in the studies. [298, 299]

I wholeheartedly agree with any sentiments that support authenticity and verifiable and duplicatable research efforts. These are critical if our goal is to find truth. I do draw the line when vaccines are mandated, safety research is absent, manipulated, or hidden from the public eye, and the choice of what is injected into one's body is removed by a totalitarian system that, by design, protects those creating the vaccines from accountability and liability which introduces unacceptable risks. That is the current status of our *"immunization"* program - a misnomer, which has set a very dangerous precedent and has already been shown by a preponderance of the evidence cited above to have killed, maimed, or otherwise permanently injured the lives and futures of too many people.

It is also well understood that having infections in early life protects against various cancers in later life. Later born children have less cancer, for instance, than firstborn children because they are exposed to more infections in early life from their siblings and the immune system is primed for maximum protection. Playing in the grass and even some dirt instead of watching TV all morning, while it may be a messy cleanup, can actually help develop a child's immune system. Children that go to daycare in early life are more protected against cancers for the same reason. Vaccinations deny a baby the opportunity to become naturally infected, and with this reduction in exposure to disease, there is a trade-off - increased rates of cancer.

People may legitimately argue over whether the reduction in disease in exchange for an increase in cancer is a good thing or a bad thing, but the trade-off is real and must be considered when weighing the honest risk-to-benefit ratio of vaccinations. Parents are entitled to know this information in order to retain true informed consent, remain free to accept or reject vaccinations, and have their human rights preserved. But that is not happening. Many parents feel that their pediatricians make them feel like idiots if they ask questions and threaten to force them out of their practices and call CPS if they don't comply.

The pharmaceutical industry is just as much to blame for deception and harming children. In August 2010, Stephen A. Krahling and Joan A. Wlochowski, former Merck virologists blew the whistle by filing a qui tam action lawsuit. The scientists alleged that the efficacy tests for the measles, mumps, and rubella vaccine *(MMR)* were faked. They claimed that by faking effectiveness tests - i.e., committing fraud - Merck misled the government about the effectiveness of the mumps component of its MMR II vaccine. The vaccine contained the same strain of mumps vaccine, which had been shown to cause meningitis and was removed from the Canadian market. In 1978, Merck introduced the MMR II, using a different strain of the rubella vaccine, but the same strain of mumps vaccine. This is a major federal case alleging fraud in vaccine testing; it encapsulates how medical research can be manipulated to achieve desired results, and why it may be wise to question the integrity and the validity of the vaccine industry's *"science-based medicine."*

The suit charges that Merck knew its measles, mumps, rubella *(MMR)* vaccine was less effective than the purported 95% level, and it alleges that senior management was aware and also oversaw testing that concealed the actual effectiveness. According to the lawsuit, Merck began a sham testing program in the late 1990s to hide the declining efficacy of the vaccine. The objective of the fraudulent trials was to *"report efficacy of 95% or higher regardless of the vaccine's true efficacy."* According to Krahling and Wlochowski's complaint, they were threatened with jail were they to alert the FDA to the fraud being committed. [300]

Robert Kennedy Jr., son of Senator Bobby Kennedy who was murdered in 1968, is an environmental attorney and activist. He recently testified before the Vermont House Healthcare Committee on May 5, 2015, discussing Big Pharma's influence in the CDC. The following is a summary of excerpts that was taken from his recorded testimony:

"The CDC is a troubled agency. There have been four separate scathing federal investigations of the vaccine division. All of these (investigations) together paint a picture of an agency that has become a cesspool of corruption. There are two divisions (related to vaccines): there is the Advisory Division and most of the people who sit on those committees are vaccine industry insiders - many of them, if not most of them, have direct financial stakes in the outcome of their decisions to add a vaccine to the schedules. In 1999, Paul Offit (M.D., pediatrician) sat on the committee that added the Rotavirus vaccine to the CDC schedule. Paul owned the patent for the Rotavirus vaccine. He sold that vaccine for 182 million dollars six years later and reportedly made 40 million dollars personally for that transaction. In 2008 the Inspector General discussed that example and said that up to 97% of the people who sit on those committees have the same kinds of conflicts that Offit does. It is very hard to believe by the people of the country that these types of decisions are being made with the health of their children in mind.

The second division is the Immunization Safety Office. Approximately 30 scientist whose job it is to ensure vaccines are safe and efficacious. They put out population (epidemiological) studies, not scientific studies. Epidemiologic studies are notoriously easy to manipulate. They never ever show safety, only harm. Those are what the CDC relies on to determine if a vaccine is safe."

In 2018, Kennedy also won a lawsuit against the United States Department of Health and Human Services for vaccine safety violations. The lawsuit brought forth evidence that vaccine safety has been neglected for over 30 years. How much this will change the vaccine landscape remains to be seen.

Dr. Viera Scheibner is arguably one of the world's most respected scientists and scholars of vaccine medical data. She is the author of Vaccination: 100 Years of Orthodox Research and Behavioral Problems in Children: The Link to Vaccination, in addition to publishing almost 100 peer-reviewed papers. During a live radio broadcast on September 18, 2009, she shared an overview of vaccine history and presented a more realistic definition of vaccination theory in light of reviewing thousands of studies, articles, and books written since Edward Jenner tested the very first vaccine in 1796. Her investigations uncover how the vaccine industrial complex, and national and international agencies who oversee vaccination policies, continue to entertain a pseudo- science that is fraught with inconsistencies, poorly designed studies, erroneous interpretations, and conclusions that are patently false.

Who Is Guarding The Hen House?

Is there a governmental conspiracy to withhold information about the harmful effects of vaccines? You betcha there is! Check out these official Government document excerpts obtained through the Freedom of Information Act.

In a letter from Leslie ball of the FDA, dated Tuesday, July 6, 1999, at 3:53 PM, to Norman Baylor, Associate Director of Regulatory Policy, CBER, in a high priority and *"confidential"* email Leslie makes comments and asks questions about the safety of thimerosal and the differences between the

FDA and CDC on exposure guidelines for Hg in thimerosal: *"[...] has the application of these calculations and exposure guidelines received the signoff by toxicologist? In prior discussions, the toxicologist seemed reluctant to state any Hg level was 'safe.' This approach leaves open to criticism that the PHS is arbitrarily designating a certain level as acceptable when there continues to be so much uncertainty about the science in this area."*

"[...] We believe that the FDA's institutional negligence can be traced back to at least 1992, perhaps further... it is highly likely that the FDA 'let slide' vaccines and biologics with Thimerosal because the manufacturers already had too much money invested in the products and it would cost money to remove the thimerosal, reformulate the product and perhaps to have to go through the process of efficacy studies..." [301]

There are many such emails secured through the Freedom of Information Act that clearly show that the FDA, CDC, and other government agencies knew of the dangers of thimerosal.

In an official document sent to Lauren Fuller, Chief Investigative Counsel for the United States Senate Health Education Labor and Pensions, Elizabeth Birt and James Moody outlined a thimerosal timeline which included the following excerpts: *"The statements by Dr. Egan (testifying under oath that thimerosal was safe) either reflect the gross incompetence of Dr. Egan or are patently false. By 1990, there was a mountain of evidence that thimerosal was unsafe and ineffective. The FDA also new that they had significant gaps in their knowledge relating to the reproductive toxicity, developmental toxicity, transformation of thimerosal following intramuscular or subcutaneous administration, and sensitization studies..."*

Individuals at FDA knew of the potential problems with thimerosal in vaccines and how to resolve it by going to single unit vaccines but chose not to do it. Do you get what happened here? The FDA knew that thimerosal was harmful and they decided to do nothing about it, except to keep the threat hidden! At the end of the letter, attorneys Birt and Moody suggested that the following charges could be brought against specific federal agencies and individuals at these agencies for criminal negligence for the following: failure to regulate the safety and effectiveness of biological products, failure to regulate and promote vaccines as provided for under the national vaccine injury compensation program, not instituting a class one recall of all vaccines administer to infants containing thimerosal in July 1999, and again in June 2000, when the results of the Vaccine Safety Data (VSD) study were discussed at the Simpsonwood meeting (discussed below), criminal conspiracy to defraud the government by deception and obstruction, and criminal obstruction of justice. [302]

Most recently, on January 6, 2019, Sharyl Attkisson an Emmy award-winning investigative journalist, host of Sinclair's Sunday morning news program, *Full Measure,* and author of the New York Times bestsellers, The Smear, and Stonewalled, threw a bombshell into the vaccine controversy. She reported that Dr. Andrew Zimmerman, a world-renowned pediatric neurologist and previous medical expert witness for the Department of Justice *(DOJ),* was used by the Feds to debunk the vaccine autism link. Through his ongoing research and clinical observations, Dr. Zimmerman eventually found that vaccines could cause autism after all. When he was acting in the capacity of an expert witness in 2007, he informed the DOJ lawyers of the connection between some vaccines and autism, and he was promptly fired. Despite this information, the DOJ continued to misrepresent Dr. Zimmerman's updated expert opinion, which would negatively impact the DOJ's defense of the vaccine industry. After collaborating with Robert Kennedy, an attorney and vaccine safety activist, Dr. Zimmerman signed an affidavit in September 2018, testifying that he and the DOJ knew in 2007 that vaccines in some individuals can cause autism.

Kennedy in an interview with Attkisson said, *"[…] that vaccines do not cause autism is one of the most consequential frauds arguably in human history."* Kennedy was instrumental in convincing Dr. Zimmerman to document the government's covering up his true opinion on vaccines and autism. Roth Hazelhurst, whose son 'Yates' has autism is a criminal prosecutor was also scheduled to be a witness at a congressional hearing on vaccine matters.

Two weeks before the hearing he briefed a congressional staff and said *"[...]*
if I did to a criminal in a court of law what the United States Department of
Justice did to vaccine injured children, I would be disbarred, and I would face
criminal charges." The hearing was abruptly canceled.

Zimmerman says that several of his own patients have autism, including
Yates. In his affidavit, Zimmerman testifies, *"I have reviewed extensive genetic,*
metabolic, and other medical records of William 'Yates' Hazlehurst. In my opin-
ion, and to a reasonable degree of certainty, Yates Hazlehurst suffered regres-
sive encephalopathy with features of autism spectrum disorder as a result of
vaccine injury in the same manner as described in the DOJ concession in Poling
(another injured child) versus HHS...In my opinion, it was highly misleading
for the Department of Justice to continue to use my original written expert
opinion (exonerating vaccines as the cause of autism) ... as evidence against
the remaining petitioners in the Omnibus Autism Proceedings (OAP)..."[303-305]

2000 Simpsonwood Meeting - The Arrogance Of Fools

In June of 2000, 51 selected vaccine authorities from CDC, FDA, universities,
private practice pediatricians, pharmaceutical industry representatives and
others met to discuss, in a closed meeting, the possibility of neurodevelopment disorders resulting from the thimerosal vaccine component. The
legality of such a meeting has been called into question, but as it turned out,
it was fortunately recorded and revealed some very important and damaging
information about the toxicity of thimerosal and aluminum in vaccines. The
transcript included over 250 pages. I have highlighted some of the more
important conversation them and included them here in a separate section.
If you really want confirmation of the cover-ups, and the frank irrational
behavior of the people who are making the decisions to inject your children with toxic chemicals, this will give you plenty of insight. Some of the
comments made at the conference are narrated by Dr. Russel Blaylock.

For starters, just to get you mad enough to read the rest, here are some tidbits from the conference. Dr. Johnson, a member of the Advisory Committee on Immunization Practices *(ACIP),* a committee within the United States Centers for Disease Control *(CDC),* said this on pages 199-200 of a transcript about his own grandson receiving a vaccine shot upon his birth: *"This association (thimerosal and autism) leads me to favor a recommendation that infants up to two years old not be immunized with thimerosal-containing vaccines if suitable alternative preparations are available. My gut feeling? It worries me enough. Forgive this personal comment, but I got called out at eight o'clock for an emergency call and my daughter-in-law delivered a son by C-section. Our first male in the line of the next generation, and I do not want that grandson to get a thimerosal-containing vaccine until we know better what is going on."*

Dr. Weil, pg. 207: *"The number of dose-related relationships are linear and statistically significant. You can play with this all you want. They are linear. They are statistically significant … You can't accept that this is out of the ordinary. It isn't out of the ordinary."* He was talking about the causal relationship between thimerosal and autism.

> The vaccine-injured cannot be swept under the carpet and treated like nothing more than statistically acceptable collateral damage.

Wow! So, let me understand this. The association between thimerosal and neurodevelopmental disorders is clear and Dr. Johnson does not want his grandson getting the vaccine, but it is okay for all the other innocent children to get it! If he chose that for his own grandson, shouldn't he also give that opportunity immediately to other parents? The vaccine injured cannot be swept under the carpet and treated like nothing more than statistically acceptable collateral damage. Too many children are catastrophically damaged by vaccines and are never able to function in any meaningful way, and he just walks away from them and stays silent because the CDC and vaccine industry's image would be tarnished if this information got out there. Isn't that called cowardice with a capital C? Does anyone else see something wrong with this picture? You can't make this stuff up. It's as real as it gets! [306, 307]

Dr. Kenneth Stoller, a pediatrician himself, is also outspoken about the propaganda and dishonesty within the ranks of the CDC and their cohorts. He writes in an open letter to the American Academy of Pediatrics:

"As a pediatrician, who has been a fellow of the AAP for two decades, I find the AAP's approach to the autism epidemic to be deeply disturbing. Not only have they allowed the myth of better diagnosing (as the reason for all the notice given to affected children) to be perpetuated, but when they were put on notice at the CDC's Simpsonwood meeting in 2000, that the mercury in the preservative Thimerosal was causing speech delays and learning disabilities, they obfuscated and hide that information. They never made good on their 1999 pledge to have Thimerosal eliminated from vaccines and almost a decade later joined in the protest against a fictitious TV show (Eli Stone) because it was critical of mercury being in vaccine. Out of 132 million doses of the worthless flu vaccine for the 2007-08 flu season, eight million doses are thimerosal-free. That means 94% contain the full amount of thimerosal... In a first analysis of the VSD datasets, Verstraeten (et al) had described a 7.6 to 11.4 fold increase of autism risk in children at one month, with the highest mercury exposure levels compared to children with no exposure." [308]

In 2004, Dr. Russell Blaylock, retired neurosurgeon and now natural health advocate reviewed the transcripts of the Simpsonwood meeting and made some very incriminating observations and comments:

"I was asked to write a paper on some of the newer mechanisms of vaccine damage to the nervous system, but in the interim I came across an incredible document that should blow the lid off the cover-up being engineered by the pharmaceutical companies in conjunction with powerful governmental agencies... It is a bombshell...

Dr. Bernier made an incredible statement (page 12). He said, 'In the United States there was a growing recognition that cumulative exposure may exceed some of the guidelines...' Now, we need to stop and think about what has transpired here. We have an important group here; the ACIP that essential plays a role in vaccine policy that affects tens of millions of children every year. And, we have evidence from the thimerosal meeting in 1999 that the potential for serious injury to the infant's brain is so serious that a recommendation for removal becomes policy.

In addition, they are all fully aware that tiny babies are receiving mercury doses that exceed even EPA safety limits, yet all they can say is that we must 'try to remove thimerosal as soon as possible.' Do they not worry about the tens of millions of babies that will continue receiving thimerosal-containing vaccines until they can get around to stopping the use of thimerosal?

The most obvious solution was to use only single-dose vials, which requires no preservative. So, why don't they use them? Oh, they exclaim, it would add to the cost of the vaccine. Of course, we are only talking about a few dollars per vaccine at most, certainly worth the health of your child's brain and future."

On page 24, Dr. William Weil, a pediatrician representing the Committee on Environmental Health of the American Academy of Pediatrics, brings some sense to the discussion by reminding them that, *"there are just a host of neurodevelopmental data that would suggest that we've got a serious problem. The earlier we go, the more serious the problem."* Here he means that the further back you go during the child's brain development, the more likely the damage to the infant . . . He also reminds his colleagues that aluminum produced severe dementia and death in dialysis cases. He concludes by saying, *"To think there isn't some possible problem here is unreal. (Page 25)"* In addition, on page 198, Dr. Rapin notes that a study in California found a 300X increase in autism following the introduction of certain vaccines. Dr. Blaylock continues:

"Dr. Clements remarks on page 248 that he wants this information kept not only from the public but also from other scientists and pediatricians until they can be properly counseled. In the next statement he spills the beans as to why he is determined that no outsider get hold of this damaging information. He says:

'My mandate as I sit here in this group is to make sure at the end of the day that 100,000,000 are immunized with DTP, Hepatitis B and if possible Hib, this year, next year and for many years to come, and that will have to be with thimerosal-containing vaccines unless a miracle occurs and an alternative is found quickly and is tried and found to be safe.'

This is one of the most shocking statements I have ever heard. In essence, he is saying, I don't care if the vaccines are found to be harmful and destroying the development of children's brains, these vaccines will be given now and forever. His only concern by his own admission is to protect the vaccine program even if it is not safe.

Dr. Chen on page 256 expresses his concern about this information reaching the public. He remarks, 'We have been privileged so far that given the sensitivity of information, we have been able to manage to keep it out of, let's say, less responsible hands...' Dr. Bernier agrees and notes, 'This information has been held fairly tightly.' Later he calls it 'embargoed information' and 'very highly protected information.'"

There are over 165 studies that have focused on thimerosal alone, an organic-mercury *(Hg)* based compound that is in the environment as well as in preservative in the flu vaccine, and found to be harmful. Of these, 16 were conducted to specifically examine the effects of thimerosal on human infants or children with reported outcomes of death, acrodynia, poisoning, allergic reaction, malformations, auto-immune reaction, Well's syndrome, developmental delay, and neurodevelopmental disorders, including tics, speech delay, language delay, attention deficit disorder, and autism. In contrast, the United States Centers for Disease Control and Prevention states that thimerosal is safe and there is *"no relationship between thimerosal- containing vaccines and autism rates in children."* This is puzzling because, in a study conducted directly by CDC epidemiologists, a 7.6-fold increased risk of autism from exposure to Thimerosal during infancy was found. [309]

But one of the biggest cover-up events is one where Dr. William Thompson, a senior scientist for the CDC, became a whistleblower and exposed the corruption in the CDC that affected countless numbers of lives. In a CDC orchestrated study, a team of researchers examined the effects of the MMR vaccine on a population of children. When the results were examined, they found that a significant number of the African American children developed autism symptoms. The research committee met in 2002 to discuss these unexpected results and chose to leave them out, which skewed the results to make it look like the MMR vaccine did not cause autism symptoms, which the evidence clearly showed it did. They decided to destroy the documents connecting the MMR vaccine and autism, and published the results in favor of the safety of the MMR vaccine. This was the defining moment that changed everything about the safety of the MMR vaccine. Pediatricians used this study to denounce the anti-vaccine crowd and to bully parents into vaccinating their children. Compensation for injuries from The Vaccine Compensation Fund became much harder to litigate, and injured children and parents were essentially put out on the street to fend for themselves. About ten years later, Dr. Thompson, who happened to save his copy of the results instead of destroying them as instructed, contacted Brian Hooker whose child became autistic, reportedly as a result of the MMR vaccine. Below is Brian's condensed account of his recorded sessions with Dr. Thompson.

"Dr. William Thompson, senior scientist at the Centers for Disease Control and Prevention (CDC) contacted me during 2013 and 2014 and shared many issues regarding fraud and malfeasance in the CDC, specifically regarding the link between neurodevelopmental disorders and childhood vaccines. Dr. Thompson and I spoke on the phone more than 40 times over a 10-month period and he shared thousands of pages of CDC documents with me. Eventually, Dr. Thompson turned this information over to Congress via Rep. Bill Posey of Florida. Among the issues discussed in the phone conversations were lies told to the public by the CDC regarding the link between thimerosal-containing vaccines and neurodevelopmental disorders (including autism) as well as the links between the MMR vaccine and autism in African American males and the MMR vaccine and "isolated" autism. Isolated autism is the term coined by CDC researchers referring to all children who received an autism diagnosis

without additional diagnoses of mental retardation, cerebral palsy, visual impairment or hearing impairment."

And below is Dr. Thompson's statement:

"My name is William Thompson. I am a Senior Scientist with the Centers for Disease Control and Prevention, where I have worked since 1998.

I regret that my coauthors and I omitted statistically significant information in our 2004 article published in the journal Pediatrics. The omitted data suggested that African American males who received the MMR vaccine before age 36 months were at increased risk for autism. Decisions were made regarding which findings to report after the data was collected, and I believe that the final study protocol was not followed . . . My concern has been the decision to omit relevant findings in a particular study for a particular sub-group for a particular vaccine. There have always been recognized risks for vaccination, and I believe it is the responsibility of the CDC to properly convey the risks associated with receipt of those vaccines."

"Oh, what a tangled web we weave, when first we practice to deceive!" (Sir Walter Scott, 1808).

Most of us are aware of the corruption within the government and how power and money promote lies, deceptions, and corruption that has no moral or ethical boundaries. With vaccines, we see it again, but at the expense of our children, whose healthy and productive lives have been stolen from them forever. Those with the power to make a difference don't see or care much about children. They only care about saving face for themselves as evidenced by several vaccine-related cover-ups, including the Simpsonwood Meetings and others mentioned above. It is clear that prospective safety studies were not performed by the manufacturers or the CDC, and the FDA was not actively engaged in protecting the public from the known damaging effects of thimerosal. They knew thimerosal was dangerous but refused to act on it, even when pressure as applied by the American Academy of Pediatrics to do so, and quickly.

Gary Null, activist and talk show host summarizes the huge web under the US Public Health Service that just reeks of corruption:

"The US Public Health Service and its various agencies - the FDA, CDC, NIAID, NIH and CBER - oversee the distribution of information to congressional committees, medical associations, state and local health officials, and the media. They are also responsible for the scheduling of vaccines, both voluntary and mandatory, and frequently working in concert with pharmaceutical manufacturers, provide research opportunities to universities and other private research group. At the end of the day, conservatively, there are thousands of individuals who make policy decisions in our vaccine industrial complex. As a result, the mainstream media has taken the position that whatever the official word is about a vaccine, it goes virtually unchallenged. Those brave enough to criticize vaccines (whether they are physicians, scientists, journalists or citizens) are considered irresponsible, are discredited, and immediately viewed with suspicion."

When the fox is guarding the henhouse, he will always be looking out for his best interests.

Real People With Real Vaccine Injuries

I will end this chapter with a few real-life stories - isn't this what it's all about? Real people, with real-life experiences where they trusted a corrupt bureaucratic governmental system who partnered with equally corrupt pharmaceutical vaccine manufacturers to produce mostly untested poisons for-profit and essentially forced compliance to inject these poisons into innocent, unsuspecting, and otherwise healthy children - without safety testing, without efficacy studies, and with full knowledge that what they were doing would harm children, then try to cover it up. God help us! What's next??

Chloe's Story

Chloe's story is one of devastation caused by a human papillomavirus *(HPV)* vaccination - at least she can speak, unlike so many others with vaccine damage who live in a mental jail of pure hell where many can't even fully appreciate what it is like to go out on a beautiful spring day and hear the birds sing.

Hello everyone!

For those who do not know me, I'm an 18-year-old girl who has a bundle of debilitating chronic conditions after being injured by the HPV vaccine. The onset of symptoms noticeably came after my second of three injections.

Before I got sick I did many things girls age 12 should do. I hiked, mountain biked, went to the park, rollerbladed to the shops, had social gatherings, went to the cinema, birthday parties, I had friends.

I was a dancer. And I think that speaks for itself. I had an artistic, busy, and athletic lifestyle. I danced six days a week; at the studio, at school and I also stretched and worked on technique religiously at home. I loved to go to after-school sport and dance clubs every night. I loved the fact that I had a regime and something to look forward to every day. I was on the right road to getting A's at GCSE. I lived life to the max, life has always been important to me, more so now I'm isolated from the real world. I danced to feel free, in control and to have the time of my life. I used my body to create a piece of art. I made memories, which I now use as a coping mechanism and a tool to guide me and help me deal with a life full of disappointment, hardship, illness, and pain.

I wanted to have a dance career; my heart bleeds with the torture knowing I may never walk again, let alone dance again.

I love art and fashion so I went into fashion design but my conditions took a downward spiral, I didn't even get a quarter way through the course.

Every day is a battle against the never-ending symptoms-against pain, random and exhausting fits, mast cell reactions, and the agony when meds, feed, and water is pushed down my tube. Then there's the war with the invisible aspects people don't see: the nausea, migraines, vision problems, light and noise sensitivity, the multiple injection wounds from injecting daily to reduce blood clots. You don't see the paralyzed stomach or delayed motility of my GI tract, the raw inflammation and ulceration in my colon, the overactive nerve endings, blocked signals in my brain and spinal cord, and of course the intense chronic pain that you don't always see in public because of the 'stay brave and cry later face'. It's all hidden until you tell the world your story.

The adverse reaction to the vaccine and the conditions I have developed over the years has had a huge impact on my life. Now my life is complicated, and that's not because I'm in a complex relationship like others my age. But because my future is uncertain. Tomorrow is another day but I never know what tomorrow or even the next hour will bring; I can't predict the future and I can't plan ahead. I don't know if I'll be able to have kids as I know many 18-year-olds who are infertile thanks to Cervarix or Gardasil.

I may have a broken body which persistently disobeys me, however I am lucky enough to be a mentally strong individual who's managed to build up her own coping mechanisms and psychological techniques despite negligence and terrible past experiences. Despite hardship I find happiness. Despite pain I find inner peace. Mindfulness may help others in my situation, and yes it will keep the demons of depression and anxious thoughts away. However, no amount of mindfulness and positivity will change the immense pain I endure and magic the mobility and loss of sensation back into my once healthy, sporty, dancing body of mine.

I guarantee my future won't be how I planned it, but it will be full of determination and dedication to continue raising much-needed awareness.

Chloe is a woman of honor and strength, unlike the faceless cowards that were responsible for her harm. In a short quote, she gives a beautiful perspective about her future.

"A successful person is a person that can build a firm foundation with the bricks that life has thrown at them" ~ Chloe

Chloe's Chronicles of Chronic Illness-My HPV Vaccine Injury Journey

Jodie's Story

A couple of months ago I watched my 10-year-old son, Lincoln, test for his black belt in martial arts. Though not unheard of, it's pretty significant considering that only eight years ago he was diagnosed with autism. He no longer made eye contact with me. He had lost his words and was unable to communicate. I was told he would never talk again. I was even told by a pediatric neurologist that I would have to institutionalize him. I was told there was no hope. But now, he has a black belt.

To me, it was symbolic of not just an accomplishment in martial arts. It was another reminder to me that he's always been a fighter; a reminder that going through the trenches with him and doing something really, really hard was all worth it.

The day that the neurologist told me there was no hope was when I decided I was not going to take this lying down. I was not going to accept that prognosis for my son, no matter what resistance I faced. When they told me there was nothing that I could do for him, that fierce mama bear instinct said, "WATCH ME." I knew I had to prepare for battle.

And I did. Today, my son no longer tests on the autism spectrum.

Watching him battle through his black belt testing reminded me of the struggle we have faced for the last eight years. It was a long, difficult journey and there were many times when it would have been easy to throw in the towel. But as his instructor said to him during testing, "Nothing comes easy. Pain is temporary."

The pain part was tough. I demanded more hours of therapy for my son so that he could get as much treatment as quickly as possible. I researched and learned all about natural medicine, food, and family history. I was thrown out of three pediatric practices for refusing to give my children vaccines. I challenged conventional medicine and found different doctors who focused on recovering my son instead of just treating his symptoms. I spent what little money we had on extra treatments and opened my mind to new ways to bring him back from that dark place.

I even changed my family's lifestyle - the way we ate, the chemicals we used to clean - everything. I even bought camel's milk. We moved our family from the only home we've known, thousands of miles north just to get away from "the rules."

One of the hardest parts for me was losing friends and family members who didn't understand the path we had chosen. Sometimes it felt lonely. Sometimes I felt like I was fighting the world, and no one was in the ring with me. Still, I wouldn't change a thing.

Maybe, like me, you've just received a diagnosis of autism or another autoimmune disease. Maybe something else devastating has happened and you don't know what to do. Maybe everything inside of you wants to fight back, but you don't know where to start. My advice to you is to just start. It's not going to be easy, but it's worth it to make the tough choices. Take that first step.

Personal Communication with Jodie Meschuk
Author of *Speak Up Buttercup*

CHAPTER 5

The Hunger Games
The Keys To Why We Are So Sick

In previous chapters, I have shared several contributing factors to the hijacking of our health. Toxic chemicals in our food, air, water supplies, vaccines, and prescription medications, all contribute to our ills causing chronic diseases such as heart disease, cancer, chronic lung diseases, stroke, and Type 2 diabetes. They account for 81% of hospital admissions, 91% of all prescriptions filled, and 76% of all physician visits. Chronic diseases also account for the vast majority of health spending with more than 75% of every dollar spent on healthcare going toward treatment of chronic disease. [310]

Honestly, in my young adult years, I thought all the talk about how toxic chemicals, pollution, etc. were killing people was a bunch of nonsense, but here we are. The evidence is pretty convincing. These diseases are responsible for seven in ten deaths among Americans each year. In 2011, 171 million people *(more than half the population)* in America had at least one or more chronic diseases. Chronic diseases can be disabling and reduce a person's quality of life, especially if left undiagnosed or untreated. For example, every 30 seconds a lower limb is amputated because of diabetes. [311 - 313]

They are the single largest threat to the health of Americans and are escalating, even amongst children and adolescents. The rate of chronic health conditions among children in the US increased from 12.8% in 1994 to 26.6% in 2006, particularly for asthma, obesity, and behavior and learning problems. Epidemiological studies show that one out of four children, or 15 to 18 million children under the age of 17 years, suffer from a chronic health problem. While the current chronic disease epidemic is grave now, the crisis is expected to worsen in the coming years. [314]

Ancel Keys - The Face Of A Movement That Ended In A Health Tragedy

While all of the toxic chemicals, pollution, and vaccines are important contributing factors in the big picture of the health crisis that we face today, there is another piece of the puzzle - perhaps the biggest piece. It involves a person who single-handedly turned the world upside down and became the face of a movement that would end in today's health tragedy. It all started with Dr. Ancel Keys, an American physiologist who studied the influence of diet on health. In particular, he hypothesized that dietary saturated fat causes cardiovascular heart disease and should be avoided. His timely hypothesis, friendship with Dr. Dudley White, America's most prominent cardiologist at the time who agreed with Keys' hypothesis, political connections, and subsequent falsification of research in the Seven Countries Study, created the perfect storm that has led to much of the health crisis that the developed world faces today. The Seven Countries Study was hugely influential, leading to congressional hearings and guidelines advising against eating saturated fat and arguing for the benefits of polyunsaturated fats. This one idea, promoted by Keys, that saturated fats caused heart disease was like setting off an atom bomb. It has changed the course of history for human health.

Curiously, Ancel Keys was also a co-author of another study that contradicted his hypothesis about saturated fats causing heart disease, but the results were never fully published. If it had been, it could have very well prevented much of the health crisis of today. That newly discovered study, Minnesota Coronary Survey, complete with tapes and documents almost 50 years old, was found stacked in the dusty basement of the principle author and research scientist, Dr. Ivan Franz. Christopher Ramsden of the National Institute of Health who specializes in the excavation of lost studies came upon an old published study referencing the research, and he contacted Ivan's son, Robert, to search his childhood home for the original study. The landmark study included 9,423 study participants, ages 20 to 97, from 1968-73, all living in state mental hospitals or a nursing home - a well-controlled environment. It was the largest experiment of its kind. Ramsden and Franz worked together and unearthed the raw data from the study, which challenged the dogma that eating vegetable fats instead of animal fats is good for the heart. The study, the largest gold-standard experiment that tested that idea, found the opposite was true. Ramsden said that his discovery and analysis of long-lost data underline how the failure to publish the results of clinical trials can undermine truth. There is no telling how this major study would have impacted the low saturated fat /high vegetable fat and carb movement had it been published. What was his motivation for not publishing the study? We will never know, but the speculation is that since the study actually contra-dicted Ancel's hypothesis that high cholesterol from saturated fats caused heart disease and that vegetable oils would lower cholesterol and increase lifespan, it got *"swept under the rug"* because the results were disappointing. Ramsden discovered another equally old and unpublished study, the Sydney Diet Heart Study, with research from 1966-73, showing similar results to the Minnesota Coronary Survey. He published those results in 2013.

On August 1, 2017, True Health Initiative released a 65-page white paper correcting many historical inaccuracies and errors that low-fat advocates have perpetuated. The paper, *"Ancel Keys and the Seven Countries Study: An Evidence-based Response to Revisionist Histories,"* focused on the manipula-tion of data from selected countries to achieve a desired outcome, not even considering sugar as a possible contributor to heart disease. In 2018, The Prospective Urban Rural Epidemiology *(PURE)* study was published in The Lancet. It was a large, epidemiological cohort study of individuals aged 35-70 years *(enrolled between Jan 1, 2003, and March 31, 2013)*. Dietary intake of 335 individuals was recorded using validated food frequency question-naires. The findings also contradicted the Keys' theory. High carbohydrate intake was associated with higher risk of total mortality, whereas total fat and individual types of fat were related to lower total mortality. Total fat and types of fat were not associated with cardiovascular disease, myocardial infarction, or cardiovascular disease mortality, whereas saturated fat had an inverse association with stroke. [315-318]

The story starts with Dwight D. Eisenhower, a man who would become Supreme Allied Commander in Europe and President of the United States from 1953-1961. He started smoking when he was a cadet at West Point. By age 59, he had reached a four-pack-a-day habit. He was known for his volatile temper and refusal to follow orders from his doctors to stay on a restrictive diet and reduce his smoking. Early in the morning of Sept. 24, 1955, 64-year-old President Dwight Eisenhower suffered a heart attack while staying at his mother-in-law's home in Denver, Colorado. The Air Force flew Dr. White from Boston to the popular president's bedside. After that initial event, Eisenhower had at least seven myocardial infarctions and 14 cardiac arrests before he died in 1969, at age 78. But it was that first heart attack that sets the wheels in motion for the health problems that we see today. Politics provided White and Keys with a golden opportunity to further publicize their message. They began to work together promoting the idea that it was Ike's high-fat diet that caused the heart attack. Never mind that he was a highly stressed, four-pack-a-day smoker, which history now shows was the most probable cause for his heart condition.

In late December 1960, Keys received a boost when the American Heart Association *(AHA)* had him draw up a statement that said reducing the amount of saturated fat in the diet was, *"a possible means of preventing atherosclerosis and decreasing the risk of heart attacks and strokes."* Nine out of 10 doctors moved forward in lockstep on the assumption that there is a relationship, and that it's a good idea to trim cholesterol levels. The American Medical Association promoted replacing butter and lard with vegetable oil and the National Institute of Health *(NIH)* mounted a National Cholesterol Education Program to persuade Americans to drastically cut back on cholesterol, which was a *"major cause of coronary heart disease."* Giant commercial interests followed suit. Vegetable oil producers began vying over whose product was better at lowering cholesterol and preventing heart attacks. Low fat is where it's at. From there, the marketing trends and political influences promoted everything fat and sugar-free, diet drinks, and every sort of non-satiating fake food. [319]

Keys was the spark that started the health revolution that ended up backfiring in such a way that we may not genetically recover for several generations. Faith in Keys' manipulated science led physicians and patients to embrace the low-fat diet for heart disease prevention and weight loss. After 1980, the low-fat approach became an overarching ideology, promoted by physicians, the federal government, the food industry, and the popular health media. Many Americans subscribed to the ideology of low fat, even though there was no clear evidence that it prevented heart disease or promoted weight loss. Ironically, in the same decades that the low-fat approach assumed ideological status, Americans in the aggregate were getting fatter. So, what is the overall damage? The top killers, including cancer, heart disease, obesity, diabetes, and brain disorders all have their roots in poor eating habits, all related to the low-fat movement.

In 1968, The Senate appointed George McGovern to chair The United States Senate Select Committee on Nutrition and Human Needs, mandated to look into the problem of hunger in America. The committee's work culminated in its early 1977 report, Dietary Goals for the United States, which promoted increased carbohydrate and reduced fat consumption along with less sugar and salt. The report recommended that Americans eat more fruits, vegetables, whole grains, poultry, and fish, less red meat *(that will reduce saturated fats)*, eggs, and high-fat foods, and that they substitute nonfat for whole milk. By 1980, the scientific consensus was emerging that a low-fat diet was needed to prevent the two leading causes of death, coronary artery disease, and cancer. By the 1980s, the food producers had begun to realize that low fat could provide profit-making opportunities. The industry began replacing fat with sugar and processed foods; leading to what would, by the 1990s, become known as the SnackWell's phenomenon, low fat foods that had just as many calories as the former high-fat versions. People end up eating more Snackwell cookies because they are fat free *(and unfortunately contain a whole bunch of bad ingredients)*. Driven by consumer demand and widespread advertising, in the '80s and '90s, low fat industrial foods proliferated to fill grocery store shelves. In 1992 the USDA released its first and long-awaited food pyramid that led full support to the ideology of low-fat. According to Nestlé, this became the most widely distributed and best-recognized nutrition education device ever produced in this country." The American Heart Association also launched its own low-fat campaign in 1998, by introducing a program to label foods with its *"heart healthy"* seal of approval. By 1997, 55 companies were participating with over 600 products certified, many of which were cereal products, including Kellogg's frosted flakes, fruity marshmallow crispies, and low-fat pop tarts. Then, in the 1990s, *"no fat"* foods were even promoted. Low fat or no fat and high carbohydrate diet became the gold standard for heart health and weight control.

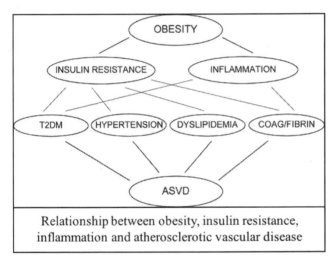

Relationship between obesity, insulin resistance, inflammation and atherosclerotic vascular disease

The *"war"* on saturated fat is considered by many to be the biggest mistake in the history of nutrition. As people have reduced their intake of animal fat and cholesterol, many serious diseases have gone up. Removing saturated fats from the diet also promoted hunger since saturated fats promote satiation. We are now in the midst of worldwide pandemics of obesity, metabolic syndrome, and type II diabetes. Studies conducted in the past few decades conclusively show that neither saturated fat nor dietary cholesterol cause harm in humans, and scientists are now beginning to realize that the entire low-fat dogma was based on flawed studies. Obesity causes insulin resistance and a state of low-grade inflammation. Both contribute to the development of several disorders, including T2 Diabetes Mellitus *(T2DM),* hypertension, dyslipidemia, and disorders of coagulation, and fibrinolysis, which are independent risk factors for the development of atherosclerotic vascular disease *(ASVD)*.

In part, being constantly hungry from low fat and high fructose laden diets may have been why people were so readily enticed by the increasingly available and unhealthy foods such as donuts, pizza, burgers, fries, pastries and some ethnic restaurant foods. The irony of the low-fat diet was that sugar, being low fat, was still officially okay. But sugar combined with fat was condemned. And while health officials were still pounding the low-fat drum, the American people were being seduced to consume foods laced with flavor enhancers including high fructose corn syrup (HFCS), sugar, msg (monosodium glutamate) and other ingredients that were sweeping the nation, causing skyrocketing obesity, diabetes, cancer, and other health problems. The choices of foods were also very confusing with so many being labeled deceptively as healthy versions.

Another crushing blow to the low fat/heart disease connection came in 2008 when a new study theorized that the main culprit in heart disease was not fat, but inflammation. In February 2010, the press reported on a meta-analysis of 21 lengthy studies, comprising 347,747 subjects, which concluded there was no association between saturated fat consumption and the risk of heart disease. That all makes sense considering all of the foods that were laced with so many pro-inflammatory ingredients, from HFCS, to high carbohydrates and *"bad fats,"* flavor enhancers made for laboratory chemicals, and more. People were toxic cesspools in many ways, and the body responded with chronic inflammation in response. Silent inflammation became the new buzzword to explain the epidemic of declining health.

High-Fructose Corn Syrup - Sweet Poison

High-fructose corn syrup was developed in Japan during the 1960s as a liquid-sugar equivalent of sucrose. Sucrose was processed from sugar cane and sugar beets, which though not terribly expensive, it wasn't exactly cheap either. High-fructose corn syrup, however, could be processed from the river of cheap corn that was flowing out of the American Midwest - and that was the decisive factor in favor of high-fructose corn syrup. It was cheap, government-subsidized, and super-sweet.

The development of high fructose corn syrup allowed fructose intake to skyrocket to 55 g/day in 1994 accounting for 10% of calories. Consumption peaked in the year 2000 by which time consumption had increased fivefold within the space of 100 years. Adolescents in particular were heavy users of fructose, often eating as much as 25% of their calories as added sugars at 72.8 grams/day. Currently, it is estimated that Americans eat 156 pounds of fructose-based sweeteners per year. The dose makes the poison.

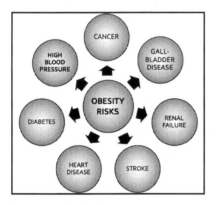

The introduction of high fructose corn syrup into the American diet was an important contribution to the obesity epidemic, currently at 39% in the United States. HFCS has become a staple ingredient of the soft-drink industry as well as numerous other foods. It interferes with several metabolic pathways, including blocking leptin, which is our main appetite suppressant hormone and promotes ghrelin hormone, which stimulates appetite. Poof! There you have it - obesity. All that excess fructose-induced fat production also leads to increased fat deposition in the liver. Excessive liver collections of fat, beginning as non-alcoholic fatty liver disease (NAFLD), are considered the liver manifestation of metabolic syndrome; up to 30% of adults now suffer from this condition. Fructose is now widely recognized as a major contributor to NAFLD, which progresses to produce non-alcoholic steatohepatitis, a precursor to liver cirrhosis and eventual liver failure. [320 - 324]

And combined with a low-fat and carbohydrate rich diet, the obesity epidemic, along with obesity-related diseases including cancer, dementia, heart disease and diabetes - has spread across every nation where sugar-based carbohydrates have come to dominate the food economy. The major trends in American diets since the late 1970s, according to the USDA agricultural economist Judith Putnam, have been a decrease in the percentage of fat calories and a *"greatly increased consumption of carbohydrates."* Annual grain consumption, full of sugars, has increased almost 60 pounds per person, and caloric sweeteners *(primarily high-fructose corn syrup)* by 30 pounds. At the same time, we suddenly began consuming more total calories: now up to about 400 or more each day since the government started recommending low fat diets. The effects of HFCS on leptin and ghrelin to increase appetite can also help to explain this trend as well as the obesity epidemic.

Your Gut Reaction

Another contributing factor that has recently become an interest of researchers is the effect of our intestinal microbiome on obesity. The idea that our gut bacteria would have anything to do with obesity was not on the radar screen in the past. But thanks to Dr. Zac Bush and others, researchers now have another piece of the obesity puzzle. Dr. Bush, a triple board-certified medical doctor, believes that there are sugar loving bacteria that reside in the gut and thrive in a carbohydrate-rich gut environment. If the sugar intake decreases, the bacteria send signals to the brain to *"feed me."* When a sugar-free, or low carbohydrate diet is started, the bacteria begin to die off, and they get pretty intense in signaling their need for us to consume some sort of carbohydrate food so they can survive. Many of the hunger pangs that people experience when starting a low-carb diet can be related to these bacteria dying from starvation. Some people give up on the diet transition because of the sometimes-intense desire to have something sweet. Knowledge of this can be very powerful in helping people understand the *"why,"* which can get them through the critical first couple of weeks.

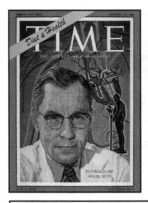 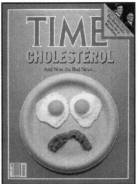 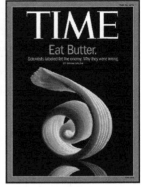

1. Ancel Keys on the cover of Time Magazine in 1961 - He claimed that saturated fats in the diet clogged arteries and caused heart disease.
2. Cholesterol 1984 – The cause of heart disease
3. Time Magazine cover story in 2014 - Scientists were wrong about saturated fats. They don't cause heart disease after all. Time has a change off heart on fat. Eat Butter!

Fat Chance

Ancel Keys appeared on the front cover of Time magazine in 1961. In the cover story, Keys claimed that saturated fats in the diet clogged arteries and caused heart disease. His theory and falsified research began a powerful movement of manipulating public perception that led to the unnecessary death and disease of millions of people around the world. In 1984, Time again influenced public perception with another article, this time demonizing cholesterol as the cause of heart disease. Known as one of Time's most memorable covers, the message was made abundantly clear: *"Cholesterol is proved deadly, and our diet may never be the same."* Time asserted that the diet-heart hypothesis - eating cholesterol and saturated fat raises cholesterol in the blood contributing to heart disease - had finally been proven. The article took the world by storm, allowing widespread fat phobia to take root for decades to come. The fallout? Over thirty years of blaming saturated fats and cholesterol and promoting a low-fat, high carb diet has created one of the worst health tragedies in history. In 2014, Time had a change of heart on fat, reportedly based on current research of course - never mind that similar research was already done exonerating fats even before the 1984 article. Decades of low-fat diets have coincided with rising rates of obesity, diabetes, and heart disease.

So where are we thirty years later? Decades of low-fat diets have coincided with rising rates of obesity, diabetes, and heart disease and it appears that Time has had a change of heart. Simply, *"Eat Butter."* Ending the War on Fats goes further. *"For decades, it has been the most vilified nutrient in the American diet. But new science reveals fat isn't what's hurting our health."* Yes, Time did give an apology of sorts, but that doesn't do much good for all of my diabetic patients in wheelchairs from leg amputation from diabetes. With greater power, comes greater responsibility for that power to end at the truth. The evidence was there, it appears that Time just didn't do its homework.

What is important to note through all this is that saturated fats in meats, butter, dairy, etc. in and of themselves are not the cause of heart disease or any of the chronic diseases. The chemicals associated with the farm to table experience can be problematic, but not the meat product itself in its natural form. Neither is high cholesterol necessarily a problem! That's right. High cholesterol is not the cause of heart disease. Even Dr. DeBakey, the famous heart surgeon and heart transplant pioneer, said as much over thirty years ago. As a matter of fact, one of his operation room assistants has said that he would routinely eat a small block of cheese for lunch back when all the other docs were convinced that fats and cholesterol were the cause of heart disease. He just ignored them. He knew what he was seeing in the operating room contradicted that idea because he was doing as many bypass surgeries on people with low cholesterol as high cholesterol.

Cholesterol - Friend Or Foe

So, high cholesterol was not necessarily causing coronary artery disease. As a matter of fact, there really is no such thing as good cholesterol and bad cholesterol per se. Docs tell their patients for the sake of simplicity that HDL *(high-density lipoprotein)* is *"good"* cholesterol and LDL *(low- density lipoproteins)* is *"bad"* cholesterol. Actually, HDL and LDL are *"taxi cabs"* for cholesterol, which cannot travel the blood stream by itself. These are two of five types of transporters. The others include chylomicrons, IDL *(interme-diate density lipoproteins)* and VLDL *(very low-density lipoproteins, mainly triglycerides)*. So, when HDL is measured for instance, the measurement is including its passenger in the taxi, cholesterol. The taxi is on a mission to take cholesterol back home to the liver after a hard day's work out in the body. HDL removes cholesterol from the bloodstream, *"lowering"* blood cholesterol. LDL does just the opposite - it takes cholesterol to the job sites in the body. They all live in the same neighborhood in the liver. When there is a call to the brain that cholesterol is needed for cellular repair or hormone production for example, the LDL taxi is called, and it goes to cholesterol's house to make the pickup. Cholesterol then goes to the address given by the brain to work. Once the work is completed, the work supervisor calls the brain and says to come and pick up the remaining cholesterol - that they are getting cranky and need to go home to see their family. The HDL taxicab then makes the run to go and pick up the remaining cholesterol and takes it back to the liver and out of the bloodstream.

This is a very sophisticated and balanced system and runs very smoothly most of the time, if we are healthy. The things that get in the way are the traffic jams caused by chronic stress, oxidation, and inflammation. Tensions are high, and there is a lot of stress. There are wrecks, flat tires, angry drivers, - five o'clock city traffic but 24/7. The normal traffic highway *"arteries"* are clogged. The more the stress, the more the damage, and the more calls to the brain to bring reparative cholesterol to the scene. LDL does that. Then, because things are such a mess and cells are dying, the immune system is activated to bring the emergency crews to help the injured cells and to clean up some of the debris. Patching things up causes further congestion and repair, so the immune system puts up *"blockades"* that may close down a lane of the highway while they do the repair, further complicating the congestion and damage. Arteries in the heart get blocked through this process. If things get too bad, the circulation highway shuts down completely.

As current research clearly demonstrates, it is the stress, inflammation, oxidation, and free radical cycle that causes so much cell damage, including damage to arteries and the cholesterol/LDL complex with triglycerides and platelet adhesion, which contribute to heart disease and stroke by clogging up the arteries. The internal cell walls of the coronary arteries become inflamed and sticky, and damaged cholesterol/VLDL sticks more easily to the arterial wall. The immune system responds to the *"wreck,"* trying to clean things up, but causes scar tissue and thickening of the arterial wall, closing it down in the process. Oxidative stress comes from various sources including diet, environmental contamination, toxic chemicals, and even medications. All contribute to the chronic diseases that are so commonplace today.

Here's an interesting note about LDL. It is actually not bad, as we have come to understand it. We are told that saturated fats raise LDL and that increases the risk of heart disease. From the discussion above, we know that oxidation is what damages the LDL/cholesterol unit and contributes to heart disease. But there is another important point to be made. LDL has several subunits - LDL large, intermediate, and small. It is the small LDL that can more easily stick to and penetrate the arterial wall, causing damage when it is oxidized. Studies show that people whose LDL particles are predominantly small and dense have a threefold greater risk of coronary heart disease. Research also shows that the large LDL subtype is more buoyant and consuming saturated fats changes the small more destructive LDL into the large benign LDL subtype. Although saturated fats increase LDL in the short-term, plenty of long-term observational studies find no link between saturated fat consumption and LDL levels. For testing purposes, the way to get a more accurate assessment of cardiovascular risk is to get HDL, LDL, VLDL, LDL-P, apolipoprotein *(apoB),* and triglycerides. Lab designation may be different but whatever the terms used in the labs, they should include these components. [325 - 328]

The Omega Fats

There are many different types of consumable fat. Some of them are good for us, others neutral, yet others are clearly harmful. The evidence points to saturated and monounsaturated fats being perfectly safe and can be healthy. However, the situation is a bit more complicated with polyunsaturated fats. When it comes to those, we have both omega-3s and omega-6s. It is important to strike a proper balance between omega-3 and omega-6 fats in your diet. They play an important role in the life and death of cardiac cells, immune system function, brain health, and blood pressure regulation. They reduce triglycerides, blood clots, arterial plaque and inflammation, depression, anxiety, they raise HDL, and improve age-related brain disorders like Alzheimer's.

Research suggests that a diet that is too high in omega-6 fats distorts the balance of pro-inflammatory agents, promoting chronic inflammation and causing the potential for health problems such as asthma, arthritis, allergies, or diabetes. Omega-6 fats compete with omega-3 fats for enzymes and will actually replace omega-3 fats. The typical western diet is characterized by excessive consumption of foods high in omega-6 fatty acids. [329]

The most common source of Omega-6s is linoleic acid, found in corn oil, soybean oil, safflower oil, cottonseed oil, sunflower oil, poultry, and some nuts and seeds. These oils are cheap to produce, so many companies use them in processed foods like candy, cookies, crackers, popcorn, granola, dairy creamer, margarine, frozen pizza, and other snacks. Soybean oil is so overused that it constitutes 20% of the calories in the average American diet. Many of the oils are also genetically modified and produced with toxic solvents. Omega-6 oils are unstable because they're made of polyunsaturated fats with multiple double bonds. Cooking at high heats, microwaving, or frying will oxidize the fats. Oxidized omega-6 does damage to your DNA, inflames your heart, and raises your risk for several types of cancer, including breast cancer. It also interferes with brain metabolism. When companies use these oils in packaged foods, they stabilize them to increase shelf life through a process called hydrogenation. Hydrogenation takes already harmful fats and converts them into synthetic trans fat. Trans fat is even worse for you.

Omega-3s are great for your cells. They are an integral part of cell membranes throughout the entire body and affect the cell receptors in these membranes. Omega-3s also provide a launch pad for making hormones that regulate blood, heart, and genetic function. There are three common types of omega-3 fatty acids: EPA *(eicosapentanoic acid)* and DHA *(docosahexaenoic acid)* - both are long-chain omega-3 fatty acids, and both come from animal sources. DHA is the really good one. It keeps your nervous system functioning and provides anti-inflammatory benefits. Higher consumption correlates with improved mood, memory, focus, greater insulin sensitivity, increased muscle growth, and better sleep. Docosahexaenoic acid *(DHA)* is an omega-3 essential fatty acid shown to play important roles in synaptic transmission in the brain. Getting enough omega-3s during pregnancy is associated with numerous benefits for your child, including higher intelligence, better communication and social skills, fewer behavioral problems, decreased risk of developmental delay, decreased risk of ADHD, autism and cerebral palsy.

ALA *(alpha-linolenic acid)* is the third type of omega-3 fatty acid. ALA comes mostly from plant sources, and most animals can't really use it, so they convert it to the super-powerful DHA but only about 8% is converted, so plant-based omega-3s like chia seeds and flaxseed oil are not the best source.

The omega-6 to omega-3 ratios should be 2-4 omega-6 to 1 omega-3. It is a good idea to eat plenty of omega-3s but most people would do best by reducing their omega-6 consumption. The average American eats a ratio of anywhere from 12:1 to 25:1 omega-6 to omega-3, respectively. The difference in structure between an omega-3 and omega-6 is where the first double bond is located. In the example, Linoleic acid is an omega-6 because the first double bond in the sixth carbon position. Both omega-6 and omega-3 are important to health. But they need to be balanced. Too much omega-6 has been associated with inflammation, liver disease, chronic pain, and other health hazards.

The best way to do that is to avoid seed and vegetable oils like soybean and corn oils, as well as the processed foods that contain them, which are high omega-6 sources. Another class of fats, artificial trans fats, is also very harmful. Studies show that trans fats lead to insulin resistance, inflammation, belly fat accumulation, and can drastically raise the risk of heart disease. Although there has been some pressure on the food industry to eliminate trans fats, they are still around. So, eat your saturated fats, monounsaturated fats and omega-3s but avoid trans fats and processed vegetable oils. Always check labels to see if there are any hydrogenated fats and stay organic whenever possible. [330-332]

Sugar - The Spice - Not So Nice!

Sugar's sweetness and seductive power have been recorded throughout history. Once considered a luxury, Christopher Columbus even brought the *"white gold"* plants with him during his 1492 voyage to North America, and the sugarcane crop thrived. But it has only been since the 17th century onward that mass distribution and consumption has taken place, contributing to the health epidemics that we see today. By the 1800s, the average American consumed four pounds of sugar a year. Today, the average American consumes between 150-170 pounds each year, about 1⁄2 pound per day or about 230 grams. The worldwide consumption is estimated at 175 million metric tons. Clearly, the global marketplace has a sweet tooth and sugar has been become a major cash crop player in the global economy, but at what cost? Globally, sugar intake per capita has increased nearly fivefold just over the past century, with recent gains driven by emerging markets in developing countries.

At the same time, diabetes and obesity - sometimes referred to as *"diabesity"* - are at epidemic proportions, and, while there are other contributing factors, sugar consumption is top among the prime reasons. It is everywhere. It's in almost all processed foods and is often added to *"nonfat"* products to enhance flavor. It coats drug pills and infuses the syrup of children's medicine.

High concentrations of both added and naturally occurring sugar are found in fruit juice and bread. Grains are hybridized to contain more sugar. It is found in canned tuna, roasted chicken, peanut butter, baked beans, cereals, meats, healthy fruit yogurts, as well as the obvious places such as biscuits, cakes, and fizzy drinks. At the writing of this chapter, a six-ounce container of Dannon All Natural Plain Low Fat Yogurt contains 12 grams of sugar. An eight-ounce glass of Tropicana Pure Premium orange juice contains a whopping 22 grams of sugar. A two-bar pack of Nature Valley Oats 'n' Honey Granola has 11 grams of sugar. (Honey is the second listed sweetener after sugar. The bars also contain brown sugar syrup.) While the label says *"natural," "pure,"* and *"nature,"* words the US Food and Drug Administration *(FDA)* doesn't regulate, these all count as sources of added sugar. [333 - 335]

Sugar and corn syrup from soft drinks, juices, and the copious, sugar-infused cold drink teas and sports drinks now supply more than 10% of our total calories. One can of Coke has about 9.5 teaspoons of sugar. The 80s saw the introduction of Big Gulps and 32-ounce cups of Coca-Cola, blasted through with sugar, but 100% fat-free. When it comes to insulin and blood sugar, these soft drinks and fruit juices, what the scientists call "wet carbohydrates," might indeed be the worst of all. Even health-conscious consumers may not realize how much sugar they ingest on a daily basis.

Sugar is addictive, more so than cocaine. Both human and animal studies have demonstrated that the consumption of sugar-rich foods or drinks primes the release of euphoric endorphins and dopamine within the nucleus accumbens, in a manner similar to some drugs of abuse. The neurobiological pathways of drug and *"sugar addiction"* involve similar neural receptors, neurotransmitters, and hedonic regions in the brain. Craving, tolerance, withdrawal, and sensitization have been documented in both human and animal studies. In an article co-authored by cardiovascular research scientist, James J. DiNicolantonio, and Cardiologist, James H O'Keefe, both from Saint Luke's Mid America Heart Institute in Kansas, together with William Wilson - a physician with the nonprofit US group practice, Lahey Health, citied rodent studies, which show that sweetness is preferred even over cocaine, and that mice can experience sugar withdrawal. They suggested, *"Consuming sugar produces effects similar to that of cocaine, altering mood, possibly through its ability to induce reward and pleasure, leading to the seeking out of sugar."* Sugar's addictive properties could also act as a gateway to alcohol and other addictive substances. [336]

There may not be the same drug withdrawal effects as with caffeine, cocaine, heroin, etc., but it is still just as addictive if not more so, and quietly destructive, like a slow growing cancer that takes over your body. As with most toxins, the dose makes the poison. The problem is that sugar seems so sweet and innocent, but let its persuasive grip take hold, and you can quickly become a victim, an addict with a higher potential for additional drug and other addiction abuse. [337]

In 2009, Dr. Robert Lustig, a pediatric endocrinologist at the University of California, San Francisco, delivered a ninety-minute lecture entitled, *"Sugar: The Bitter Truth,"* emphasizing how toxic sugar is. He says that the food industry is manipulating people to consume more sugar specifically high fructose corn syrup *(HFCS)*, about 39 grams or 9.5 teaspoons of sugar in a sugar-based drink. Those similar beverages with HFCS have been tested to show that there is 50% more fructose *(60/40 ratio)* than glucose. Sucrose is 50/50. Americans drink an average of 50 gallons of sweetened soda a year. [338] Too much sugar can also make you more prone to illnesses. If you are sick several times throughout the year, you may want to look at your sugar consumption because excess sugar consumption depresses your body's immunity. Studies have shown that consuming 75 to 100 grams of simple sugars *(about 20 teaspoons of sugar - the amount found in two-and-a-half average 12-ounce cans of soda)* can suppress the body's immune responses considerably. These sugars are known to create a 40 to 50% drop in the ability of white blood cells to kill bacteria and germs within the body. The immune-suppressing effect of sugar starts less than thirty minutes after ingestion and may last for five hours. By consuming 150 to 170 pounds of simple sugars each year, a person may have up to 80,000 hours of immune suppression! [339]

Sugar *(Glucose)* - Tipping The Scales To Energy Or Fat

The concentration of glucose in your blood is the critical upstream switch that places your body into a *"fat-storing"* or *"fat-burning"* state. The carbohydrates you eat, with the exception of indigestible forms like most fibers, eventually become glucose in your blood. Assuming your metabolism is functioning normally, if the switch is on, you will store fat. If the switch is off, you will burn fat. Therefore, all things being equal, *"diets"* are just ways of hacking your body into a sufficiently low-glycemic state to trigger the release of a variety of hormones that, in turn, result in a net loss of fat from long-term storage.

When your blood has a high concentration of glucose for a sufficient period of time, your pancreas kicks insulin into gear, which tells your cells to open the door and take in glucose, put it in a temporary storage *(like RAM in your computer)* called glycogen, and put everything else into long-term storage inside your fat cells. On the other hand, when your blood has a low concentration of glucose for a sufficient period of time, this process is reversed. Your pancreas releases a protein called glucagon, glycogen is depleted, a bunch of other hormones *(epinephrine, cortisol, testosterone, etc.)* is introduced into your system, and TAGs are thereby pulled from your fat cells and converted into Acetyl Co- A, which is the key precursor for the process your body uses to generate *"energy"* *(i.e. ATP)* for your cells.

Ok, so we know that glucose gets into our blood quickly and is used by all cells,

Nutrition Facts

Serving size   1 potato (148g/5.2oz)

Amount per serving

Calories **110**

	% Daily Value*
Total Fat 0g	**0%**
Saturated Fat 0g	**0%**
Trans Fat 0g	
Cholesterol 0mg	**0%**
Sodium 0mg	**0%**
Total Carbohydrate 26g	**9%**
Dietary Fiber 2g	**7%**
Total Sugars 1g	
Includes 0g Added Sugars	**0%**
Protein 3g	
Vitamin D 0mcg	0%
Calcium 20mg	2%
Iron 1.1mg	6%
Potassium 620mg	15%
Vitamin C 27mg	30%
Vitamin B$_6$ 0.2mg	10%

* The % Daily Value (DV) tells you how much a nutrient in a sering of food contributes to a daily diet. 2,000 calories a day is used for general nutrition advice.

stored temporarily in glycogen, and stored long-term in fat cells. But what about fructose? Fructose does not stimulate insulin like glucose does, so in small amounts fructose is *"good for us"* in that it helps with our normal energy storage and supply. But, indeed, part of the reason why soft drinks, fruit juices, and other processed foods with HFCS are so *"bad for us"* is because it's easy for us to consume too much, which thereby sends a significant percentage of it into our fat cells and does other unhealthy things referenced above. [340, 341]

So, when we eat any type of carbohydrate, simple sugars like sucrose and fructose being the worst, it is converted by the body to glucose, which stimulates insulin to be released. It doesn't matter whether it is a fizzy drink, sweets, table sugar, or a complex carbohydrate such as whole-grain bread, pasta, rice, or potatoes; the process of insulin release is the same. Some are more easily converted into simple sugars than others. The more complex the carbohydrate and the more fiber that is present, the less will be absorbed. You know when you read the ingredient label of a product such as bread or spaghetti sauce, and the total carbs are more than the sugars and fiber added up, and you wonder why? The remainder is starch, which doesn't have to be labeled, but nonetheless, they are still digestible carbohydrates that add to the total. One canned potato for instance, is very high in starch. It has about 26 grams of carbohydrate – that's a lot! But someone unfamiliar with how to read labels might not realize how much convertible sugar is in just one potato. There are three grams of fiber, and one gram of total sugars. But the rest is sugar starches.

It also doesn't matter if it is 'natural' or 'processed.' Honey, raw sugar, dates, fruit, etc. all raise your blood glucose levels equally as processed sugars. Saying that, if you are able to tolerate carbohydrates, then your choice should always be natural, unprocessed carbs, with a higher fiber profile. Always go for nutrient dense, real food, whole food such as berries, non-starchy vegetables, etc. Choose complex colorful carbs where possible. They are absorbed slower and are packed with vitamins, minerals, antioxidants, and phytonutrients. Eat a rainbow! Also, it has been well documented that increased fiber in the diet reduces the concentration of glucose in the blood. The mechanisms behind this are not completely known, however, but it is likely because of a binding effect that prevents the degradation of carbs into free glucose. [342]

By maintaining a lower blood sugar level, you require lower insulin levels. Insulin is the major regulator of metabolism and by controlling insulin you stop fat from being stored, lose weight, allow fat to be utilized as fuel, improve your blood lipid profile, increased energy, reduce hunger, reduce risk of developing Type II diabetes and reduce inflammation that leads to cardiovascular disease, dementia, and cancer.

Diabetes

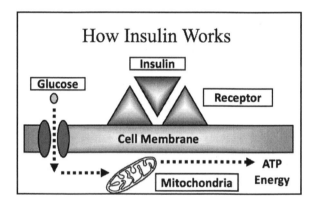

Diabetes, also called diabetes mellitus, is a condition that causes blood sugar to rise. When your digestive system breaks down food, your blood sugar level rises. The body's cells take up the sugar *(glucose)* in the bloodstream and use it for energy. The cells do this using a hormone called insulin, which is produced by the pancreas *(an organ near the stomach)*. Insulin docks on the cell's insulin receptor, and in doing so, a door is opened, and glucose can enter into the cell, then to the mitochondria where it produces energy for the cell to use. When your body doesn't produce enough insulin and/or doesn't efficiently use the insulin it produces, sugar levels rise in the blood-stream. Right away, the body's cells may be starved for energy. Over time, high blood glucose levels may damage the eyes, kidneys, nerves, heart and other circulatory arteries, and the brain.

There are several types of diabetes, but Type 1 and 2 are the most common and of more importance on a global scale. Type 1 diabetes is also referred to as insulin-dependent diabetes. Those with Type 1 diabetes must take insulin or other medications daily. This compensates for insufficient amounts of insulin, a hormone required to bring blood glucose into the cell and produce energy for the body. Type 1 diabetes was previously known as juvenile diabetes because it's usually diagnosed in children and young adults. However, this chronic disease can strike at any age, more so in recent history. Those with a family history of Type 1 diabetes have a greater risk. As already discussed in the vaccine chapter, there is compelling evidence that Type 1 diabetes can be caused by viruses, some associated with vaccines given at a young age. The viruses can attack the insulin-producing cells in the pancreas and destroy their capacity to produce insulin.

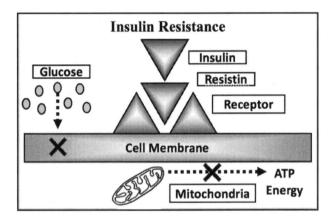

Type 2 diabetes *(T2DM)* is the most common form of diabetes. Historically, Type 2 diabetes has been diagnosed primarily in adults. But adolescents and young adults are developing T2DM diabetes at an alarming rate because of higher rates of obesity, environmental chemicals, and physical inactivity risk. This type of diabetes can occur when the body's cells develop *"insulin resistance."* In subclinical milder forms, this type of diabetes can go undiagnosed for many years. That's cause for concern, since untreated diabetes can lead to many serious medical problems. [343]

What does obesity have to do with diabetes? In obesity, adipose *(fat)* tissue not only stores and releases fatty acids but also synthesizes and releases a large number of other active compounds such as angiotensin 2, Resistin, TNF-α, interleukin 6, interleukin 1-β and others. Some of these compounds, when infused in large amounts, can produce insulin resistance by blocking its ability to dock on the cell's receptor site so the cell door is never opened to receive glucose for energy.

Insulin resistance is a condition that affects more than 60 million Americans. It occurs when the body makes insulin but does not use it efficiently. This means that glucose builds up in the bloodstream and creates havoc instead of being used by cells to produce energy *(ATP)*. To compensate for the high blood sugar levels, the insulin-producing cells in the pancreas release more and more insulin to try to keep blood sugar levels normal. Gradually, these cells fail to keep up with the body's need for insulin. Consequently, blood sugar levels begin to rise. When a fasting individual has too much glucose in the blood *(hyperglycemia)* or too much insulin in the blood *(hyperin-sulinemia)*, that person may have insulin resistance. People with insulin resistance are at greater risk of developing pre-diabetes, Type 2 diabetes, and other metabolic disorders. Those with insulin resistance are also more likely to have a history of being obese and physically inactive, and likely to have other cardiovascular risk factors such as dyslipidemia, high triglycerides, and high blood pressure.[344]

But insulin also regulates fat metabolism. We cannot store body fat without it. Think of insulin as a switch. When it's on, in the few hours after eating, you burn carbohydrates for energy and store excess calories as fat. When it's off, after the insulin has been depleted, you burn fat as fuel. So when insulin levels are low, you will burn your own fat, but not when insulin levels are high. The fatter you are, the more insulin your pancreas will pump out per meal, and the more likely you'll develop insulin resistance, which is the underlying cause of Metabolic Syndrome or Syndrome X, high blood sugar, high blood pressure, high cholesterol/triglycerides, and excess fat around the abdomen. These can lead to cardiovascular disease, diabetes, stroke, and obesity.

The United States has the highest prevalence *(11% of the population aged 20-79 years)* of diabetes among developed nations including countries of the European Union plus Canada, Australia, New Zealand, Singapore, South Korea, Israel, Andorra, Norway, Switzerland, and the US itself. And in terms of estimates of absolute numbers of people with diabetes in these nations, the US, with almost 30 million people with diabetes, has around two thirds the number of cases of all the other 37 nations in the developed nation league combined *(46 million)*.

The individual country data follows the release of the Diabetes Atlas summary, revealing that an estimated 415 million people globally have diabetes in 2015. This figure is expected to increase to around 642 million by 2040. Some 75% of people with diabetes live in low-income and middle- income countries, and every six seconds there is a diabetes-related death, with five million such deaths each year globally. While the US leads the league of developed nations, in terms of the global league, it is in 60th position. This is because diabetes is sweeping through the Middle East, Caribbean, and Latin American regions, as well as the multiple nations making up the Pacific Islands. [345]

Fueled by rapid urbanization, nutrition transition to empty processed foods, and increasingly sedentary lifestyles, the epidemic has grown in parallel with the worldwide rise in obesity. Asia's large population and rapid economic development have made it an epicenter of the epidemic. Asian populations tend to develop diabetes at younger ages than Caucasians. Several factors contribute to accelerated diabetes epidemic in Asians, including high prevalence of smoking and heavy alcohol use, high intake of refined carbohydrates, and dramatically decreased physical activity levels. Poor nutrition in utero and in early life, combined with over-nutrition with poor quality foods in later life, may also play a role in Asia's diabetes epidemic.

In addition to the 30.3 million or 9.4% of Americans who have been diagnosed with diabetes in 2015, there are another 84.1 million who have pre-diabetes, meaning their blood sugar levels are higher than normal but not yet high enough to be considered Type 2 diabetes. Even more alarming, there are approximately 7.1 million Americans who have diabetes, but don't know it. This 9.4% + is in stark contrast to .2% of the population with diabetes in the 1890s. [346 - 348]

Diabetes has a greater health impact on Americans than heart disease, substance use disorder, or COPD. In addition to the complications of diabetes including cardiovascular disease, nerve damage *(neuropathy)*, kidney damage *(nephropathy)*, eye damage *(retinopathy)*, foot damage, skin conditions, or hearing impairment, there is compelling preclinical and clinical evidence that supports a pathophysiological connection between Alzheimer's disease *(AD)* and diabetes sometimes called Type 3 Diabetes. Altered metabolism, inflammation, and insulin resistance are key pathological features of both diseases. A variant of the so-called Alzheimer's gene, APOE4, seems to interfere with brain cells' ability to use insulin, causing the symptoms of Alzheimer's disease. [340, 350]

The vast majority of diabetes cases are associated with obesity. There are epidemiological data, plausible mechanisms, and clinical data from diet intervention studies that provide strong support for a direct causal/ contributory role of sugar in the epidemics of metabolic disease, and for an indirect causal/contributory role mediated by sugar consumption promoting body weight and fat gain. The following example may be extreme, but there are so many other obesity and diabetes cases that end in a similar tragedy. When I first started my medical practice, I remember a 20-year old woman who was taken to the emergency room in an ambulance in response to a 911 call. She was transferred to the ICU where she died shortly after - the result of a do not resuscitate *(DNR)* order by her parents. She weighed approximately 750 pounds - 20 YEARS OLD! She was living in the back of a van because one day she just couldn't get out of the van so her parents left her there. They fed her an unbelievable amount of unhealthy foods every day according to the medical residents caring for her in the ICU. Because she was so big and heavy, they had to transfer her to the ICU by using the freight elevator. The beds in the ICU were too small so she slept on egg crate foam mattresses on the floor. She didn't last very long. She came in to the ER with a massive infection complicated by diabetes. The infection was located under a huge belly fat apron that hung down to her knees. The bacteria were breeding there undetected. The infection was so massive that she had a cardiac arrest and died.

Diabetes And Personality Type

There are other factors as well that contribute to diabetes including environmental chemicals and even chronic unhealthy emotional responses *(or lack of healthy responses)* in some people, especially men, with quiet and reserved personalities. They tend to manifest their unreleased stress in the gut with disorders like Irritable Bowel Syndrome *(IBS)*, colon cancer, diabetes, and other gastrointestinal symptoms. These *(melancholy personality)* men give 110% of who they are to whatever they do. They are non-conflict background players, not interested in accolades from others, just doing the best job possible. When the storms of life come, they do not overreact, and may not emotionally react at all - at least on the outside. You generally don't know how they are feeling about things. Men tend to be this way, but it is especially true of this personality type. They are just quiet about life on the outside, but inside the battle to perform *"perfectly"* rages on, and they become their own worst critic when that 110% effort does not produce the intended results. That internal stress generally manifests its physical symptoms in the gut. While they may not cry out for it, they really need the support and appreciation of others around them. If there is an unsupportive *(choleric personality especially)* wife or boss always criticizing them for being too slow, too methodical, or too whatever because they are generally non-conflict, they may not argue or even respond, but inside they are ripping themselves apart even more because of the criticism. They are hard enough on themselves and any criticism from others just drives the knife deeper. They don't so much see the big picture but focus more on details of life, which become their whole world.

This personality type is all about truth. If someone thinks they are a terrible person, an emotionally unhealthy melancholy *(1 on the enneagram)* will most likely think that it must be true, because that is the lens through which they view the world. They already half drown in their own self-criticism, and now it is being confirmed by others around them. The stress and negative self- image begins to destroy them from the inside out, starting with the physical manifestations in the gut. They also tend to blow up emotionally - big time - when it all gets too much for them to handle. Like, shaking up a carbonated beverage and spewing it out over everyone within range. Not to leave out the women here, they can experience many of the same manifestations, but they tend to do better overall because they are much better communicators about their feelings and tend not to hold things in as much as men. When women have diabetes, it can be for the same reasons, but just not as much as with men. [351]

Type 2 Diabetes Is Curable

The good news about diabetes, obesity, and the rest of the life-stealing diseases is that they don't have to own you. And, despite the lockstep marching tune of the medical community to the contrary, diabetes can be cured in most people willing to take ownership of their lives! Most can recover and lead very healthy, happy, and productive lives. People just need their toolbox filled with the right *"how-to"* information. Not just the what and how, but the why, which will help carry them through when the temptations come knocking. The *"why"* is the anchor that keeps us all grounded.

Back in the early 2000s, I conducted a study with diabetic patients through my office. I approached a well-known essential oils company that also has nutritional and most other healthy lifestyle products, to see if they would partner with me and provide the nutritional products that I needed for the study. There was no hesitation on their part. The study lasted for three months. I included nine diabetics in the study. All had metabolic syndrome with increased blood pressure, high blood sugar, excess body fat around the waist, and abnormal cholesterol or triglyceride levels. I told them that their diabetes could be cured. They looked at me bewildered because their primary care docs never mentioned that a cure was possible, but quite the opposite. I also told them that they would lose weight, and the high blood pressure and high triglycerides would go away as well. Now, they really thought I was from another planet. But they all agreed to participate. I instructed them - this is what you do, this is what you don't do, and these are the supplements that you are to take for three months. I asked them to monitor their blood pressure, and weight, and make sure that they worked with their primary care doctor to monitor blood glucose, cholesterol, and triglyceride levels. At the end of three months, seven of the nine were completely off their medications; all were losing weight, had more energy, and felt much better. Their faces were filled with that glow that accompanies a healthy lifestyle. The other two were cheating, so they didn't quite get off all of the medications, but they were getting there. The point is that diabetics and most others are not stuck in their poor health dilemma like they were told.

The answers are not in medications, but in caring for the precious life force within us, using what nature provides. Our cells are designed to thrive on nature's food, not on man-made alterations or synthetic substitutes. Nature's foods also include essential oils, the lifeblood of plants. Many essential oils help balance blood sugar, reduce inflammation, and are very effective in weight management strategies. Black pepper, ocotea, lavender, clove, coriander, helichrysum, grapefruit, and cinnamon bark all have been shown to help with blood sugar control, inflammation, and weight management. It is all there for us - we just need the educational tools to implement the fix. A more comprehensive list is given in the New Beginnings chapter. It is not hard and is very complimentary to your body.

How To *"Just Do It"* With A Healthy Body Diet Plan

Over the years, I have been actively engaged in many organized sports activities including triathlons, basketball, baseball, football, and others. That has done a lot to keep me fit and healthy over the years, but there is a limit to how much exercise is needed before it becomes destructive to cells. You don't need to do triathlons or even run for long distances. Working out and moderate aerobic and anaerobic exercise goes a long way. Studies now suggest that fast/ slow interval walking is the best cardiovascular health. While we are younger, we don't readily recognize how much damage is being done with intense physical activities. I've been there! But the truth of the matter is when there is a large cell turnover from high-stress physical activity; the DNA telomeres shorten with every cell turnover. You have only so many turnovers and the more that takes place, the quicker your body ages.

Where I failed most was in not providing my body with the proper nutrition. I was younger and just didn't know. I remember years ago, when four of us from med school decided to do an 800-mile bike ride in one week through the mountains of New England then down the coast from Maine to Massachusetts. It was a blast! But one thing happened that would not have happened if I had known how to nutritionally handle the metabolic stress from the extreme physical exertion. I was climbing a mountain on the bike in Vermont when I *"bonked" (a biker's term for I'm done)*. The others were ahead of me, so they didn't know what had happened. The bike was just to heavy to peddle up that steep grade. I had to get off my fully loaded bike and push it very slowly for a long way up the rest of the mountain. My legs were toast. Yes, people in cars stared as they went by. It was an embarrassing moment in my life, and I committed to never walk my bike like that again. I broke several of Velocio's Seven Commandments of riding, and I paid the price. Even after that, I still unnecessarily struggled at times during high-performance activities, but that was because I didn't understand the simplicity, nor the art and science of a balanced diet to meet my nutritional needs, whether sitting at home writing a book, or getting after it with some physical activity. [352]

Years later, I finally got *"educated"* and found my way to a healthy home and nutritional lifestyle that compliments my body and my very busy life. I feel like I have the same energy that I did when I was twenty-five. Running my medical practice, a blueberry farm, and a large direct sales organization, teaching nationally on healthy lifestyle practices, working out, playing basketball, biking, swimming, and raising a family all take their toll. But you know what, I hardly miss a beat. Yes, personality type and genetics play a small part, but I wouldn't be able to do what I do if it were not for providing my body with the high-octane natural food, fuel, and supplements that allow me to purr down the highway of life. It really makes a difference. I know because I experienced what bad fuel can do to my body - it's like having water mixed with the gas in your car. You stutter, gyrate, and throw nasty black discharge out the tailpipe as you press down to go 60 mph but can only manage 30. Clearly your car is messed up. If this is you or someone that you know, let's pull off the highway and get into the garage for an overhaul.

Let's begin by talking about choosing a healthy macronutrient profile - a diet. What I am recommending is not a *"fad"* diet plan. First off, fad diet plans usually fail. The cigarette diet *(reach for a Lucky [cigarette] instead of a sweet),* the Hollywood diet, Banana and Skim milk diet, Zen macrobiotic diet, Pritikin, Beverly Hills, Enter the Zone, Sleeping Beauty, Dash diet, and many more are rightly considered fad diet plans unless they are based on current science and have stood the test of time.

I am not talking about just changing your eating habits. I am talking about changing your life, forever. It is a much bigger picture but changing your eating habits based on solid science is a great place to start. To most people, a *"diet"* is a plan to lose weight. I am talking lifestyle, longevity, enjoying your foods *(I am a "foodie"),* and passing on those good epigenetic habits to future generations.

Healthy Diet Options

According to the current research and epidemiological observations, a low carb diet is fundamentally sound. But what about the rest - the fats and proteins? There are various plans that address combinations and percentages of fats and proteins in a low carb diet. One option is Trim Healthy Mama *(THM)*. It consists of a plan that in a nutshell combines carbs and protein or fats and protein, but not carbs and fats together in a meal. It is relatively flexible and is based on some solid science. We used the plan successfully for several years. The carbs are to be complex, and refined sugar is not allowed. Another is the Mediterranean diet emphasizing proportionally high consumption of olive oil, legumes, unrefined cereals, fruits, and vegetables, moderate to high consumption of fish, moderate consumption of dairy products *(mostly as cheese and yogurt),* moderate wine consumption, and low consumption of non-fish meat products. A good plan if the carbs are monitored. It does restrict saturated fats so the foundational principles should be adjusted to accommodate research showing that saturated fats can be beneficial to overall health. Paleo is another low carb, high protein diet that philosophically focuses on how our ancient ancestors must have eaten. The protein intake for meats is not restricted and generally takes center stage, tubers such as sweet potatoes *(high carbohydrate - 27 gram mostly starch)* are okay according to the diet parameters, but grains and dairy are restricted or eliminated. The health profile of foods can also depend on how they are prepared. The sweet potato can have a safe Glycemic Index of about 44-60/100 when boiled, but when baked it rises to 94/100, which is very unhealthy, especially for diabetics. Glycemic Index is important for people with Type 2 diabetes, because they often have a delayed insulin response. If glucose goes up fast, the body does not respond quickly enough, and glucose levels can get way too high after meals. So, we want low-Glycemic Index foods. [354, 355]

We prefer to consume even fewer carbs then those allowed on THM and the Mediterranean diet, more healthy fat, and a moderate amount of protein. Some plans like the Adkins and the keto diets have the right idea according to what we know today about the science of food consumption. Despite their many similarities, keto and Atkins have their differences. Firstly, Atkins is easy to follow because it allows for moderate carb intake at specific points in time. Keto, on the other hand, can be difficult for some people because it drastically restricts carbs and is very different from your standard healthy diet. Secondly, weight loss is the primary goal of Atkins while the goal of keto is better overall long-term health, with weight loss being a natural consequence. And lastly, the goal of keto is switching to ketosis and burning fat for fuel, while Atkins does not lead to drastic metabolic changes.

There are several versions of the Atkins diet, which was first introduced in 1972, but the one that is most like the keto diet is the induction phase of the Atkins 20 plan and the Modified Atkin's diet. The difference between the keto and Atkin's plans is that the Atkin's diet does not restrict the amount of protein consumed. That can be a problem in that through gluconeogenesis *(making new glucose)* too much protein can end up increasing fat storage.

The keto *(ketogenic)* diet is a high-fat, adequate-protein, and low- carbohydrate diet. This is the diet plan that has a lot of research, and the one that I mostly prefer, especially if there are specific health issues to address. Like anything else, there are nuanced variations of the plan. Doctors originally developed this diet to treat unmanageable epilepsy in children. This was way back in the 1920s after several studies found that reducing carbs causes nutritional ketosis, which was long considered a cure for epilepsy. Later on, the diet became popular for weight loss and overall health. The goal of the keto diet is ketosis - a metabolic state of enhanced fat burning and greater ketone levels, which become high-octane fuel for the cell. Ketones are molecules that replace the glucose from carbs. They're a more efficient and cleaner fuel source than carbohydrates. Studies also show that ketones provide health benefits beyond weight loss. While the goal of Atkins is mainly weight loss and the prevention of obesity-related diseases, the keto diet provides benefits beyond weight loss. Some of these benefits include enhanced mental clarity, greater energy levels, reversal of Type 2 diabetes, reduction of cardiovascular disease, cancer prevention, appetite control, and increased longevity.

The keto diet is very strict when it comes to macronutrient intake. The macronutrient ratios of ketogenic diets are based on years of research. This research shows that our metabolism changes drastically on carb intake below 50 grams per day. The macronutrient ratios on keto look something like this:[356]

- 5-10% of energy from carbs

- 20-30% of energy from proteins

- 65-80% of energy from healthy fats

By following these nutrient ratios, you are more than likely to enter nutritional ketosis. Nutritional ketosis is a direct result of carb scarcity and resulting drops in insulin. In turn, drops in insulin stop fat accumulation. After a few days of eating this way, you don't have enough glucose in your body to fuel the brain or even to burn fats. That's why your body makes ketones as replacement fuel. One of the goals of the keto diet is also to make you metabolically flexible. This means that your body can easily switch from sugar burning to fat burning and vice versa. Most people aren't metabolically flexible which makes it hard for them to lose weight through the burning of fat. There are several versions of keto as well depending on the goal. Bodybuilders may use a different formula because of the different physical stresses they experience. Here are some main differences:

Keto leads to ketosis and the burning of fat for fuel. Because of the flexibility and reintroduction of more carbs in the Atkin's diet, the burning of fat does not occur as readily. Atkins focuses on weight loss, keto on long-term healthy lifestyle. Weight loss is a natural benefit with keto.

With no ceiling on the amount of protein consumed in Atkin's, ketosis is hindered or prevented when more than 700 calories of protein is consumed which activates gluconeogenesis and the production of glucose for fuel instead of fat for fuel through ketosis. Keto's primary focus is high fat, medium protein, and low carbs.

Both can cause weight loss, but because of reintroduction of up to 100 grams of carbs later in the Adkin's Lifetime Maintenance phase, the keto plan, which generally restricts carbs to 30 grams or less keeps weigh loss more sustainable.

Sugar and honey spike blood sugar and are restricted in both. Remember, there is some wiggle room in these plans. It is a mindset. You have to know your body.

The biggest problem with Atkin's is the reintroduction of carbs. So, it is a short-term weight loss plan, but not necessarily a healthy long-term lifestyle plan.

While a superior lifestyle plan, the biggest problem with keto is that it can be difficult to maintain, so it may not be right for everyone. However, it can be modified to accommodate certain preferences. Everyone's metabolism is different so just experimenting to see what works the best for your body is a reasonable approach.

Keto plans can be very powerful and have some dramatic effects. They can cause you to basically reverse all the processes of environmentally and epigenetically induced premature aging. It regulates your mitochondria; it improves your gene expression, reduces inflammation, improves all your cardio-metabolic risk factors, and reduces all the things that interfere with normal metabolic function. Gram for gram, the oxidation of fats for fuel produces much more released energy compared to the oxidation of carbohydrates. For instance, one molecule of glucose releases 38 ATP for energy, and one molecule of palmitic fatty acid releases 129 ATP. Longer carbon chain fatty acids produce even more ATP for energy. This is a big difference and may help explain why those on keto seem to have more energy and sharper brainpower. Keto can also lead to the reversal of diabetes and stop epilepsy where nothing seems to work. They can also effective in autism, Alzheimer's, neurocognitive disorders, other behavioral issues, and possibly even cancer. A higher, good fat diet plan also stimulates muscle building. This has been shown over and over again in human and animal studies. Lean body mass increases with good quality protein and fat, and it decreases with sugar and starch.

Do fruits work well with keto? Again, it depends on what you are trying to accomplish. Fruits can be fine, but the lower sugar, and higher fiber fruits fit much better with a keto plan. Some fruits, like berries, are powerful antioxidants. Any foods that are anti-inflammatory, like most whole foods, are great with keto. Get away from processed foods, from a lot of sugar and starch *(which are all inflammatory)*, and too much protein, which can be converted to glucose for fuel. If you insist of having bread available, German rye is an option. It is very dense and relatively low carb. There are nut and seed breads, which you can make. Recipes are online that are low carb, keto-friendly. We use cauliflower bread mostly to make sandwiches, which is keto-friendly.

Finally, if you choose a keto lifestyle, you should plan to drink plenty of water and be sure to take in adequate minerals. When you are on a low- carbohydrate diet, you will have lower insulin and glycogen levels and higher ketone levels. This will cause your body to retain much less water and fewer minerals than it did before. This is why it is imperative to maintain adequate fluid and mineral intake, especially at the beginning of a low-carbohydrate diet. Whether you are strictly keto, Atkins, or use some other form of modified low carbohydrate diet, you are in the right ballpark. Just modify it to achieve your ultimate health goals. [358 - 360]

The Vitamin Connection

Vitamins *(A, Bs, C, D, E, K)* and minerals *(calcium, magnesium, zinc, iron, etc.)* are also key components and regulators of many of the processes described above. Notable examples are B1, B2, and B5, which are all involved in the various stages of deriving energy from fat, proteins, and carbohydrates. Furthermore, Iron, Niacin, and B6 help metabolize L-carnitine, which is essential for the transport of fatty acid components to energy-producing areas of cells. B9 Folate and B12 are critical to the methylation cycle, formation of neurotransmitters for cognitive performance, and reducing inflammation.

The list of similar examples is extensive, but what is key is that if you are deficient in any vitamin and/or mineral, it can mess up all your other efforts.

For example, being low in vitamin D or calcium can affect your ability to stop eating and being low in magnesium can seriously mess with your insulin sensitivity. There are many medications that deplete your body of magnesium. In this toxic world, it is very important to supplement our nutrition with a good multivitamin to cover the oxidative stress and inflammation caused by environmental chemicals and poor food quality. In my family, we choose to supplement using a multivitamin complex called Master Formula. Made with whole foods, it provides a very well-balanced nutritional micronutrient formula. Nutritional supplementation is a cold reality, necessary in today's world of toxins that cause increased levels of stress, inflammation, oxidation, free radicals, and cellular damage. [361, 362]

You don't have to be a scientist to understand what your body needs, not only to survive but also to thrive. Combining a healthy diet profile that suits your needs and adding food-based supplements can be the ticket to health and longevity, not just for you, but also for your future generations.

CHAPTER 6

Total Home Makeover
A Fresh And Clean Start To A Healthy Home

Rise and shine! Wouldn't it be nice to wake up *"clean"* - your body, your home, and your family, all safe from toxic chemicals? If you said yes to that, then get ready for a total home makeover! Creating an environmentally safe home and learning to make healthy food choices are the two things that we can all do to prevent sickness and diseases like cancer, autoimmune diseases, obesity, heart disease, diabetes, Alzheimer's, etc. And as you learn to environmentally makeover your home, imagine the impact as your lifestyle silently encourages others who may be struggling to do the same.

Creating that environmentally safe home doesn't have to be overwhelming, though it may feel that way when you first get started. Like most everything else, it gets easier the more you do it. The most important thing, though, is to get started. You may be tempted to feel guilty and say, *"I already messed up."* But be encouraged, because you are now on a different path. In the past, you did what you knew how to do. I was there too, and I am still learning - but now I have fun doing it because I can help others experience the joy, health, energy, and the zest for life that they longed for but didn't know how to achieve. Remember, an expert in anything started out as a beginner!

Setting The Stage

As part of your Total Home Makeover, I will cover each main room of the house to identify the things that need to be eliminated, and I will finish with a fairly comprehensive list of dos and don'ts. But to jump-start this discussion, I want to share the personal story from a friend that I feel will set the stage for important changes that may need to be made.

> I was told that I could not see him or call him for the *first 24 hours he was at* the facility. As I said *"goodbye"* there was so much hurt behind his beautiful blue eyes, so much uncertainty of *"Where do I fit in, why am I like this? When will my life be normal, and when will I feel at peace inside?*

Joshua was having severe behavior problems, medicated 24/7 with nine pills a day, 365 days a year, for seven years. His behavior was so out of control that he was rejected from local daycare facilities, asked to leave two private schools, placed in a *"severely emotionally handicapped"* program, and was put on medications, all starting before the age of five. He was diagnosed with ADHD, OCD, Tourette's, and mood disorders. In the fourth grade, he was institutionalized for five weeks in an outpatient facility for depression and suicidal thoughts *(in fourth grade!!)* and then in a psychiatric facility by fifth grade for threatening to kill others and harm himself. Even though testing indicated that Joshua was extremely gifted, his emotional and behavioral problems kept him labeled as emotionally handicapped. As his mother, Taunya, said goodbye to him at the psychiatric facility, she looked into his eyes and saw the pain and uncertainty that he was feeling. She shared her thoughts as she felt them at that moment of separation.

"The immense pain I felt for my child left me numb and hopeless. I wanted so badly to take him in my arms, hug him, and tell him that everything would be okay, but I didn't know that to be so. I would go to the ends of the earth for him but felt as though I was already there and didn't know where to go from there. Despite all the avenues I took, all the endless hours of searching, every year continued to grow darker and darker. After being released from the hospital, the doctor recommended weaning him off the medications, since they did not seem to be helping. The doctor assured me that by weaning Joshua off the medicines slowly there would be no problems with withdrawal. The opposite was true! We went through three weeks of severely out-of-control behavior.

Several times Joshua became extremely violent, and I came close to calling 911 for help. His reaction to withdrawal from the many drugs was a nightmare."

A mom's love for her children goes beyond comprehension. Inside, they never give up. That is not always appreciated by the children or even the father, but it is real. This situation was no different. When Joshua's childhood was stolen from him because toxic chemicals in his food changed his life, his mom never gave up. She searched numerous alternatives to help her son and happened upon the Feingold behavior treatment program that focuses on removing toxic synthetic food chemicals and dyes from the diet to improve overall health and behavior. It totally transformed Joshua's life. He was finally free, eating healthy, and responding brilliantly to life compared to where he was. Taunya writes:

"During Joshua's seventh grade year he became involved in athletics, and I watched with admiration as he showed dignity and self-control with each competition. Joshua demonstrated a wonderful balance with athletics and academics. In football, he was cool under pressure and always showed good sportsmanship. As a basketball player, he illustrated great coordination and superior instincts handling the ball. He was awesome on the court, scoring a majority of the points at nearly every game. In track, he surprised everyone when he went to district in pole vaulting and won first place. This was a sport he'd never attempted, yet he was smooth with style and grace. On the swim team, he enjoyed the meets and swam his heart out, going to district with his team and placing 2nd in several relays."

As we saw in Joshua's story, toxins can enter our homes and bodies from any number of places. When it comes to choosing safe products for your home, it can sometimes feel overwhelming. With small changes however, or one room at a time, a healthy home makeover is simplified. It is really a three-step process. Decide whether or not changes are necessary, then identify the products and lifestyle habits that need to be changed, then simply *"ditch and switch"* the bad for the good. Once you get the train moving, the momentum will carry you through, and it will start to look easy.

Setting Goals

Write down your goals based on where you need the help. Is it nutrition, cleaning out toxins, or both? Then pick where you want to start - what is most important? Detox your home one room at a time, reduce your risk of disease with a chemical-free approach throughout the house, reduce the monthly expenses by learning to make some of your own household cleaning products *(it's easy),* reduce electromagnetic frequencies *(EMF)* with some easy-to-do habits, and make your kitchen a culinary sanctuary for fine dining with healthy foods. If you happen to periodically go out for a meal that is not so healthy, don't sweat it, just come home, and detox with special herbs and essential oils. As long as you are characterized by a healthy lifestyle and your liver is doing its job, you should do very well.

Another important fact in the total home makeover is that in general, the worst air that you can breathe is in your home. As you already know, indoor air is two to five times more polluted than outdoor air, and we spend roughly 90% of our time indoors. A shocking 2009 study that examined the air inside 52 ordinary homes near the Arizona-Mexico border found indoor air was far more contaminated than previously imagined. A whopping 586 chemicals were identified, including the pesticides diazinon, chlorpyrifos, and DDT. Phthalates were also found in very high levels. Even more disturbing, they detected 120 chemicals that the researchers couldn't even identify!

Here are some general sources of toxic chemicals to consider in your home detoxification efforts: laundry soaps, dryer sheets, cleaning products, air fresheners, perfumes, cosmetics *(sorry ladies, this is one of the most polluted categories),* pet products, personal care products, pest control products, food and water, toxic chemicals, and even the air that you breathe. Think about this disturbing fact: the breathing zone of a baby *(less than two feet above ground)* can be more contaminated than an adult's *(four to six feet above ground)* because many contaminants weigh more than air *(mercury, pesticides, etc.).* For example, in one study, the pesticide, chlorpyrifos, was found to be nearly four times more concentrated at about 5-10 inches from the floor compared with the air two feet or more above the floor in a room with a window open for ventilation. Other studies have been published detailing the toxic load in homes that are harmful to your health. No two homes have exactly the same air quality issues, but you can do many things to reduce your own exposure to the worst environmental contaminants. [363 - 366]

As far back as 1989, a House Subcommittee asked The Occupational Safety and Health Administration *(OSHA)* to analyze 2,093 chemicals used in personal care products. They found 884 were toxic - 778 caused acute toxicity, 146 caused tumors, 218 caused reproductive complications, 314 caused biological mutations leading to cancer, and 376 caused skin irritations and eye development problems. That was 1989! It has been estimated that about 1000 new chemicals are introduced each year. So, is this really a big deal? If these ingredients were truly bad, why are they in our commonly used products? Good question and hopefully I have answered that throughout this book. It is easy to understand why so many are skeptical about the detrimental effect toxins have on our health. But it is true, and the impact on our health after long-term use is becoming more evident. Some of the more common health disorders resulting from personal care products for example include:

- Sleep Problems
- Migraines
- Hormone Imbalances
- Mood Swings
- Fertility Issues
- Heart Rate Issues
- Blood Pressure Issues
- Asthma
- Low Energy
- Skin Disorders
- Allergies
- Cancer
- Add/ADHD
- Auto Immune Disorders

Identifying Products Room By Room

In each room of the house, there are products that you definitely want to ditch and switch to more healthy versions. Most are those used regularly and some are stashed away in a cupboard or drawer. We tend not to think about these until they are needed. But going through these lists of items will prompt you to be on the lookout when the time comes to deal with each room.

Laundry Room: Household cleaners, laundry detergents, dryer sheets, insecticides, stain remover, bleach, air fresheners, and fabric softeners.

- Dryer sheets are among the most toxic products in your laundry room. You smell those artificial fragrance and softener chemicals all day long on your clothes, and your skin absorbs them. Wool dryer balls with essential oils dripped on them replace toxic dryer sheets beautifully. Static cling is reduced with vinegar in rinse cycle and/or damp drying.

- *"Dirty"* cleaning products known to be hormone disruptors, carcinogens, and liver toxins include phthalates, phosphates, perfumes, DEA *(diethanolamine),* ethylene glycol, propylene glycol *(also in antifreeze and cake mixes),* and butoxyethanol used in window cleaners.

Kitchen: Counter dish soap, automatic dishwasher soap, hand soap, lotion, fruit and veggie wash, scouring powder, all-purpose cleaner.

Living Room: Furniture polish, dusting spray, carpet deodorizer, carpet cleaner, air freshener, candles, fabric freshener.

- Most air fresheners interfere with your ability to smell by coating your nasal passages with a nerve-deadening agent. The toxic chemicals include camphor, phenol, ethanol, formaldehyde, and artificial chemical fragrances. They can cause headaches, rashes, dizziness, migraines, asthma attacks, mental confusion, coughing, and more. Some of the substances are also linked to cancer and hormone disruption.

Bedroom: Furniture polish, dusting spray, carpet deodorizer, carpet cleaner, air freshener, laundry detergents and softeners on bedding, candles, and personal lubricants.

- FYI: You and your children may be snuggling with poisons from laundry products! These are chemicals that can linger in bed sheets, blankets, pillows, etc.

- Alpha-Terpineol - Linked to disorders of the brain and nervous system, loss of muscle control, depression, headaches

- Benzyl acetate - Linked to cancer of the pancreas.

- Benzyl alcohol - Linked to headaches, nausea, vomiting, dizziness, depression and disorders of the brain and nervous system

- Chloroform - On EPA's hazardous list

- Ethanol - Listed on EPA's hazardous waste list - brain and nervous system disorders

- Ethyl Acetate - Listed on EPA's hazardous waste list, causes headaches

- Pentene - Causes headaches, nausea, dizziness, fatigue, drowsiness and depression

- Quarternary ammonium Compounds - Causes contact dermatitis and respiratory disorders

Baby and Children's Room: wipes, diaper rash cream, baby lotion, baby shampoo, baby oil, baby wash, chemicals in bedding from laundry, air fresheners, diaper pail freshener, soothing scents, linen spray, toys.

- FYI: Hazardous substances in consumer products are a constant worry. Because children have less body mass and are developing rapidly, toxic chemicals in toys are of particular concern. Recent studies have revealed alarming levels of cadmium and lead in products intended for children, including compounds in plastics, such as phthalates and Bisphenol A, that have harmful effects. For instance, in a first-of-its-kind study published by the American Chemical Society, researchers analyzed 59 baby teethers commonly sold in the United States, and found 100% of them contained Bisphenol A *(BPA)*, Bisphenol S *(BPS)* or Bisphenol F *(BPF)*, and most contained various parabens, as well as the antimicrobials, triclosan and triclocarban, known carcinogens. This is a serious problem and regulations should be much stricter. [367, 368]

Bathroom: bleach/mildew spray, cosmetics, chemical cleaners, air fresheners, toothpaste, skin care, perfumes/fragrances, hair spray, make-up, shampoos and conditioners, mouthwash.

- Certain chemicals in shampoos, toothpaste, lotions, etc., which hinder the proper development of the eyes to which children under the age of six are very vulnerable. No More Tears shampoo, a well-known product marketed for babies contained a formaldehyde-releasing ingredient called Quaternium, a known carcinogen. In 2014, due to public pressure, its makers announced that quaternium and a few others ingredients would be removed, which they were. But the shampoo still contains toxic chemicals including dyes and others that should be avoided.

Cosmetics

Since cosmetics are REALLY big business, I am including this special section to give an overview of an under-regulated industry that uses some very toxic chemicals in their products. Almost 13,000 chemicals are used in cosmetics and only about 10% have been evaluated for safety. The average US woman uses 12 personal care products a day, containing 168 different chemicals. Also, in the report, *"Heavy Metal Hazard: The Health Risks of Hidden Heavy Metals in Face Makeup,"* Environmental Defence tested 49 different makeup items, including foundations, concealers, powders, blushes, mascaras, eyeliners, eye shadows, lipsticks, and lip glosses. Their testing revealed serious heavy metal contamination in virtually all of the products:

- 96% contained lead

- 90% contained beryllium

- 61% contained thallium

- 51% contained cadmium

- 20% contained arsenic

There are other chemicals risks as well. In 2000, the EWG *(Environmental Working Group)* released a study showing that 37 nail polishes from 22 companies contained dibutyl phthalate *(DBP)*. DBP is known to cause lifelong reproductive impairments in male rats and has been shown to damage the testes, prostate gland, epididymis, penis, and seminal vesicles in animals.

It's used in nail polish because it increases flexibility and shine, but research by the US Centers for Disease Control and Prevention *(CDC)* revealed that all 289 people tested had DBP in their bodies. Worse still, this chemical, which is linked to birth defects in animals, was found at the highest levels in women of childbearing age. [369]

Many have *"secret chemicals"* that have been identified but are not listed on the label because they are *"exempt"* from labeling regulations. The FDA does not require reporting on any flavor, fragrance, or trade secrets. Under the Federal Food, Drug, and Cosmetic Act and the Fair Packaging and Labeling Act, the FDA can regulate cosmetic chemicals. But it only steps in if it has *"reliable information"* that there is a problem. In practice, that has often meant that nothing is done until a public outcry forces them to be involved to regulate or remove the harmful chemicals. From the FDA website on cosmetics: *"Companies and individuals who manufacture or market cosmetics have a legal responsibility to ensure the safety of their products. Neither the law nor FDA regulations require specific tests to demonstrate the safety of individual products or ingredients. The law also does not require cosmetic companies to share their safety information with the FDA. . . . FDA's legal authority over cosmetics is different from our authority over other products we regulate, such as drugs, biologics, and medical devices. Under the law, cosmetic products and ingredients do not need FDA premarket approval, with the exception of color additives. . . . However, FDA can pursue enforcement action against products on the market that are not in compliance with the law, or against firms or individuals who violate the law."*

There are some natural makeup lines out there, just do your homework. These chemicals will take their toll and, while you think ladies that they may make you pretty and sexy, what happens to your skin and insides down the road won't be so pretty. [370 - 373]

Here is some additional information on household products that should be assessed for safety - just to give you an idea of the pervasiveness of toxins throughout the house.

Other Household Products

Shower Curtains - Vinyl shower curtains are made with polyvinyl chloride *(PVC)*, otherwise known as plastic number 3 or vinyl, a plastic that can release hormone-disrupting phthalates into the air. These gases can linger in your home for up to four months. Purchase no-chemical cloth shower curtains instead of the plastic.

Water Filters - Reverse osmosis water filters are a good alternative. No tap water is okay without a good quality filtration system. Tap water is filled with toxic chemicals and medications that have been poured down the drain or urinated into the toilet that go into the drinking water system. For the most part, these do not get filtered out by the municipal water filtration systems. Any filter system is better than none, but get a proven system to insure that it will remove the chemicals that you are concerned about. We also have a very large Berkey that we keep around for emergencies. This removes fluoride and all chemicals and heavy metals from your water.

Bedding - Sadly, our pillows, mattresses, and blankets are full of chemicals and flame-retardants that can interfere with our health.

Air Filters - Keep air filters inspected and changed frequently. They can significantly reduce the toxins inhaled in your home on a daily basis. Cigarette smoke, dust, pet dander, lead, off-gassing from carpets, formaldehyde from particle board, chemicals in aerosol sprays, unclean air ducts, fumes from cleaning products, benzene, carbon monoxide, asbestos, flame retardants, and more can all contribute to air that's unhealthy to breathe.

Plastics - Remove any containers, bowls, cups, plates, bowls, etc. that are plastic and replace them with glass or ceramic. If you use paper plates know that if they have a shine on them, they have a plastic coating that can come off with acidic or hot food products. Even the ones without that shine, and you think are safe, are treated with chemicals to bleach them white and make them pleasing to your eye.

Mold - Mold is common in any damp area in the home, such as bathrooms and basements. Be sure to keep these areas dry and check regularly for mold. Mold is the cause of numerous health issues. We had an undiagnosed mold problem from a shower leak into the bottom of a towel closet next to the shower. There was a sort of sweet smell in the bathroom that was unusual but we just couldn't identify. Someone mentioned mold, and we freaked! The whole bathroom was sealed, and a mold remediation team came in to clean it up. There are some simple DIY preparations that can kill mold so always have these on hand. Vinegar, essential oils, soap, and water can do the job.

Carpets - Look for natural carpet options without any chemical treatment. They are out there, but you may have to spend some time searching. Better to limit carpet in the house as much as possible. Carpets contain harmful chemicals, including volatile organic compounds *(VOCs)*, flame-retardants, anti-stain ingredients, and other harmful chemicals.

Pots and Pans - It is best to stay away from Teflon-coated nonstick pans, which can release small chemical toxins into the air and particles into your food when the pans are heated. They also have perfluorochemicals *(PVCs)*, which are used to coat carpets, clothes, furniture, and food packaging, among other things. They can persist in the human body and have been associated with lower birth weight for babies, cancer, infertility, elevated cholesterol, and liver problems. Safe options include titanium/ceramic, cast iron pans, high quality, stainless steel, and glass bakeware.

Microwave Ovens - We had a microwave oven BC *(before children)*. We just didn't pay much attention to the various health risks of microwaves, or most other foods. We were young and indestructible - most of you can relate. But then the kids started to come, five of them! And life took on a whole new meaning. It wasn't just us that we were responsible for. So, we started to shift perspective in a number of health-related ways. One of those was regarding microwave ovens. After doing a fair amount of research, we decided to remove our microwave oven from our house. That was about twenty years ago, and we haven't missed it. I highly recommend that you do the same. The research shows several disturbing facts about the impact of microwaves on our health from various sources such as ovens, Bluetooth, and cell phones.

Contrary to popular belief, microwaved foods don't actually cook from the inside out. Microwave cooking begins within the molecules where water is present. Since not all areas contain the same amount of water, the heating is uneven. When thicker foods are cooked, microwaves heat the outer layers, and the inner layers are cooked mostly by the conduction of heat from the hot, outer layers, inward. Also, besides depleting your food's nutritional value, microwave ovens can produce carcinogenic toxins, which can be of concern. Also, when heating packages, carcinogens like dioxin, benzene, toluene, and xylene can leach out into your food. When plastic is heated, toxic chemicals like BPA and phthalates can leach out of the containers or covers, contaminating your food with endocrine and hormone disruptors. Even acidic foods like spaghetti sauce can leach out plastics into your foods especially when heated in a microwave oven. Microwave ovens also damage food, producing carcinogens and destroying nutrients.

While there is still some controversy over the totality of microwaves on health from the various sources, I believe it is better to remove the ovens because they are just not needed, and why take the risk for you and your family? [374 - 375]

Dyes

Dyes - Can be natural or synthetic, harmless or very harmful. Synthetic dyes permeate the food and cosmetic industry because they are cheap to make, but like the rest of the manufactured chemical world, the human toll seems to be ignored unless the industry is forced to make changes. Synthetic food dyes originally made from coal tar and now petroleum, have long been controversial. Many dyes have been banned because of their adverse effects on laboratory animals. It is said that we *"eat with our eyes as much as with our mouths,"* and that's certainly the case when we walk down the aisles of a supermarket. The brightly colored oranges are made that way with a toxic synthetic dye, and Fruit Loops boxes with cereal that contain synthetic dyes, and so many others entice us to purchase otherwise unattractive processed foods. Synthetic dyes are a lot cheaper than natural dyes, but most are also health hazards waiting to happen.

There are other more natural and healthy options such as beta-carotene *(a precursor to vitamin A),* paprika, beet juice, and turmeric. But the changes won't take place unless there is consumer pressure to do so. While the European Union has placed regulations on labeling food dyes to inform consumers of the health risks, the United States has no such requirement. Synthetic food dyes are one of the most widely used and dangerous additives. For example, the Center for Science in the Public Interest *(CSPI)* reported the following: *"The three most widely used dyes, Red 40, Yellow 5, and Yellow 6, are contaminated with known carcinogens . . . Another dye, Red 3, has been acknowledged for years by the Food and Drug Administration to be a carcinogen, yet is still in the food supply."*

I have highlighted the dyes that are most used and their side effects. My recommendation is to stay from all food and cosmetic synthetic dyes and to make some noise to force changes in labeling regulations and to remove those synthetic dyes that are harmful to your health. [376]

- **Blue #2** *(Indigo Carmine)* Causes a statistically significant incidence of tumors, particularly brain gliomas, in male rats. What it's in: Colored beverages, candies, pet food, & other food and drugs.

- **Citrus Red #2** It's toxic to rodents at modest levels and caused tumors of the urinary bladder and possibly other organs. What it's in: Skins of Florida oranges.

- **Green #23** *(Fast Green)* Caused significant increases in bladder and testes tumors in male rats. What it's in: Drugs, personal care products, cosmetic products except in eye area, candies, beverages, ice cream, sorbet, ingested drugs, lipsticks, and externally applied cosmetics.

- **Red #3** *(Erythrosine)* Recognized in 1990 by the FDA as a thyroid carcinogen in animals and is banned in cosmetics and externally applied drugs. What it's in: It's in Sausage casings, oral medication, maraschino cherries, baked goods, and candies.

- **Red #40** *(Allura Red)* This is the most-widely used and consumed dye. It may accelerate the appearance of immune system tumors in mice. It also causes hypersensitivity *(allergy-like)* reactions in some consumers and might trigger hyperactivity in children. What it's in: Beverages, bakery goods, dessert powders, candies, cereals, foods, drugs, and cosmetics.

- **Yellow #5** *(Tartrazine)* Yellow 5 causes sometimes-severe hypersensitivity reactions and might trigger hyperactivity and other behavioral effects in children. What it's in: Pet foods, numerous bakery goods, pickles, beverages, dessert powders, candies, cereals, gelatin desserts, and many other foods, as well as pharmaceuticals and cosmetics.

- **Yellow #6** *(Sunset Yellow)* Caused adrenal tumors in animals and occasionally causes severe hypersensitivity reactions. What it's in:

Colored bakery goods, cereals, beverages, dessert powders, candies, gelatin deserts, sausage, cosmetics, and drugs. [377 - 380]

I recommend making checklists that can be referred to along the way. They can serve as reminders, encouragements, check-off lists, to help you as you grow into your New Beginnings lifestyle. My wife and I couldn't make all the changes at once, so we started with the things that were most important at the time and when we got that done, we moved to the next goal. We even offered to go through someone's house and help them know where to start. Sometimes we recommend going through the pantry and just throwing everything into the trash can that had toxic chemicals. That may leave the cupboards bare in some houses, but that's okay. It forces you to go to the store and get something healthy for the family. Then the cleaners, nutritional supplements, personal care products, makeup, essential oils . . . the works. Get it so clean that you would feel safe inviting someone over with environmental illnesses who can't visit other people because of the toxic load in the home. That's the goal! It may take some time to get there, but you will if it is important to you. There is no failure here - it just is!

My Top Evidence-Based Healthy Lifestyle Habits

Food Based Habits

- If you are consuming simple carbohydrates, don't drink sugar calories, and minimize other edible sugar calories. Use stevia, xylitol, erythritol, and occasional honey and molasses as sweeteners. Do not use Splenda or other artificial sweeteners. They can be neurotoxic.

- Eat plenty of nuts. Buy organic when you can. They are high and good fats and are very nutritious and healthy and can help you lose weight, fight diabetes, and heart disease.

- Eat real food instead of processed food and snacks. They are filled with toxic chemicals, high fructose corn syrup, dyes, and other designer chemicals to keep you hooked. These are major contributing reasons why the world is sicker than ever before.

- Don't consume caffeinated coffee. There is a 40% loss of oxygen to your brain with just one cup. Caffeine it is a major vasoconstrictor affecting most organ systems in the body. It interferes with adenosine receptors in the brain, causes addictive responses similar to cocaine, severely alters brain wave activity, increases risk of heart attack, stroke, and high blood pressure, and is a diuretic causing loss of water.

- Drink home brewed organic tea. It is filled with healthy ingredients especially catechins and L theanine. There are many varieties from which to choose. Just don't buy the typical *"cheapo"* teas. Green, white, and oolong tea leaves tend to have the most health benefits.

- If you eat fish, eat small fatty fish with short life spans. They are full of DHA and EPA and are less likely to be contaminated with mercury and other toxins. Close to shore, wild Alaskan salmon is very healthy as well.

- Take care of your gut health. Remember from the previous chapters, your gut houses your immune system. Prebiotics, probiotics, enzyme supplements, organic foods that help reduce glyphosate load, sauerkraut, and plenty of veggies and fiber.

- Drink at least two quarts of *"healthy"* water per day, especially before meals. Make it reverse osmosis, no plastic water bottles, use rubber-coated glass bottles, and filtered deep well water that has been tested for contaminants. Also, reverse osmosis removes most of the minerals in water, so make sure you replace them with a pure sea salt (not Himalayan which has radioactive and other elements that are not beneficial to the body – we use Redmond Real Salt)). Anything but straight city or municipal treated tap water which can be contaminated with chemicals, prescription medications, cancer drugs, and much more.

- One study in Obesity journal in 2010, *Water Consumption Increases Weight Loss...* showed that drinking 16 ounces of water before a meal has also been shown to help with weight loss by 44%.

- Take food-based vitamins, not synthetic.

- Always have fresh vegetables on the table. Cruciferous and colored veggies give you a variety of nutrients. Cooking vegetables can destroy the vitamins that you are hoping to consume. They are okay to eat but have fresh on the table as well. No microwaved foods.

- Organic fruits are good, but fruit juices can be detrimental to your health. Processed fruit juices have high sugar content, and nutrients are destroyed in the heating/pasteurization process, and then some vitamins will be replaced with artificial. A couple of large pieces of fresh fruit are good but watch the sugar content. Complex fruits like berries are more nutritious with less simple sugar.

- Consuming fats can be very healthy for you as long as they are not trans fats or vegetable oils. Fatty oils like olive, avocado, hemp seed, palm, and coconut are all healthy. Purchasing MCT *(medium-chain triglyceride)* oils and adding it to shakes is very healthy as well. Most of these are extracted from coconut oil, but as mentioned previously, when purchasing MCTs make sure that it has caprylic *(C8)* and capric acid *(C10)* and very little lauric acid *(C12)*, C6, C8, and C10 MCTs. Saturated animal fats can be healthy too, just make sure they come from healthy sources.

- Make essential oils a part of your healthy lifestyle plan. They are an integral part of our healthy lifestyle efforts and have been responsible for solving many health challenges, physical and emotional. I cover this in greater detail in the New Beginning chapter. The quality and source of essential oils are very important. Do your homework. Lavender for instance is one of the most adulterated oils in the marketplace. It may smell like lavender, but that $5 bottle of oil is not real lavender - it is synthetic or has been adulterated with additives. EOs can be used in many household, nutrition, and personal care products, and can help ward off nasties that can interfere with your overall health.

- Don't diet. Many fad diets are not based on science. Change lifestyle habits with a why instead. You can tweak your lifestyle habits to lose weight with a sustainable science-based weight control program.

- Buy organic. While not perfect, like growing your own, it is still the best choice. Find local co-ops that order in bulk. We order from Azure Standard. It is cool because we order online, and a truck comes from across the country to a drop-off point and everyone goes and picks up their order. They cut out the middleman saving a lot of money for healthy foods.

- Consume home-prepared meals as much as possible. Most everything else will have mystery chemicals.

- Fix your kid's lunches. Don't let them eat that chemical-laden cafeteria food which can be devoid of many needed nutrients, contributes to obesity, allergies, and other medical disorders.

- Learn to respectfully say no when offered unhealthy food by others. Or, if it is a must, just pray over your food.

- Eat healthy snacks. Learn to be creative with healthy smoothies, juicing, and blending.

- Enrich your diet with whole food vitamins, minerals, and prebiotics. Eat wild fermented foods such as sauerkrauts and kimchi. Probiotics are good, but take breaks, so the gut does not become overrun with the same bacteria colonies. Wild fermented kombucha is good too but watch the sugar content and caffeine. Water kefir is a good choice as well.

- Dairy can be good depending on the source. Avoid milk and other dairy products that contain the genetically engineered recombinant bovine growth hormone *(rBGH or rBST)*. If you drink dairy, find an organic farm. Raw milk products from A2A2 cows can be a much better choice than A1A2 for some, and certainly a better choice over pasteurized milk, which is essentially colored water. Farm fresh milk will have more good bacteria and enzymes, which have all but been destroyed from the pasteurization process. Make sure that no glyphosate is used on the farm. Glyphosate-free yogurt and cream can be good too.

- Coconut, organic unsweetened almond milk, goat's milk and even camel's milk are great alternatives to cow's milk as long as they do not have added ingredients like carrageenan - which is carcinogenic and inflammatory.

- Grow an herb and vegetable garden. Got a small space? Square Foot Gardening is a book that I used when we lived in a suburb neighborhood with smaller lots. It will show you how to best utilize your space.

- Slow cookers are great for preparing meals for the working mom.

- If you are supplementing, be sure to use supplements from whole foods. If MTHFR positive, supplement with 6S-5-methyltetrahydrofolate. For additional support in making neurotransmitters along the folate pathway, you can add SAMe if needed. There are a number of suppliers to choose from. And, it is best to stay away from high doses of folic acid, especially if you are MTHFR mutation-positive or deficient in another enzyme, dihydrofolate reductase *(DHFR)* that takes synthetic folic acid and converts it into a form that puts it onto the folate highway to be further converted to bioactive folate.

Action Habits

- Buy products that come in glass bottles rather than plastic or cans as much as possible, as chemicals can leach out of plastics *(and plastic can linings),* into the contents; be aware that even *"BPA-free"* plastics typically leach other endocrine-disrupting chemicals that are just as bad for you as BPA. Store your food and beverages in glass, rather than plastic, and avoid using plastic wrap as much as possible but don't let it touch your food. Use glass baby bottles to reduce exposure of BPA and other plastics.

- Replace your non-stick pots and pans with ceramic or glass cookware.

- Filter your tap water for both drinking AND bathing. To remove the endocrine-disrupting herbicide Atrazine, make sure your filter is certified to remove it. According to the EWG, perchlorate (covered in *The Killing Fields* chapter) can be filtered out using a reverse osmosis filter.

- Look for products made by companies that are friendly to your body and the environment. This applies to everything from food and personal care products to building materials, carpeting, paint, baby items, furniture, mattresses, and others.

- Do not use fluoride. It is totally unnecessary in water and toothpaste and has been shown to cause cancer and interfere with thyroid function and other systemic effects. Toothpaste can also contain triclosan, a carcinogen like fluoride. Maintain good oral hygiene with essential oil-based products such as toothpaste and mouthwash.

- Use a vacuum cleaner with a HEPA filter to remove contaminated house dust. This is one of the major routes of exposure to flame-retardant chemicals. When buying new products such as furniture, mattresses, or carpet padding, consider buying flame-retardant-free varieties, containing naturally less flammable materials, such as leather, wool, cotton, silk, and Kevlar.

- Avoid stain-resistant and water-resistant clothing, furniture, and carpets to avoid perfluorinated chemicals.

- Make sure your baby's toys are BPA-free, such as pacifiers, teething rings, and anything your child may be prone to suck or chew on - even books, which are often plasticized. It's advisable to avoid all plastic, especially flexible varieties.

- Use natural cleaning products or make your own. Avoid those containing 2-butoxyethanol and methoxydiglycol - two toxic glycol ethers that can compromise your fertility and cause fetal harm. Don't expect to always find that information on the ingredients list. You may have to contact the manufacturer for a full list of ingredients if you want to continue using that specific product. Best solution? Go natural with essential oil-based cleaning products. That is what we do.

- Switch over to organic toiletries, including shampoo, toothpaste, antiperspirants, and cosmetics. EWG's Skin Deep database can help you find personal care products that are free of phthalates and other potentially dangerous chemicals.

- Replace your vinyl shower curtain with a fabric one.

- Replace feminine hygiene products *(tampons and sanitary pads)* with safer alternatives. Do not use non-organic cotton tampons. They are filled with pesticides, fungicides, and other nasty chemicals.

- Look for fragrance-free products. One artificial fragrance can contain hundreds - even thousands - of potentially toxic chemicals. Avoid fabric softeners and dryer sheets, which contain a mishmash of synthetic chemicals and fragrances.

- Stay away from manufactured chemical perfumes. They don't have to tell you all of the toxic chemicals that are in that alluring fragrance. And don't use plug-in fragrances.

- Avoid both active smoking and passive second-hand smoke. If you can't avoid it because of your job, get another job that is physically and emotionally safe and healthy. Your body deserves the respect.

- Use all-natural bug repellents. Again, essential oils do a fantastic job without the nasty chemicals seen on most OTC bug repellents.

- Use only chemical-free deodorants. No antiperspirants. Baking soda, coconut oil, and some water mixed with essential oils works great. Some essential oils are very antibacterial so body odor can be eliminated.

- Good quality sleep is critical. Sleep quality is also one of the strongest risk factors for obesity and heart disease. Your body repairs itself at night and the cleanup crew can't do its job well if you are not getting enough quality sleep.

- Interval fast/slow walking is a great way to exercise. It conditions the heart and causes less oxidative stress to the body compared to other strenuous routines.

- Work out and stretch daily. Yoga can be a good choice for some, but there are many others out there as well. Go to the gym with a friend. It increases the accountability factor. [381 - 386]

Have a forward-thinking plan and implement only as much as you think you can handle at one time. If you overload yourself with too many changes at once at the expense of other priorities such as family, there will be negative consequences as well. Meet with the family, tell them how much you love them and that you want a healthier lifestyle in the home, so some changes are coming. One thing that children love is to see humility and vulnerability in parents. We all make mistakes so, don't hesitate to apologize for past lifestyle practices if that is appropriate. They appreciate your caring about them, and apologizing may teach them a good life lesson. Then make it family team effort. Put the kiddos in charge of some aspect of your transformation.

CHAPTER 7

New Beginnings

And suddenly, you just know it's time to start something different, and trust the magic of new beginnings. Meister Echart

New beginnings are relevant - they give us hope. They may even ignite spunk in us that has been long buried. We sometimes get so caught up in the routine that we forget the fresh passions and new beginnings that drove us to curiosity and exploration in years past.

Spring is a great time of new beginnings here on our 70-acre farm. We moved here several years ago from the hustle and bustle of a rapidly growing and upscale suburban community. Farm life is so much more chill and soothes the soul. I love walking, exploring, and finding new life almost on a daily basis. A new flower catches my eye and invites me in for a nose kiss to enjoy its fragrant bouquet, a bird greets the farm in the early morn with its sweet song of hope: life is good. All of nature sings its gift of new life. It is also a time of letting go of the past. The winters of life serve their purpose. But we can't stay there. When we feed the energy of pain from winters past, we don't have enough energy to feed our new beginnings in the springs of life. We can't grow; we just exist. New beginnings may signify a whole host of changes unique to each of us. They are inevitable and can be as simple as spring-cleaning, a new wardrobe, a new hairstyle, or as momentous as a change in careers, new lifestyle choices, or dusting off old dreams. We do have a choice in how to redefine ourselves to make the most of these transitional moments in life. Have courage and embrace them! [387]

New Beginnings is about you - personally - first and foremost. Because when you are physically, emotionally, and spiritually healthy, you become wise, equipped, confident, beautiful, fresh and radiant, tempered with humility, and it magnifies your strength, creating endless possibilities for growth. You are ready to get out there with a life-giving message and make a difference for yourself and others. As you grow and thrive, you can help others do the same, setting that example for the rest of the family, your friends, and community. What speaks louder than a changed life?

Growth is where you walk alone, move out of your comfort zone and take risks. It cannot be delegated and is a continuing process of exploration and change. Humility drives the quality of that growth. There is also no failure in growth - all failure is success because you grow from it - the willingness to fail in the process is a strength. If you make it weakness, if you keep telling yourself that you are a failure, then like an echo in a chambered valley, that will resonate back on you many times over and you become what you believe about yourself. I will for sure help you on the what and how, but that will not carry you through. You will also need a why - your own personal why. Your why - your purpose - will help define you and your success. It makes you special - and you are special! If there is no why, it won't end well. If you know the why, your vision is clear - a magnificent blend of colors and life and energy for the journey.

Before we get too far though, let me offer you some encouragement. Some of you may be living in chronic despair. You cope, but honestly, life is miserable, and you just seem to exist and not much more. Maybe it's poor health, broken relationships, unfulfilled dreams, children that have gone astray or are even hateful towards you, or some other event that is stealing your joy and zest for life. Sometimes life stinks. Been there, done that. While unpleasant for now, that doesn't define you unless you choose to let it. As a matter of fact, that stinky stuff of life is actually good and will help you grow. It is like manure fertilizer. Those of you who have put manure around your plants know what I mean. For the rest of you, trust me, it smells really bad. But the stink is only for a short while and once it settles, it is great to help plants thrive. It gets deep down to the roots and provides critical nutrients for healthy plant growth. The stinky stuff of life, while unpleasant, promotes personal growth - it is a necessary part of life and helps us to thrive. But, when you're up to your eyeballs in the manure of life, it is certainly hard to see that it's going to help us thrive. The bottom line is that there is a tension between where you are now and where you know you should be. It comes down to wanting versus choosing. Wanting keeps you where you are. It is a non-active term. Choosing moves you toward where you should be - and it changes everything.

As you step forward into your new beginnings, I want to encourage you to keep your mind open about many things. Choosing to live the life you were meant to live is going to require change, perhaps much change, and in some ways it may be difficult emotionally, spiritually, and physically. But you are ready, or you wouldn't still be reading.

PART ONE

Discovering The Real You - Understanding The Emotional Matrix

There are three basic things that human interactions crave: safety, a sense of belonging, and to feel like they matter. Safety includes security, stability, and freedom from fear. It's a primal need that begins very early in life. Belonging includes being part of a tribe, having equal value, and connecting in meaningful ways to others. That passion is very strong. Feeling like we matter includes doing something in life that makes a difference; some call this *"purpose."* Reactions to situations run deep into the subconscious, and part of our emotional health journey is to flush out and discard the old stuff that may interfere with our ability to trust others, to feel safe, to love and understand others, and have healthy and productive relationships.

New beginnings should start with an accounting of our emotional health. Living in the emotional matrix can be a blessing or a nightmare and many places in between. My hope is to give you enough tools to help you evaluate your emotional wellbeing and then perhaps begin to look at interpersonal relationships in a new way.

I think most of us would agree that our emotional responses to the world in which we live are complicated to say the least. And, for me, while I am finally feeling comfortable in my own skin, I am still learning about others, and at the same time still learning more about myself *(a lifelong process)*. People process their experiences through so many filters; it is often not easy to gauge how they really feel. Heck, they don't even understand their own feelings. I don't always understand mine either. You know why? Because about 90% of emotional responses come from the subconscious. They are based on genetic and epigenetic experiences throughout life, most of which can occur prenatally to about six to eight years of age, and are then embedded as learned responses. The immediate emotions we feel as human beings are ultimately protective and survival messages delivered via the subconscious. 388, 389

Your Basic Personality Framework

So, where do we start in this matrix and how do we make reasonable sense of it all, and maybe encourage some emotional healing and new beginnings for you and family and friends? Just getting an overview of personality types might be the best place. Personality describes the defining characteristics that make you, YOU! We all have our own *"personality language."* We use this language to speak to and understand the world in which we live. The way we perceive the world is heavily influenced by our inborn temperament and shaped by our life experiences. Hippocrates, The Father of Medicine, *(c 460-c.370 BC)* first advanced the Theory of Personalities, that one's own persona is based on four distinct temperaments. Personality describes temperament *(which is comprised of the person's abilities, motivations, defense mechanisms, values)* influenced by life experiences. There have been many adaptations of this basic system throughout the centuries.

The Hippocrates/Galen Personality Model

Based on the four-temperament model, Greek physician Aelius Galenus *(Galen)* devised the terms sanguine, choleric, melancholy, and phlegmatic to describe the impact of The Hippocrates' Four Humors of personality. They are based on observable external behavior unlike the Enneagram Personality inventory which is based on internal motivation. Here is a brief description.[390]

Choleric:

- Basic Tendencies: Fast-Paced, Task-Oriented, Extroverted, Optimistic

- Strengths: Decisive, Takes Action, Good Delegator, Self-confident, Takes Risks, Good Debater *(actually energized by conflict!)* Movers/ Shakers

- Weaknesses: Bossy, Impatient, Harsh, Blunt

Sanguine:

- Basic Tendencies: Fast-Paced, People-Oriented, Extroverted, Optimistic

- Strengths: Fun Loving, Enthusiastic, Emotional, Great Communicators

- Weaknesses: Disorganized, Can't Remember Names or Details, Gullible, Poor Time Managers

Melancholy:

- Basic Tendencies: Slow-Paced, Task-Oriented, Introverted, Pessimistic

- Strengths: Accurate, Analytical, Attentive to Details, High Standards, Intuitive, Controlled, Organized, Gives 110% to whatever they do.

- Weaknesses: Too critical, Perfectionist, Easily Depressed, Too Focused on details and preparation

Phlegmatic:

- Basic Tendencies: Slow-Paced, Other-Oriented, Introverted, Quiet, Background Players

- Strengths: Patient, Easygoing, Team Player, Calming Influence, Steady, Balanced, Dry Sense of Humor.

- Weaknesses: Indecisive, Over-accommodating, Too Passive, Conflict Avoider

We are all wired differently, and most of us are a blend of two personalities. Perhaps that explains why there have been so many different personality profile tests developed over the years. Most will measure external behavior - how someone will respond to the world around them, which helps a lot in understanding what to expect in outward behavior.

The Enneagram Of Personalities

What is even more important is the *"why"* of behavior. Internal motivation is what really drives behavior. That can be measured using an even more ancient and sophisticated system called the Enneagram of Personalities. Covering the Four Temperaments and the Enneagram in some detail gives a big picture for your further study. These tests are an excellent tool in developing effective communication skills for yourself and others, which are critical for emotional health.

The Enneagram of Personalities is a powerful gateway to self-awareness and understanding of others. A schematic diagram describes the structure and dynamics of nine personality types, opening a path to a more integrated and rewarding life. [391] The Enneagram's exact ancient history is uncertain, although the system first appeared in both Asia and the Middle East several thousand years ago or longer. Because it evolved as an oral tradition, it is difficult to know its precise origins, though its roots spread out over several thousand years, culminating in the Enneagram diagram and tests that are very popular today. It uses a nine-point diagram that represents nine distinct strategies for identifying self and for relating to other. Each Enneagram type has a different pattern of thinking, feeling and acting that arises from a deeper inner motivation. And that is the main difference between the standard temperament/personality models, which only describe external behaviors. This is a huge distinction and totally rocked my world after teaching the four-type personality model for over twenty years. It is so much more important to understand the why, but being a student of both models is important in order to have well-rounded, mature identity and communication skills. We all have some common experiences in life, but how we process and respond to those experiences will be different - not better or worse, just different. And, there are some group commonalities in motivations and external responses. Both models help to paint a picture of those differences and commonalities. The Enneagram just gives us a much broader understanding of ourselves and others. We can have much more fulfilling relationships that way.

Let's begin with an overview of the nine basic personality types.

Type 1 - The Reformer gains worthiness and love through being good, correcting errors in self, others, and the world. Ones have an emphasis on personal integrity and self-control. Their attention goes toward seeing and correcting what is wrong and doing the right thing. They are known for their honesty, dependability, and common sense. They have high standards and tend to see the world in black and white, right and wrong. It's easy for them to be critical, of themselves as well as others. Ones can suffer anxiety about *"getting it right,"* and often delays action until it is right. They may suppress personal needs, delay pleasure, and can become engulfed in detail that impairs productivity.

- Gifts: honesty, industry, responsibility, ethical and fair - they will work hard for vision of improvement.

- Goal: embody integrity through perfection.

- Strengths: Honest, responsible, improvement-oriented.

- Problems: Resentful, non-adaptable, overly critical.

- Speaking style: Precise and detail-oriented, with a tendency to sermonize or preach.

- Lower emotional habit: Resentment, which comes from getting angry, but holding it in.

- Higher emotion: Serenity, which comes with letting go of anger about the way things are and accepting imperfection.

- Archetypal challenge: To change what can be changed, to accept what cannot be changed, and to develop the wisdom to know the difference.

Type 2 - The Helper seeks approval, love, and fulfillment of needs through giving to significant others and alters their own needs to meet the needs of others. They focus on relationships, making connections, and empathizing with the needs and feelings of other people. Usually good at supporting others and helping bring out their potential which can lead to denial of own needs and authentic self which leads to feeling controlled and longing for freedom. They want to be accepted and liked by others and will adapt or change to earn this approval. Setting personal boundaries can be challenging.

- Gifts: Giving, supportive, sensitive to others needs and feelings, energetic, and romantic.

- Goal: Stay connected through partnership.

- Strengths: Caring, popular, communicator.

- Problems: Privileged, naive, dependent.

- Speaking style: Being nice and sympathetic, giving advice, sometimes militant for a cause

- Lower emotional habit: Pride about being special, important, or indispensable in relationship, poor self-esteem when approval is not forthcoming

- Higher emotion: Humility, which is being able to know and hold on to the experience of self-worth with neither self-inflation nor excessive judgment

- Archetypal challenge: To find oneself in relationship, balancing dependency and autonomy

Type 3 - The Achiever believes love and approval will be the reward of performance, achievement, and success. They channel their emotional energy into getting things done. They take the initiative and work hard to accomplish their goals. Highly adaptable, they excel at *"feeling out"* and meeting the expectations of others when that will lead them to success. They equate self- worth with performance, keeping busy, and looking good. A danger for Threes is concentrating on external praise or material rewards while losing contact with who they are inside. It's difficult for them to step out of their roles.

- Gifts: Optimistic, accomplished, leadership, efficiency, positive and confident.

- Goal: Be productive though efficiency.

- Strengths: Successful, energetic, high achiever.

- Problems: Overworked, impatient, competitive.

- Speaking style: Enthusiastic, motivating themselves and others for success Lower emotional habit: Vanity, based on keeping up a good image and always being successful.

- Higher emotion: Truthfulness - the willingness to go beyond appearances and develop personal authenticity.

- Archetypal challenge: To let go of image and social persona and find one's inner essence.

Type 4 - The Individualist or Romantic often experiences a sense of longing or melancholy, with intense emotional highs and lows. They fear abandonment and loss and are driven to search for an ideal love. They seek meaning and depth in their relationships, their work, or their quest for personal creativity. They tend to be dissatisfied with life as it is and long for the unavailable, so they can live in the past or future, and succumbs to sadness, a melancholy demeanor, and can create dramatic crises at times. Fours feel unique and special, *"on the outside looking in."* While they are good at creating an image, it's most important for them to be authentic. Often passionate, sometimes overly emotional, their attention moves back and forth from empathizing with others to their own inner experience. Individualists at heart, Fours need time alone. To heal and grow, they must balance sadness with the capacity for happiness and satisfaction, even if the relationship or the experience seems flawed or incomplete.

- Gifts: Depth and intensity of feeling, creative desire to express the essence of life, and is empathetic.

- Goal: Become authentic through personal expression

- Strengths: Compassionate, idealistic, emotional depth.

- Problems: Moody, withdrawn, uncooperative.

- Speaking style: Sometimes warm and full of feeling, sometimes flat and dry, they tend to be subjective and try to be aesthetically correct. Often a tone of sadness or dissatisfaction.

- Lower emotional habit: Envy or melancholy arising from the experience of disappointment or deficiency.

- Higher emotion: Equanimity, which means keeping the heart open and welcoming all feelings yet staying in balance.

- Archetypal challenge: Living with an open heart while integrating joy and suffering.

Type 5 - The Investigator or Observer focuses on intellectual understanding and accumulating knowledge. They are often scholars or technical experts because of their keen perception and analytical ability. Many people of this type are intellectually brilliant or knowledgeable, while feelings and relationships present an enormous challenge. They defend against intrusion and feelings of inadequacy through protecting privacy. They hold back strong feelings, limit desires and needs, and their security comes through knowledge and information. Fives enjoy living in their own mind in a world of ideas.

Fives need to balance their tendency to withdraw or withhold from people by reaching out to others, even if that means discomfort.

- Gifts: Knowledgeable, respectful, mental clarity, dependable, thoughtful.

- Goal: Achieve total knowledge through objectives.

- Strengths: Scholarly, perceptive, self-reliant.

- Problems: Isolated, overly intellectual, stingy.

- Speaking style: Rational and content-oriented, most comfortable in their area of expertise, not big on *"small talk"*.

- Lower emotional habit: Avarice or hoarding, which means holding on to information or other resources based on the fear of shortages, either in oneself or the environment.

- Higher emotion: Non-attachment, which is letting go in order to be available for replenishment.

- Archetypal challenge: Participating in life with feelings and integrating the inner and outer worlds.

Type 6 - The Loyal Skeptics have too much fear of fear and use perception and intellect to understand the world and figure out whether other people are friendly or hostile. They focus on guarding the safety of the group, project, or family. Sixes are good at anticipating problems and coming up with solutions. Knowing the rules and making agreements with other people is important, yet at the same time they tend to doubt themselves and question others. They can oscillate between skepticism and certainty, rebel, or true believer. Sixes seek safety from harm in a dangerous world through vigilance by imagining the worst-case outcome in order to prepare. They look for hidden agenda, mistrusts others and are both obedient and rebellious with authority. Additionally, they are ambivalent and indecisive for fear of error. As Sixes learn to trust themselves as well as other people, they become more flexible and develop the courage to act, even in the presence of doubt or ambivalence.

- Gifts: Warm, loyal, intuitive, imaginative, usually great sense of humor.

- Goal: Achieve security through careful observation and alertness.

- Strengths: Loyal, courageous, attentive to people and problems, often strategic thinkers.

- Problems: Suspicious, pessimistic, doubtful.

- Speaking style: Setting limits on themselves and others, having serious questions, and playing devil's advocate - by contrast, sometimes they are ideologically zealous.

- Lower emotional habit: Suspicion or distrust, which can lead to either fearfulness and holding back or an aggressive and pushy attitude.

- Higher emotion: Courage, which is not bravado but rather means feeling the fear and moving forward anyway.

- Archetypal challenge: To sustain faith in other people and the life force, and to overcome the mind/body split.

Type 7 - The Enthusiasts or Epicureans are forward thinkers and movers. They usually bring an optimistic and positive attitude to all of their activities, which reflect an interest in many different subjects. Not wanting to be limited to doing one thing, they prefer to keep their options and possibilities open. Although they can be excellent communicators, Sevens are less concerned with image and other people's approval than other types. They put a priority on having fun, whether that's found in travel and adventure or more intellectual pursuits. Sevens attempt to avoid fright and pain by escaping into fun, pleasure, and imagination, and see life as limitless possibilities with many options. They avoid boredom, enjoy freedom, variety, and interesting experiences. Sevens have difficulty with commitment and follow-through. Because their attention shifts so quickly, it's challenging for Sevens to focus in depth and to stay the course in work and relationships. Their motto is don't worry, be happy.

- Gifts: Outgoing, playful, creative imagination, optimistic, idealistic, love of life .

- Goal: Stay upbeat through current enjoyment and positive future

- Strengths: Adventurous, fun-loving, quick-thinking

- Problems: Self-absorbed, dispersed, uncommitted

- Speaking style: Personal storytelling, which can be either highly entertaining or simply self-absorbed - they also focus on the positive and tend to ignore or quickly reframe the negative.

- Lower emotional habit: Gluttony, which is not just about food, but rather a kind of intoxication or over-consumption of ideas, fun experiences, or substances

- Higher emotion: Sobriety, which means both limiting consumption and calming the mind to be present in the moment

- Archetypal challenge: To make idealism practical, integrating optimism and positive thinking with the shadow side or problems

- **Type 8 - The Challenger or Protector** believes being strong, powerful, and domineering is the only route to safety. Aggressive and impulsive, they take charge of situations, express anger readily, and have difficulty feeling dependency or *"softer"* emotions. Eights admire strength, place high priority on truth, fairness, and justice, and often deny their own weakness or fear.

- Gifts: Courageous, good leadership qualities, powerful, straightforward, protective of the weak

- Goal: Embody power through control and dominance, their challenge is to combine assertion and control with interdependency and cooperation, as well as learning how to curb their often excessive appetites.

- Strengths: Enthusiastic, generous, powerful.

- Problems: Excessive, angry, dominating.

- Speaking Style: Eights usually speak assertively and exert strong leadership - they tend to be bossy and often get angry when something goes wrong.

- Lower emotional habit: Anger and excessiveness, with a revengeful attitude toward people.

- Higher emotion: Innocence, which means to face life with an open heart and without cynicism.

- Archetypal challenge: To harness the life force in productive ways, integrating self-assertion with vulnerability.

Type 9 - The Peacemaker or Mediator seeks acceptance and comfort by *"forgetting the self"* and attending to others and ends up out of touch with own feelings, desires, and life direction. They merge with others to gain a sense of belonging and harmony. They have a problem with priorities and find it difficult to change directions or shift attention to what is most important. They are self-forgetful, meaning they forget their own agenda. Nines excel at seeing all points of view, so while it might be difficult for them to make personal decisions, they can be excellent mediators and peacemakers for others. They seek harmony in their environment. They avoid conflict and anger but can be passive/ aggressive when upset.

- Gifts: Nonjudgmental, supportive, accepting, good mediators, empathetic, positive, trusting.

- Goal: Seeks peace through understanding and acquiescence.

- Strengths: Balanced, accepting, harmonious.

- Problems: Stubborn, ambivalent, conflict, avoidant.

- Speaking style: Inclusive and welcoming at their best, Nines may have trouble getting to the point. They can be linear and controlled, or quite scattered.

- Lower emotional habit: Laziness of attention, or heedlessness, makes it hard for them to face priorities or conflict.

- Higher emotion: Right action, which is the willingness to do what needs to be done and take care of oneself well in the process.

- Archetypal challenge: Waking up to priorities in the present moment, integrating harmony with conflict [392 - 396]

Real Life Comparisons Of The Two Models

To give you an idea of how the two personality profiles work in real life, I will use my wife and myself as examples.

In the four-temperament model, I have primarily choleric and secondarily sanguine traits. In my choleric, I am generally a fast-paced, task-oriented, bottom line, a no excuses, just get it done personality type. That works very well for getting tasks done, but not necessarily for fostering relationships. The *"task"* is just not that important to everyone, especially sanguine and phlegmatic temperaments unless there is social relevance to the task - relationships are more important to them. And if tasks are important to others, the pace at which the task is done may be different - melancholy types for example are task-driven, but they tend to drive at a much slower and methodical speed. Cholerics will drive 90 to nothin' to get it done.

As a choleric, where I have failed in the past is running over people in the process of completing the task, especially with the strength of my tone or ignoring how someone else may feel or think about the situation. In the past, I have been bossy, impatient, and harsh sometimes in my responses. While my sanguine side can make it fun and encouraging sometimes as well, my overriding tendency has been to operate in my primary choleric language. Other cholerics completely understand and are not offended, but other personality types can be taken back by this overpowering communication style.

That is where understanding the Enneagram shines. When understanding the internal motivation instead of just external behavior, a different picture emerges. I am an Eight with a Seven wing on the Enneagram. It has been said that an Eight is the most misunderstood temperament mostly because of their aggressive style. People think Eights are mad at them when they're not. They just don't come across as very friendly at times and can be bossy and blunt. But behind it all is a very deep caring for others and they place a high priority on truth, fairness, and justice, and are not afraid to fight for it as necessary. They stand up for others and can be counted on to get things done. Knowing that about them can change the relational landscape. Others can be more understanding and appreciative of an Eight's *"heart"* when they are confronting the battles of life - and most everything is a battle to overcome in an Eight's life. Also, once Eights realize that about themselves, they can start on the journey towards healing and softening their communication style. When at peace, an Eight will gravitate to some of the characteristics of a Two on the Enneagram. Eights then feel they have the freedom to focus on relationships, making connections, and empathizing with the needs and feelings of other people, helping to bring out their full potential.

My wife Angel is a phlegmatic with a secondary melancholy on the four temperaments profile. She is a Nine with a One wing on the Enneagram. Like most husband and wife relationships, we are fairly opposite in the way we see and react to the world, but also have many common interests. For example, while I can actually be energized by conflict *(the challenge is sometimes too great an enticement to resist),* she is a peacemaker and tries to avoid conflict. She is softhearted, easy to like and believe, and since she can see all sides of a disagreement, she can be excellent mediator.

As you can see, my wife and I do not have the same personality traits, and without good communication and a strong understanding of our differences, we could be a mess, and as with most couples, have had our relational challenges over the years. There can still be obvious disagreements and misunderstandings about how to proceed in life, but a healthy difference between us is also complimentary and a very powerful asset for achieving safety, belonging, and mattering. Because we understand the *"why"* of one another's behaviors, we are better able to have an open heart and mind toward one another. I highly encourage you to take the Enneagram Personality test. It is well worth the investment.

PART TWO

Faith And Its Role In Health

There are many sources from which we can receive encouragement when dealing with life's most unpleasant circumstances. Family and close friends are often our typical encouragers, but self-help and life strategy coaches are also very popular choices. It has been said that the advice of one grandmother is better than the advice from ten doctors. I have certainly seen where that has been true. Sometimes an outsider can even help with a perspective shift that friends just can't give for some reason.

Something Bigger Than Self

Everyone is on his or her own journey, but for me, belief in a higher power is what grounds me. Not that I don't seek advice from others, it's just that I have to measure that advice against my core grounding. I know I am not alone here because studies have shown that those who believe in a higher power in this universe, something bigger than themselves, tend to be healthier, more loving, and more productive.

Researchers from the Mayo Clinic said, *"Most studies have shown that religious involvement and spirituality are associated with better health outcomes, including greater longevity, coping skills, and health-related quality of life (even during terminal illness) and less anxiety, depression, and suicide. Several studies have shown that addressing the spiritual needs of the patient may enhance recovery from illness."* [397]

This chapter is not a treatise about the reality of the providence of God, but for those who may be skeptical, my hope is that you will be curious enough to explore the possibilities. And if you are a science-minded skeptic, there is so much out there from quantum physics, to the origins of the universe, time dilation, the indisputable math of equidistant letter sequencing and gematria in the Hebrew manuscripts that comprise the Old Testament, and more . . . that all unequivocally point to God, as we can best understand Him with our four-dimensional thinking. But know this too, science doesn't explain God, science confirms God and His majesty over all things. *(Check it out in the Quantum Physics section at the end of this chapter.)*

At the end of the day though, understanding the science of God won't be what matters most. If it provides a roadmap to get to the doorway of belief, then great. But you have to decide to step through the door and into a different reality, one based on love and trusting in something beyond your own understanding. I am confident that if you open the door and step through it, what you will find is a peace that surpasses all understanding, something that we all desire but don't necessarily know how to access.

You Are A Masterpiece Of Design

Let me try to explain it this way. Most of us remember the days when film was used in photography *(not so much today with digital photography)*. The images, which were created on film, were not the true picture - they were negative images that had to be developed. We have a similar spiritual transformation that takes place. Hidden in our negative without God, is the life that we long for, a positive picture of you, taken long before you came to be. But you have to be developed to become everything you were created to be.

So what were you created to be? God says you are excellent in every way, a Masterpiece of design. You have royalty in your blood. But it is easy to believe otherwise, and that is often a big part of why we cannot get truly healthy because we believe we are less than, unworthy in some way. Bury those old tapes that tell you otherwise. It is the present that matters. Each day is a new day, and God doesn't focus on the past, so why should you?

As you take steps toward your new beginning, building a relationship of faith in a higher power, God, is proven to change your health for the better. And, don't think that you are not worthy of a relationship with God. Nothing you have done in the past can hold you hostage or keep you from the love of God. Shake off the guilt, the condemnation. When you have a relationship with God, you are growing and are not who you were. Not perfect but trying. Take off the mask. God doesn't bless who you pretend to be. He blesses who you are, faults and all.

While driving one day, I was very distraught about a matter and talked to God about it - actually it was a monologue of my rants. I knew I was going down the wrong emotional path in an area of my life but just couldn't manage to get free of the anger I was feeling. As I was having my conversation with God, he stopped me in the middle of my complaining. It's difficult to explain how He communicated with me, but as clear as the words before you, He just said, *"Thomas." (I know it's Him when I hear Him use my formal first name in my mind).* No other words were necessary. A wave of love swept over me, and I felt Him within me. His presence permeated every cell in my body and the emotional pain simply went away. THAT was a really cool experience!

A relationship with God is upside down and inside out compared to the world we face when we get up to the alarm. To be spiritually intuitive may be different from what we would expect: if you want to be a leader, have a servant's heart. Spiritual maturity doesn't come from life's experiences but from your response to those experiences. Maturity always comes with conflict and struggle. We think that our strength can carry us through. In some context, that may be true. But not in our spiritual lives, because our strongest link is where we feel we don't need God. We have been brainwashed into thinking that God only wants strong people, but it is in our weakness that we are made strong. God's power is perfected in our weakness. Don't misunderstand weakness! It takes a lot of strength to overcome our desire for self-serving power. His grace is sufficient for us. So, be thankful for both strengths and weaknesses and give both over to be used by God who will amplify it all through you and for His divine purposes.

Perhaps the most crucial aspect of spiritual maturity is the act of forgiveness. I read a quote somewhere once that said, *"Holding unforgiveness in your heart is like swallowing poison and waiting for the other person to die."* We hold onto grievances and offenses because we think it gives us power over the offender in some way. What other possible reason could we have for holding that grudge? But holding a grudge does not give you power. It diminishes you and gives power to the other person. They are not the ones in bondage. They are most likely living their lives, completely unconcerned with whether or not you forgive them. *(Often times they are unaware they even need to be forgiven!)* Forgiveness is like unlocking the door to set someone free and realizing that you were the prisoner all along. And forgiveness brings with it true joy and peace.

Overcoming Mountains

In addition to my medical practice, I am a farmer/gardener. I love being out among the plants. One thing that a gardener knows is that there is a time for pruning. Sometimes God, the Master Gardener, will prune you back so far that you think that you look ugly inside, but you're not. It is a purposeful pruning to prepare you for new and fruitful growth. Energy is going to your roots to create a deep solid feeding system, and you are being prepared for new a beautiful blooming season. I know it is hard in the moment; I have been there. Sometimes we get so full of ourselves that the fruit that we do produce may be weak and bitter. Or, we are so full of ourselves that we are too heavy, and we break off from the branch that sustains us. Pruning needs to take place - there is a bigger plan in the works.

That is why it is good to draw your best cards from God's truth to keep you anchored and to hang with like-minded people who can be there to walk alongside you. If things don't work out, don't put a question mark where

God has put a period. Just move forward. God has something better. You may not understand it, but quiet and still your soul and dwell on God's truth and whatever is noble, right, pure, loving, admirable and whatever else is complimentary to God's nature. [398]

One person that has impacted my life for overcoming obstacles is Nick Vujicic, an internationally recognized author and speaker with a very encouraging message. Nick was born without arms or legs, one of seven known worldwide with Tetra- Amelia Syndrome. Author of DVDs and books including his first, Life Without Limits: Inspiration of a Ridiculously Good Life, he has wide appeal to young and old around the world, including frequent speaking engagements in prisons and traveling to the world's hell holes to bring his message of hope through a relationship with God.

> "I never met a bitter person who was thankful, or a thankful person who was bitter."
> "I have the choice to be angry at God for what I don't have or be thankful for what I do have."
> "There's no point in being complete on the outside when you're broken in the inside."
>
> Nick Vujicic

At a very early age, Nick had thoughts of suicide amidst the bullying, jokes, and taunts about his condition. After all, what good in life is someone without arms and legs? He grew through his depression in adolescence and found a deeper meaning to life through his relationship with God, and he stopped letting others or his circumstances define who he was. He is now married with several children and is a highly sought-after inspirational speaker. He can do most of what everyone else does. He surfs, golfs, plays cricket, skateboards, swims, has skydived and generally defies the limits one might expect of a person with no limbs. His message is not about comparing suffering, limitations, or other obstacles and saying, "See, I did it - just think positive and you can too!" His message is about hope beyond what we can see.

What are your mountains? Small or large, we all have them. How do we handle the obstacles, the challenges that tend to try and take us down? Does God really intervene? Yes, he does, and in more ways than you may realize

- sometimes small and sometimes big. He has in my life - many times. Some may chalk up unusual experiences that may seem like miracles to chance or just unexplainable circumstances, and they just move on. I believe God used my struggles growing up as honing and prep work by His design. Taking a bad situation and turning it into good is His specialty. We just aren't always able to see it that way at the time.

I remember Angel and me renting a sailboat for a week on the Chesapeake Bay. It was great! Sailing with friends, anchoring overnight at popular bayside ports - what a blast. The last day there, we were anchored about five hours from our dock of origin. It was a beautiful day for sailing, and I was anxious to get going. Angel reminded me that we were low on gas and that we should fill up before we left. I told her that we would be okay because the weather was so nice and we had enough to get us from the river entrance to our dock. *(You see where this is going.)* We didn't have cell phones in those days so it was not that easy to check on the weather patterns for the day on such short notice. So we took off and sailed our way back. We were in the middle bay next to the shipping channel where the big ships lined up to enter into Annapolis when a rare storm kicked up. There was lightning everywhere. We could not see in front of us, the sails were up, and we were destined to either run aground or run into a tanker in the middle of the bay. I sent Angel down below and all she could do was look up at me crying while the lightning was striking all around me. It came up so quickly that I couldn't even take down the sails and start the motor. After securing myself to the boat so I wouldn't get thrown overboard, I managed to take down the sails in the middle of the storm after she came up for a few minutes to take the wheel. She went back down after I started the motor, but we didn't have much gas. It was a very dangerous situation. I prayed, *"Lord if you are real, show me the Thomas Lighthouse so I can get my bearings."* No sooner did I pray that then the Lord turned my head and like a curtain, the fog move apart, I was able to see the lighthouse very clearly, then the fog curtain shut again. I adjusted my heading and about five minutes later the storm passed about as fast as it started. The intensity of the storm even caught the attention of the local news channels. As it turns out, this storm produced one of the heaviest downpours in one hour ever recorded.

The acceptance of miracles is often counterculture and complicated by life-altering tragedies that can also occur in life. Like me, I am sure most of you have experienced your share of life-altering tragedies as well and wondered where God was in the midst of that? When my mom committed suicide, I was so angry with God. I wondered how He allowed it to happen. That anger ate me up inside well into my adult years, and I paid the price through some of my behaviors and responses to other stresses. Then, when I was ready, and honed enough for His purposes, He gave me healing, and a platform to share with others how He brought me out of that shadow of doubt. Doubt is just part of our human nature, part of the four-dimensional world in which we live. Nothing is ever perfect. People do tend to remember more of the bad things that have happened than the good. That is why God instructed several times in the Bible for *"memorials"* to be built so people will not forget how He loved them and has intervened in their lives.

Really strange and wonderful healings and other unexpected things occur every day. We just may be too busy to notice. Keep track of special events with your own memorial box in your home. Tell your story; keep a clear memory of what God did for you. Keep telling your stories to your children so that your family for generations to come never lose the memory of your own sense of awe and wonder for what God has done in your life. If you want to know about an actual recorded miracle that occurred with over 200 people as witnesses, check out the story of Duane Miller in his book, Out of Silence, A Personal Testimony of God's Healing Power. Got mountains in your life that you can't seem to traverse in your journey? Don't talk to God about how big your mountains are, talk to your mountains about how big your God is.

Quantum Physics - What In The World?

I want to introduce you to Quantum Physics because I believe that this information can help give an additional healthy perspective into life's journey and our connection with God. But before doing so, I have a story to tell. I was in the greenhouse one day checking on some plants. It's a big greenhouse and a bird was stuck inside flying back and forth trying to find a way out. My presence didn't help. He was obviously not happy. I was trying to encourage him towards the doors, but he just didn't get it. He seemed to be getting a bit exhausted. At one point, he landed on a table and just sat there. I decided to try and catch him to see if I could help him get out. So, I slowly approached him and said *(I can't believe that I was talking to a bird - I don't even chirp that well!)* that I was only trying to help him get out, and that if he would just let me pick him up, I could set him free. As I moved closer, he closed his eyes, and he let me pick him up without struggling or flapping his wings. He just trusted me? I picked him up and carried him outside and put him on a rock. He opened his eyes, I backed off, and after about a minute of staring at me, he flew off.

Now, I don't know what you may think about that, but I believe I was given the privilege of entering into a world that was not my own. That experience makes me appreciate the fact that there really is a lot more going on than we realize, that we draw to ourselves that which compliments the way we think, feel, and process the world around us. But we can't see through the glass clearly until we wash the windows. Then we can observe our world with a new clarity.

Seeing through the glass more clearly involves appreciating the way quantum physics impacts our lives on a daily basis. Max Plank, considered Father of Quantum Physics, writes, *"All matter originates and exists only by virtue of a "force" which brings the particle of an atom to vibration and holds this most minute solar system of the atom together. We must assume that behind this force is the existence of a conscious and intelligent mind. This mind is the Matrix of all matter . . . Both Religion and Science require a belief in God. For believers,*

God is in the beginning, and for physicists He is at the end of all considerations . . . He is the "DIVINE MATRIX" that holds all things together."

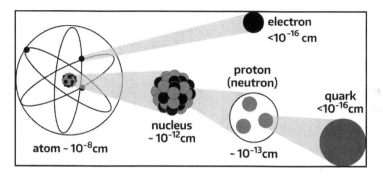

Take an atom for instance. The quantum particles of an atom are super small - the protons, neutrons, quarks, and electrons are made out of quantum waves with constant frequency and amplitude moving in one direction. They are wave and particle - a paradox - both are true. When they are stopped and observed, they enter into our four-dimensional world and are particles. Otherwise, they are waves. The wave/particles can be here and there at the same time. I know; it's weird. I am leading up to something so be patient. [399] Quantum physics tells us that the invisible energy realm *(wave)* collectively referred to as the field, is the primary governing force of the material realm - what we do see. It's the blueprint that forms reality. It connects everything. What is the source of the force? It is God. Science doesn't explain God - it can't. Science just confirms the observable and the conclusion that He is at the end of all observations and considerations.

> *Science doesn't explain God. Science CONFIRMS God and His authority over all things.*

Quantum physics says our consciousness affects the behavior of subatomic particles. Particles and waveforms move backward and forward in time and space and appear in all possible places at once. This is called non-locality. Our free choices affect the physical and conscious world in which we live. This is called the observer effect. Our intention and *"way of being"* affects physical space. Our perception of ourselves plus how we manage our daily experiences controls our body. If we change our perception, we change our biology. You become the master of your life instead of a victim.

Austrian physicist Erwin Schrodinger said you're only aware of the reality you choose to observe. Like a TV with a hundred channels, you can only watch one channel at a time. You're completely unaware of what is happening on the other 99 channels. We spend so much time talking about what doesn't work that we missed the whole point: namely, that we have the ability to produce something that does work. Opposites, for example abundance/lack, are both true. It's a question of which reality we choose to believe. Tune in only to your intent and don't give any airtime to the reality from what you're trying to escape.

The law of entanglement in quantum physics states that relationship is the defining characteristic of everything in space and time. Relationship is independent of distance and requires no physical link. That has been proven experientially. Praying for someone with whom we have a relationship is an example. But the relationship does not have to be direct. Working backwards throughout history, the principles of quantum physics suggests that we are all related, no matter how remote it may seem in our four-dimensional thinking. We affect each other, and we don't have to be aware of it necessarily. The closer we lean into the Creator, the Source, the more discerning we become in relational matters.

Everything made is made of things not visible at the subatomic level. If your thoughts dwell on failure, sickness, and disaster, that is probably what you will manifest. If you live and breathe and dwell in the love of God, you will manifest the benefits of that reality. What you manifest during your lifetime will also epigenetically have an influence on future generations. You can take that to the bank. Words are energy and energy affects matter. If you believe and speak words long enough they can become true. No, you won't grow another set of arms to handle all of those kids, but your reality in dealing with the stresses of life can be clean and have the fresh aroma of contentment and gratitude.

There are many historical and religious texts including verses in the Christian Bible that directly parallel quantum physics principles. There are important connections here about living a wholesome physical, emotional, and spiritual life. It is important not just to us but to future generations as well. Here are some examples:

John 1:1-5 *In the beginning was the Word, and the Word was with God, and the Word was God. He was with God in the beginning. Through him all things were made; without him nothing was made that has been made. In him was life, and that life was the light of all mankind. The light shines in the darkness, and the darkness has not overcome it.*

Col 1 16-17 *For in Him all things were created: things in heaven and on earth, visible and invisible, whether thrones or powers or rulers or authorities; all things have been created through Him and for Him. He is before all things, and in Him all things hold together. The Son sustains all things by His powerful Word.*

Romans 1:20 *For since the creation of the world God's invisible qualities - His eternal power and divine nature - have been clearly seen, being understood from what has been made, so that people are without excuse.*

Romans 12:2 *Do not conform to the pattern of this world but be transformed by the renewing of your mind. Then you will be able to test and approve what God's will is - his good, pleasing, and perfect will.*

1 Timothy 6:15-16 ... *God the blessed and only Ruler, the King of kings and Lord of lords who, alone is immortal and who lives in unapproachable light, whom no one has seen or can see.*

Psalm 104:2-3 *The Lord wraps himself in light as with a garment; he stretches out the heavens like a tent...*

So, how do we then live? If you believe that no one likes you, and if you admit that rejecting type of energy, people will be driven away from you.

If you love yourself and others and demonstrate that you care about them, they feel that and will be drawn to you. The energy of love is a powerful drawing card for good in your life.

God is constantly holding, sustaining, and directing the vibrations and inter-ference of non-physical waves. Controlling waves control what they make up - everything. *"Unseen"* waves come together to form particles like quarks, photons, neutrons, electrons, which form DNA, genes, chromosomes, cells, and us. God knows every hair on our head. He knows how many atoms, electrons, quarks, and waves are in every hair. By faith, we have the power to call things that are not as if they were by our words. It is not instant, although it can be. It is not magic. But it is real. It is by God's design not ours and will manifest as He sees fit, not as we see fit. By speaking life, we access God. If we speak life-giving words, we call life-giving things into being, if we speak death-giving words; we call in death-giving things into being. Speak Life!

PART THREE

Healthy Lifestyle Tips

Your brain is a powerhouse and consumes more energy than any other organ, accounting for about 20% of the total energy requirements - two-thirds for electrical impulses and one-third for cleaning.

One of the cleanup mechanisms that keeps all cells healthy and the trash off the streets, so to speak, are antioxidants. Antioxidants are extremely important for healthy brain function because of how much energy the brain uses. But people throw that term around like a Frisbee and not many really understand the importance of good antioxidants any more than they understand the aerodynamics of what makes one Frisbee better than another. So let me break down the science a little bit for you.

"Oxidative stress (associated with brain disorders, cancer, diabetes, obesity, and heart disease, to name a few) occurs when an oxygen molecule splits into single atoms with unpaired electrons, which are called free radicals... Electrons like to be in pairs, so these atoms, called free radicals, scavenge the body to seek out other electrons so they can become a pair. This causes damage to cells, proteins and DNA."

Harmful free radicals are generated in the body during normal metabolism and upon exposure to environmental insults such as infectious agents, air pollution, man-made chemicals in food and household products, UV light and radiation, negative emotions and so on. Anything that causes stress automatically moves the mind and body into a fight and flight stress response, which can produce excess oxidation and free radicals, which produces cell damage. When free radicals are not neutralized by the body's primary and secondary defense mechanisms, an excess occurs. If harmful radicals have exceeded the body's capacity to effectively neutralize these radicals, then these harmful radicals will damage cell proteins, lipids, and DNA. Therefore, we need antioxidants to ensure that our defense mechanisms for neutralizing harmful radicals will not be exceeded. Numerous epidemiological studies have demonstrated an association between higher intakes or higher blood concentrations of certain antioxidants and a lower incidence of certain degenerative diseases. [400, 401]

Antioxidants neutralize free radicals, while a lack of antioxidants keeps the number of free radicals in the body higher than normal. That's the nutshell version. But I want to go into a little more depth, so you understand the gravity of their role in your overall health.

Antioxidants are nature's way of providing your cells with adequate defense against attack by reactive oxygen species *(ROS)*. Cellular antioxidant defense mechanisms can be classified into primary and secondary systems. The primary defenses include familiar nutrients such as vitamins *(vitamin E and vitamin C)*, carotenoids *(b -carotene, lycopene)*, thiols *(glutathione, lipoic acid)*, ubiquinols, flavonoids and polyphenols *(from herbs, teas, grape skins)* and so on and a variety of enzyme systems *(catalase, superoxide dismutase, glutathione peroxidase)*. Primary defense mechanisms are thought to interact directly with harmful free radicals. Some are made by the body (endogenous) and others must be consumed from food or supplements (exogenous). The secondary defenses include enzymes that breakdown proteins and lipids. Secondary defenses are primarily involved in repair of already damaged proteins and lipids.

There are many real foods that you can eat and drink that are filled with natural antioxidants. With so many choices, you should learn to pick your favorites out of the categories that suit your lifestyle. But it is crucial that you DO NOT stick to getting just one or two types of antioxidants. You need a wide array to provide you with optimal benefits. When classified according to their solubility, antioxidants can be categorized as either soluble in lipids/ fat or water. Both of these are required by your body in order to protect your cells, since the interior of your cells and the fluid between them are composed of water, while the cell membranes themselves are mostly made of fat. Since free radicals can strike either the watery cell contents or the fatty cellular membrane, you need both types of antioxidants to ensure full protection from oxidative damage.

Lipid-soluble antioxidants are the ones that protect your cell membranes from lipid peroxidation. They are mostly located in your cell membranes. Some examples of lipid-soluble antioxidants are vitamins A and E, carotenoids, and lipoic acid. Water-soluble antioxidants are found in aqueous fluids, like your blood and the fluids within and around your cells). Some examples of water-soluble antioxidants are vitamin C, polyphenols, and glutathione. Let's learn a little more about endogenous and exogenous antioxidants.

Endogenous Antioxidants

Glutathione - Known as your body's most powerful antioxidant, glutathione is a substance produced naturally by the liver and is found in every cell in your body. It is also found in fruits, vegetables, and meats. It is called a *"master antioxidant"* because it is intracellular and has the unique ability of maximizing the performance of all the other antioxidants, including vitamins C and E, CoQ10, alpha-lipoic acid, as well as the fresh vegetables and fruits that you eat every day. Glutathione's primary function is to protect your cells and mitochondria from oxidative and lipid peroxidative damage. It is also essential for detoxification, energy utilization, and preventing the diseases we associate with aging. Glutathione eliminates toxins from your cells and gives protection from the damaging effects of radiation, chemicals, poor diet, infections, medications, trauma, and environmental pollutants. Your body's ability to produce glutathione decreases with aging. However, there are other nutrients that can promote glutathione production, such as high-quality whey protein, curcumin, raw dairy, eggs, and grass-fed meat. Orange, lemon, and other citrus essential oils, potent antioxidants, are known to be very high in d-limonene, which is a powerful stimulant of glutathione production. Many trials have shown the anticancer properties of d-limonene as well as its ability to modulate inflammation and oxidative stress.

Alpha-Lipoic Acid *(ALA)* - Your body produces alpha-lipoic acid naturally, but it's also found in a variety of foods and as a dietary supplement. Lipoic acid is one of the most potent, versatile, and longer-acting antioxidant vitamins known. Of all the major antioxidant vitamins, only ALA possesses the unique ability to work in both water-soluble and fat-soluble environments in the body. This ubiquitous property means that lipoic acid has access to all parts of our cells to neutralize damaging free radicals, which are implicated in many age-related diseases including heart disease and diabetes. [402]

Aside from its free radical scavenging abilities, this powerful antioxidant is also a great modifier of gene expression to reduce inflammation, a very potent heavy metal chelator, and enhancer of insulin sensitivity. ALA is the only antioxidant that can be easily transported into your brain, which offers numerous benefits for people with brain diseases, like Alzheimer's disease. ALA can also regenerate other antioxidants, like vitamins C and E and gluta-thione. This means that if your body has used up these antioxidants, ALA can help regenerate them. Studies also show that lipoic acid in combination with acetyl-L-carnitine *(also made by the body and is a supplement)* can reverse mitochondrial decay and restore mitochondrial function to youthful levels. As the amount of lipoic acid produced by the body decreases with aging, supplementation may be necessary to maintain adequate levels.

CoQ10 - Used by every cell in your body, CoQ10 *(ubiquinone)* is converted by your body to its reduced form, called ubiquinol, to maximize its benefits. CoQ10 has been the subject of thousands of studies. Although CoQ10 is cycled between the ubiquinone and ubiquinol forms it is ubiquinol that is the antioxidant or protective form of CoQ10. This is because its reduced state allows it to neutralize free radicals and thereby prevent them from damaging cellular DNA, lipids, and proteins. Therefore, CoQ10 supplements that contain ubiquinone must first be metabolized into ubiquinol in the body in order to exert their antioxidant effects.

Aside from naturally protecting you from free radicals, it also helps produce more energy *(ATP)* for your cells, provides support for your heart health, immune system, and nervous system, helps reduce the signs of normal aging, helps maintain blood pressure levels within the normal range, and is a major antioxidant. . If you're under 25 years old, your body can convert CoQ10 to ubiquinol without any difficulty. However, when you get older, your body becomes more and more challenged to convert the oxidized CoQ10 to ubiquinol. Therefore, you may need to take a ubiquinol supplement.

Beneficial effects of CoQ10 supplementation have been reported in patients who take statins. Statins are a family of drugs that are used to lower cholesterol. They function by inhibiting an enzyme called HMG-CoA reductase, which plays a key role in cholesterol synthesis. However, statins also inhibit the production of mevalonate, which is a precursor for both cholesterol and CoQ10. As mentioned previously, statin use has been associated with increased muscle pain, and CoQ10 supplementation decreases the severity of pain and the amount to which it interfered with patients' daily lives. I see these effects from statins routinely in my office certainly not everyone, but way too many. Because of the side effects, there is also an increased risk of heart attack from a drug that is marketed to prevent heart attacks. Also, statins have been reported to cause liver damage, kidney damage, cancer, and dementia. In my opinion, statins are dangerous medications with no inherent benefit to longevity but have definitely been shown to produce side effects interfering with quality of life. [403]

Superoxide Dismutases *(SODs)* are a class of closely related enzymes that catalyze the breakdown of the superoxide anion into oxygen and hydrogen peroxide. SOD enzymes are present in almost all aerobic cells and in extracellular fluids. Superoxide dismutase enzymes contain metal ion cofactors that, depending on the isozyme, can be copper, zinc, manganese, or iron. In humans, the copper/zinc SOD is present in the cytosol, while manganese SOD is present in the mitochondria.

Catalase *(CAT)* works by converting hydrogen peroxide into water and oxygen, using iron and manganese cofactors. It finishes up the detoxification process started by SOD.

Glutathione Peroxidase *(GSHpx)* and glutathione reductase are selenium-containing enzymes that help break down hydrogen peroxide and organic peroxides into alcohols. They are most abundant in your liver.

What has become clear in the current research is that these systems are dependent on several mineral cofactors, which are all too often deficient in today's western diet. Eating vegetables and nuts can provide the proper amounts of minerals. [404]

Exogenous Antioxidants

There are antioxidants that cannot be manufactured inside your body and must be obtained from antioxidant-rich foods or potent antioxidant supplements. Some of these you may not be familiar with, and it is very important to add them to your nutritional profile. Vitamins in general will be covered in more detail in a separate section of this chapter. It is important to understand however, that testing for antioxidant capacity of exogenous foods and supplements has been done in vitro *(in test tubes for example)* and not in vivo *(in the body)* which is very difficult to assess. It is better to focus on whole food phytonutrients *(other healthy components)* along with antioxidant capacity to develop a more comprehensive understanding of the health benefits of certain foods and supplements. Exogenous antioxidants can include:

Vitamin A Carotenoids are a class of naturally occurring pigments that have powerful antioxidant properties. They are the compounds that give foods their vibrant colors and have antioxidant properties. There are over 750 naturally occurring carotenoids, and right now, you probably have at least 10 different kinds circulating through your bloodstream. These richly colored molecules are the sources of the yellow, orange, and red colors of many plants. Fruit and vegetables provide most of the 40 to 50 carotenoids found in the human diet. alpha-carotene, beta-carotene, beta-cryptoxanthin, lutein, zeaxanthin, and lycopene are the most common dietary carotenoids. Alpha-carotene, beta-carotene and beta-cryptoxanthin are *"pre-vitamin"* A carotenoids, meaning they can be converted by the body to retinol *(vitamin A)*. Lutein, zeaxanthin, and lycopene are non-pre-vitamin A carotenoids because they cannot be converted to retinol. They are selectively taken up into the macula of the eye, where they absorb up to 90% of blue light and help maintain optimal visual function. Carotenoids have been studied for their effects in reducing cardiovascular disease and certain cancers. [405]

Vitamin C - Vitamin C is a well-known antioxidant and has a wide range of important health benefits. As an antioxidant, vitamin C can help combat oxidation by protecting proteins, lipids, and other vital molecular elements in your body. Vitamin C is also essential for collagen synthesis, which is an important structural component of your bones, blood vessels, tendons, and ligaments. You can get vitamin C from raw, organic vegetables and fruits, but you can also take it as a supplement, or have it administered intravenously *(IV)*. Vitamin C antioxidant supplements are not as bioavailable as you might think. The effectiveness is more dependent on *"complex"* of structures associated with the natural form. When taking a vitamin C supplement, choose a whole food vitamin C complex or one made with liposomal technology, which makes the nutrient more absorbable to your cells. More on Vitamin C below.

Vitamin E - Natural vitamin E is a family of eight different compounds: four tocopherols and four tocotrienols. You can obtain all these vitamin E compounds from a balanced diet composed of wholesome foods. However, if you take a synthetic vitamin E supplement, you may only get one of the eight compounds, which is inadequate for your needs.

(More on vitamins below under the heading Vitamins and Nutrients)

Non-Vitamin Exogenous Antioxidants

There are other antioxidants consisting of herbs, spices, and essential oils that are a must for your dietary antioxidant profile. There are many studies confirming their value, but just make sure that you are purchasing quality products. These heavy hitters include:

Astaxanthin - Although it's technically a vitamin A carotenoid, this dietary antioxidant deserves its own recognition and category due to its superb nutritional advantage. It is similar to the category for zeaxanthin. It is a red fat-soluble pigment that does not have pro-vitamin A activity in the human body, although some of the studies reported that astaxanthin has more potent biological activity than other carotenoids. Astaxanthin is a marine carotenoid produced by green microalgae and is in several fish species. The natural sources of astaxanthin are algae, yeast, salmon, trout, krill, shrimp, and crayfish. Sockeye salmon has the highest reported source of astaxanthin from seafood. Krill is very high as well. As a supplement, the absorption is enhanced with additional fish or other fatty dietary oils. The current research data on astaxanthin is encouraging and has resulted from well-controlled trials in in-vitro and in-vivo models. [406]

Astaxanthin has been touted by some as the most powerful carotenoid in terms of free radical scavenging. How much antioxidant activity does astaxanthin have? Per 100 gram, which you wouldn't necessarily consume, it has been shown to up to 6,000 times the antioxidant power of vitamin C, 800 times that of CoQ10, and 550 times that of vitamin E, according to laboratory testing. Contrary to popular belief, fish and other seafood do not produce astaxanthin themselves. Rather, they obtain this phytonutrient from certain species of microalgae they eat *(or from the smaller fish and marine life they eat, who eat that microalgae)*. It's similar to how fish obtain EPA and DHA, as those too are nutrients they do not produce. The original source of all Omega-3, DHA is vegan, as it comes from algae. [407]

Astaxanthin, used as an antioxidant nutritional supplement, is reported to have wide-ranging benefits showing potential benefits on various diseases including cancers, hypertension, diabetes, cardiovascular, gastrointestinal, liver, neurodegenerative, and skin diseases. Effects are reported such as:

- supporting your immune function

- improving your cardiovascular health by reducing C-Reactive Proteins *(CRP)* and triglycerides and increasing beneficial HDL

- protecting your eyes from cataracts, macular degeneration, and blindness protecting your brain from dementia and Alzheimer's

- reducing your risk of different types of cancer

- promoting recovery from spinal cord and other nerve injuries

- reducing inflammation from all causes, including arthritis and asthma improving your endurance, workout performance, and recovery

- relieving indigestion and reflux

- helping stabilize your blood sugar, thereby protecting your kidney

- increasing sperm strength and sperm count and improving fertility

- helping to prevent sunburn, and protecting you from damaging radiation effects

- reducing oxidative damage to your DNA

- reducing symptoms of diseases, such as pancreatitis, multiple sclerosis, carpal tunnel syndrome, rheumatoid arthritis, Lou Gehrig's disease, Parkinson's disease, and neurodegenerative diseases

In order to get the 12 mg per day, which is what many supplement manufacturers recommend as a dosage, you would need to consume about four servings of nature's most potent source; wild sockeye salmon. *(If you are consuming astaxanthin in capsules, be sure to use a reputable manufacturer.)*

Fish sources can be problematic today because they are a source of heavy metals which can be harmful to our health. In layman's terms, when you eat a fish, you are also eating all the contaminants in the fish it ate over its lifetime. Wild sockeye salmon that stay close to pristine inlets are a good safe source.

Actually, the natural form of astaxanthin is derived directly from the source, the microalgae species, Haematococcus pluvialis. Unlike spirulina, which is sometimes grown in outdoor ponds or harvested directly from the ocean, making it subject to environmental pollutants, the largest manufacturers of natural astaxanthin grow the algae in climate-controlled tanks and using other sophisticated operations to ensure safety, purity, and consistency.
408 - 411

L-Theanine is an amino acid seldom found anywhere in nature other than tea. It easily crosses the blood-brain barrier and exerts subtle changes in biochemistry by increasing levels of dopamine and serotonin that cause a tranquilizing effect improving mood, reducing mental and physical stress, and improving alertness and cognitive performance in a synergistic manner with caffeine. The production of GABA, the brain chemical known for its calming effect, is also increased after taking theanine. Increased GABA can also put you in a better mood and create a sense of well-being. [412]

There have been many recent clinical trials conducted by various organizations proving that the combination of L-theanine and caffeine found in tea increases the ability to focus without the over- stimulating effects of caffeine alone. [413]

In a paper by Eschenauer and Sweet, it was concluded, *"increased alpha activity in the brain induced by L-theanine has been associated with increased creativity, increased performance under stress, and improved learning and concentration as well as decreased anxiety."* A 2001 study suggests that the combination of L-theanine and caffeine *"improves the ability to multi-task and reduces task-induced fatigue."* [414]

Brain waves are classified into four categories *(Delta, Theta, Alpha, and Beta)*, each with an associated mental state. Stimulants, like caffeine, (in coffee, OT C meds, energy drinks, and sodas), promote Beta waves and suppress the others, leading to increased stress, anxiety, and over-excitement. It can be very difficult to focus and concentrate when you are emitting Beta waves. Delta waves are only seen in the deepest stages of sleep and Theta waves are seen in light sleep and drowsiness. Alpha waves are present during wakefulness where there is a relaxed and effortless alertness. L-theanine directly stimulates the production of Alpha brain waves. [415]

Polyphenols are a large class of chemical compounds synthesized by fruits, vegetables, teas, cocoa, and other plants that possess certain health benefits. Polyphenols have antioxidant, anti-inflammatory, anti-carcinogenic and other biological properties, and may protect from oxidative stress, free radicals, and some diseases. Many studies have been carried out that strongly support the contribution of polyphenols to the prevention of cardiovascular diseases, cancer, osteoporosis, neurodegenerative diseases, and diabetes mellitus, and suggest a role in the prevention of peptic ulcers.

Polyphenols are divided into several groups, one of which is represented by flavonoids, the largest subgroup. There are several subclasses of flavonoids including anthocyanins, flavanols, flavanones, flavones, and isoflavones. The richest sources of polyphenols in the diet are fruits, vegetables, and beverages such as tea. Some plants may contain several different polyphenols from various classes.

Consumption of fruits and vegetables has been shown to improve health and directly or indirectly reduces the risk of numerous chronic diseases. Increasing one serving of fruit and vegetable intake per day could reduce the risk of coronary heart disease by 4%. It is believed that the nutrients and non-nutrient bioactive compounds present in fruits and vegetables are responsible for these health benefits. Among numerous plant-based bioactive compounds, flavonoid polyphenols have been studied extensively and have shown promising results improving various disease aspects. Certain plant-based food groups are known to be much higher in flavonoids than others including some fruits, vegetables, spices, and grains. As water-soluble nutrients, flavonoids can be lost through water contact, and in some cases, up to 80% of specific flavonoids can be lost into cooking water during the boiling of foods.

They are susceptible to damage by heat, and as mentioned earlier, they are also susceptible to damage over prolonged periods of time. This issue of time brings us to the benefits of fresh fruits and vegetables, which are likely to be more flavonoid-rich the fresher they are at the time of purchase. The issue of heat is one of the reasons we caution against frying or lengthy cooking even in medium heats. [416]

Although flavonoids have shown countless health benefits, their low bioavailability has been a concern, so quality and amount in the diet can play a factor. Flavonoids are metabolized in the gut and then the less active metabolites *(but still very important)* travel into the bloodstream. Most of the flavonoids however pass through the small intestine, reach the colon, and get extensively metabolized into phenolic acids by the colonic microflora and are then absorbed. The healthier the intestinal and colon flora, the more conversion and absorption. Nevertheless, consumption of flavonoids, however the body decides to metabolize and utilize them, has shown to produce tremendous health benefits. [417]

Catechins are a powerful flavonoid antioxidant belonging to the "flavanol" subgroup of flavonoids. Teas as well as dark chocolate and other cocoa products contain various catechins. In the US, the largest single source of flavonoid catechins is in black, oolong, and green tea, and over half of all flavonoid intake comes from the flavanol subgroup that includes catechins, epicatechins, gallocatechins, and theaflavins, all important to our healthy lifestyle efforts. [418, 419]

Apigenin is a naturally occurring plant flavonoid "flavone" abundantly present in common fruits and vegetables including parsley, onions, oranges, apples, tea, chamomile, wheat sprouts, basil, oregano, tarragon, cilantro, endive, broccoli, cherries, leeks, onions, tomatoes grapes, beans and barley, and some spices. Apigenin crosses the blood-brain-barrier and has been shown to possess remarkable anti-inflammatory, antioxidant, and anti-carcinogenic properties. In the last few years, significant progress has been made in studying the biological effects of apigenin at cellular and molecular levels. Apigenin is particularly abundant in the flowers of the chamomile plant *(68% apigenin of total flavonoids)* and may even be one reason why drinking chamomile tea has been found to reduce thyroid cancer risk by up to 80%.

Curcumin is another powerful antioxidant, beneficial for both brain health and cancer prevention/treatment, much like apigenin. Turmeric, a spice that has long been recognized for its medicinal properties, has received interest from both the medical and scientific worlds. Turmeric is the major source of the polyphenol curcumin. The medicinal properties of turmeric, the source of curcumin, have been known for thousands of years. It aids in the management of oxidative and inflammatory conditions, neurodegenerative disorders like Alzheimer's, cancer, metabolic syndrome, arthritis, anxiety, and hyperlipidemia. It may also help in the management of exercise-induced inflammation and muscle soreness, thus enhancing recovery and performance in active people. In addition, a relatively low dose of the complex can provide health benefits for people that do not have diagnosed health conditions. Most of these benefits can be attributed to its antioxidant and anti-inflammatory effects. Curcumin is poorly absorbed when consumed. There are several components that can increase bioavailability. For example, piperine is the major active component of black pepper and, when combined in a complex with curcumin, has been shown to increase bioavailability by 2000% in 45 minutes after oral administration of the 2 grams curcumin to 20 mg piperine combination. Curcumin combined with enhancing agents provides multiple health benefits. The same effect can be seen with tea catechin flavonoids EGCg and apigenin previously discussed. [420 - 423]

To increase the bioavailability and also direct nose-to-brain drug transport, nasal delivery of curcumin has also been used. In a study, the pharmacokinetics results showed that the absolute bioavailability of curcumin in the microemulsion-based in situ ion-sensitive gelling system was 55.82% by intranasal administration. And the distribution of curcumin in the brain versus blood following intranasal administration was higher than that following intravenous administration. Other options for longer circulation, better permeability, and resistance to metabolic processes of curcumin include several formulations that have been prepared using nanoparticles, liposomes, micelles, and phospholipid complexes. [424]

These studies reflect the use of the piperine component of black pepper and not the essential oil. Piperine inhibits intestinal and liver glucuronidation, which metabolizes curcumin fast thereby increasing serum concentration of curcumin. There are no established amounts but is has been suggested that 1/4 teaspoon black pepper per teaspoon of curcumin is a good ratio. Supplements may have 100:1 ratio of curcumin to black pepper extract *(piperine, the active component)*. In any case, while the effect is real, individual response may vary so finding the balance based on general parameters is the best approach.

In the brain, the anti-inflammatory effect can be quite profound. Microglial cells in the brain are important effectors of the immune system with a major role in chronic neurodegenerative diseases. They respond to inflammation and attacks, sometimes being overzealous in the attack and taking out brain cells in the process. Curcumin is a potent modulator (puts the brakes on) of the microglial cell activation. Curcumin reduces microglial migration and anti-inflammatory and neuroprotective properties. How cool is that! Thus, curcumin could be a nutraceutical compound to develop immuno-modulatory and neuroprotective therapies for the treatment of various neurodegenerative disorders like Alzheimer's and autism. [425]

Curcumin as an antioxidant, anti-inflammatory, and lipophilic action improves the cognitive functions in patients with Alzheimer's disease. A growing body of evidence indicates that oxidative stress, free radicals, beta-amyloid deposits in the brain, cerebral deregulation caused by bio-metal toxicity (like thimerosal and aluminum) and abnormal inflammatory reactions contribute to the key event in Alzheimer's disease pathology. Due to various effects of curcumin, such as decreased beta-amyloid plaques, delayed degradation of neurons, metal-chelation, anti- inflammatory, antioxidant, and decreased microglia formation, the overall memory in patients with AD can improve.[426, 427]

Resveratrol - Is a polyphenol found in certain fruits like grapes, vegetables, cocoa, and red wine, this antioxidant can cross the blood-brain barrier, providing protection for your brain and nervous system. Resveratrol has been found to be so effective at warding off aging-related diseases that it was dubbed the *"fountain of youth."* Aside from providing free radical protection, this antioxidant can help inhibit the spread of cancer, especially prostate cancer, lower your blood pressure, keep your heart healthy, and improve elasticity of your blood vessels, normalize your anti-inflammatory response and help prevent Alzheimer's disease.

Like other antioxidants and phytonutrients, such as lycopene found in toma-toes, or lutein found in carrots, resveratrol is a powerful compound that regenerates the body all the way at the cellular level. Resveratrol works by modifying inflammation in the body, in addition to having other positive effects on hormone production, blood circulation, and fat storage. Studies demonstrate that it specifically seems to have been found to lower insulin levels, which is key to staying young and at a healthy weight, and fighting diseases like diabetes. Resveratrol helps the *"powerhouse"* part of cells *(the mitochondria)* that supplies cells with energy to work optimally. It is import-ant in the repair of damaged blood vessels. Finally, as a potent antioxidant, resveratrol is constantly fighting damage from free radicals that can increase cancer risk. Red grapes and red wine are said to be rich in resveratrol, but with the poor absorption seen with flavonoids, you probably need much more wine than is good for you. In case you're wondering, white wine has some too but much lower amounts since the grapes' skins are removed earlier in the winemaking process.

Superfoods

Goji /Wolfberries: The superfood of superfoods, goji berries are a gold mine of nutrition. As a mixture of active polysaccharides, goji berries have shown multiple pharmacological activities, including anti-aging, antioxidative, antifatigue, anticancer, antidiabetic, antiviral, hepatoprotective, cardioprotective, neuroprotective, hypolipidemic, radioprotective, anti-osteoporosis, anti-inflammatory, and immunomodulating effects. The mechanisms for these beneficial effects are multifaceted, involving a number of signaling molecules and pathways. [428]

As a traditional Chinese highly celebrated medicinal herb and super-food supplement, Gogi berries, Lycium barbarum *(also named Wolfberry, Fructus lycii, Gouqizi, and Goji berries)* have been used in the People's Republic of China and other Asian and European countries for more than 2,000 years of recorded history. The berries have become increasingly popular in Western countries as an anti-aging and antioxidant product. The fruits, which are red-colored and mildly sweet in taste, are found throughout regions of Europe and China, however the best berries are said to come from the Ningxia Province in the People's Republic of China. These berries are consumed raw, as a juice, or as brewed tea and are also be processed to tinctures, powders, and tablets. Wolfberry inhibits the proliferation of various types of cancer cells and has also drawn attention because of its polysaccharide, betaine, lutein, and zeaxanthin content. The fruit contains 18 types of amino acids, eight of which are essential amino acids, such as isoleucine and tryptophan. It is also the source of 21 trace minerals including zinc, iron, copper, calcium, selenium, and phosphor, and also thiamin *(B1)*, riboflavin *(B2)*, pyridoxine *(B6)*, vitamin E, and vitamin C. [429] The NingXia wolfberry from the NingXia Province in China has a centuries-old history of reported health benefits. I consume this in a puree form mixed with essential oils and other high-quality berry juices as a super nutritive beverage. The NingXia wolfberries by themselves are an excellent tasting treat as well. In recent years, the magazine Domestic and Foreign published a story about a great herbal master who lived over 200 years and died in 1930. He attributed his health and longevity to this berry. According to a test known as ORAC *(Oxygen Radical Absorbance Capacity)* developed by USDA researchers at Tufts University, at 31,000 μmol TE/100 g, the NingXia wolfberry is a powerful antioxidant food with the inherent ability to neutralize cell damaging and disease-causing free radicals. The numerous health benefits of the wolfberry have been studied extensively and published in medical and other health journals around the world.

Tea: Made from the leaves of Camellia sinensis, tea is one of the most widely consumed beverages worldwide. Tea has been used as a medicinal herb, dating back 4700 years to China, and in Asia. Catechin antioxidants are the predominant component of tea's health benefits but there are other important health-promoting substances as well including L-theanine, caffeine, GABA, and others. Catechins and their derivatives are thought to contribute to the beneficial effects ascribed to tea. Green tea has more catechins than oolong tea. Both help prevent heart disease and cancer and are very potent antioxidants. Especially abundant in green tea, epigallocatechin 3-gallate *(EGCG or EGC3G)* is found to be the most potent tea polyphenols for anti-oxidative, antimutagenic and anti-pathogenic effects. The many bioactive compounds in tea appear to impact virtually every cell in the body to help improve health outcomes.

Since ancient times, it has been said that drinking green tea brings relaxation. The substance that is responsible for a sense of focus and relaxation is L-theanine and the health benefits were described above. The benefits of L-theanine have also become particularly prominent in recent years. One cup of green tea contains approximately 8-30 mg of L-theanine. In recent years, many health benefits of consuming green tea have been reported, including the prevention of diseases associated with free radicals and reactive oxygen species, such as cancer, or cardiovascular and neurodegenerative diseases. In addition to the antioxidant properties of the catechins, their anti-diabetic, antibacterial, anti-inflammatory, and anti-obesity activities also have been reported. The health benefits of green tea are mainly attributed to its antioxidant properties, including the ability of catechins to scavenge reactive oxygen species or chelate with metal ions. [430, 431]

Teas other benefit includes weight management. Oolong teas have gained some recent recognition as weight-loss teas. In a 12-week study done in the US basing on 132 healthy but over-weight individuals, people who drank 625 mg of tea catechins *(about 48-60 ounces of tea)* daily AND exercised three times a week took on average 7.7% *(11.7% max, 3.8% min)* off of their abdominal fat, compared to 0.3% in those who exercised but did not have the tea drink. [432]

The results suggest that oolong tea increases metabolism through its polyphenols rather than just through caffeine. Increased metabolism results in reduced body fat. Most notably is the reduction in visceral body fat - the type of fat found between internal organs, which creates the *"beer belly."* Tea is a perfect complement to healthy eating and exercise for weight management.

Chamomile: One of the most ancient medicinal herbs known to mankind. It is a member of Asteraceae/Compositae family and represented by two common varieties viz. German Chamomile *(Chamomilla Recutita)* and Roman Chamomile *(Chamaemelum Nobile)*. The dried flowers of chamomile contain many terpenoids and flavonoids contributing to its medicinal properties. Essential oils of chamomile are used extensively in cosmetics and aromatherapy. Many different preparations of chamomile have been developed, the most popular of which is in the form of herbal tea, which is consumed to the tune of more than one million cups per day.

Chamomile has been used for centuries as an anti-inflammatory, antioxidant, mild astringent, and healing medicine. As a traditional medicine, it is used to treat wounds, ulcers, eczema, gout, skin irritations, bruises, burns, canker sores, neuralgia, sciatica, rheumatic pain, hemorrhoids, mastitis and other ailments. Externally, chamomile has been used to treat diaper rash, cracked nipples, chickenpox, ear and eye infections, disorders of the eyes including blocked tear ducts, conjunctivitis, nasal inflammation, and poison ivy. Chamomile is widely used to treat inflammations of the skin and mucous membranes, and for various bacterial infections of the skin, oral cavity and gums, and respiratory tract. Chamomile in the form of an aqueous extract has been frequently used as a mild sedative to calm nerves and reduce anxiety, to treat hysteria, nightmares, insomnia, and other sleep problems. Chamomile has been valued as a digestive relaxant and has been used to treat various gastrointestinal disturbances including flatulence, indigestion, diarrhea, anorexia, motion sickness, nausea, and vomiting. Chamomile has also been used to treat colic, croup, and fevers in children. It has been used as an emmenagogue (stimulates menstrual flow) and a uterine tonic in women. It is also effective in arthritis, back pain, bedsores, and stomach cramps. [433]

Ginseng: An important herbal antioxidant is which has been used for countless generations, especially within the protocols of traditional Chinese medicine. Herbal ginseng exists as three distinct varieties: Oriental varieties, Siberian, and American. Ginseng is considered an *"adaptogen"* which means that the benefits provided by the herb will adapt to the stresses the person experiences, whether it is mental or physical, the difference in the stimulation of both male and female hormones being an example. It is in this area that all three ginsengs excel. Oriental, or panax ginseng, is grown mainly in China and Korea, where it is harvested for its roots. Chinese ginseng root is dried naturally and turns a whitish color, whereas Korean *(red panax)* ginseng root is treated differently and turns a reddish color, which is why it is sometimes referred to as *"red panax."* All ginsengs are used medicinally, usually in efforts to boost energy and enhance vitality and derive their pharmacological properties from ginsenosides, the major and bioactive constituents.

Korean ginseng is considered the most potent, which in Asia is said to improve circulation, revitalizes the body, and aids recovery from weakness after illness, increase vitality and stamina, improve work efficiency, combat fatigue, and enhance libido. In Western countries, it is taken more sporadically as an energy booster, although a review article published in a 2005 edition of *"Phytotherapy Research"* concluded that herbal *"adaptogens"* such as ginseng, may benefit people diagnosed with fibromyalgia, chronic fatigue syndrome, depression and Alzheimer's disease by reducing pain levels, boosting energy and cognition, and restoring sleep cycles. Other studies suggest that ginseng stimulates the immune system; has anti fatigue, anti-stress, antitumor, anticancer and anti-aging properties; balances blood sugar levels; enhances mental performance and memory; lowers cholesterol; strengthens the heart muscle; and protects against radiation damage. The main difference between Korean and Chinese ginseng is potency. Chinese ginseng has milder energy-boosting effects, so it is thought to be better suited for young children, the elderly, and the very ill. Modern research provides some support for use of ginseng for diabetes, hypertension, hyperlipidemia, and heart failure when administered in the doses recommended in Asia. [434-436]

American Ginseng, Panax quinquefolium is indigenous to the eastern woodlands ranging from Georgia to Quebec and was used by many American Indian tribes. Ironically, American Ginseng is highly sought after in China, while Americans chase after Chinese. While having much the same adaptogenic qualities of Chinese, American is believed have cooler or milder effects. What this means is that American Ginseng is excellent for the high-paced, stressed, not enough time culture that we live in. While still energizing the system, American Ginseng calms the central nervous system, quiets the brain, and lowers blood pressure. Also because of its more subtle nature, it is generally better to use on a day-to-day, long-term basis than Chinese.

Siberian Ginseng, Eleutherococcus senticosus, cousin to Panax ginseng, is native to Siberia, Japan, Korea and China with the Siberian grown being the highest prized. As with its cousins, Siberian Ginseng was traditionally used to promote longevity and general health. Research, mostly from Russia, confirms its abilities to increase mental and physical performance; stimulate the immune system increasing phagocytosis; increase circulation and vasodilation. Ginseng is anti-inflammatory and will increase the benefits of medical radiation treatments while lessening the negative side-effects. It is neutral energetically and so is appropriate for daily use. [437-439]

Avocado: In addition to being an excellent source of healthy fats, avocados also have other unique health benefits, including enhancing your body's absorption of nutrients and inhibiting production of an inflammatory compound produced when you eat beef. Avocados have a very impressive healthy fat content. They also contain compounds that inhibit and destroy oral cancer cells and being very high in potassium avocados will help balance your potassium to sodium ratio. Avocados are one of the safest fruits you can buy conventionally-grown, so you may not need to spend the extra money for organic ones. Their thick skin protects the inner fruit from pesticides.

Nuts: Tree nuts are nutrient-dense foods with complex matrices rich in unsaturated fatty and other bioactive compounds: high-quality vegetable protein, fiber, minerals, tocopherols, phytosterols, and phenolic compounds. By virtue of their unique composition, nuts are likely to beneficially impact health outcomes. Epidemiologic studies have associated nut consumption with a reduced incidence of coronary heart disease and gallstones in both genders and diabetes in women. Limited evidence also suggests beneficial effects on hypertension, cancer, and inflammation. Interventional studies consistently show that nut intake has a cholesterol-lowering effect, even in the context of healthy diets, and there is emerging evidence of beneficial effects on oxidative stress, inflammation, and vascular reactivity. Blood pressure, visceral fat, and the metabolic syndrome also appear to be positively influenced by nut consumption. Thus, it is clear that nuts have a beneficial impact on many cardiovascular risk factors. Contrary to expectations, epidemiologic studies, and clinical trials suggest that regular nut consumption is unlikely to contribute to obesity and may even help in weight loss.

Safety concerns are limited to the infrequent occurrence of nut allergy in children, but some nuts such as almonds can be high in pesticides. The best consumer safety practice overall is be sure and purchase organic nut. Nuts are nutrient-rich foods with wide-ranging cardiovascular and metabolic benefits, which can be readily incorporated into healthy diets. Walnuts for example, are satisfyingly crunchy, and they're also rich in potentially brain-protective compounds such as vitamin E, folate, omega-3 fatty acids, and antioxidants. A preliminary study published in the British Journal of Nutrition in 2011 revealed that a diet supplemented with walnuts produced an 11% improvement on inferential reasoning tests in young adults.

Sprouts and Microgreens: Many of the benefits of sprouts and microgreens relate to the fact that, in their initial and early phase of growth, plants contain more concentrated amounts of nutrients. As a result, you need to eat far less, in terms of amount, compared to a mature plant. Sprouts may be harvested within just a few days or a week of growth, while microgreens are typically harvested after two to three weeks when they've reached a height of about 2 inches.

Essential fatty acids heighten, and the protein quality of several vegetables improves when sprouted. Sprouts can also contain up to 100 times more enzymes than their full-grown counterparts and help protect against chemical carcinogens. Watercress may be the most nutrient-dense of all. Sprouts and microgreens are easy and inexpensive to grow at home. They're a particularly excellent choice during winter months when outdoor gardening is limited or ruled out. Another major benefit is that you don't have to cook them. A simple way to dramatically improve your nutrition is to swap out lettuce for sprouts and/or microgreens in your salad, or on burgers, sandwiches or tacos. Even a few grams of microgreens per day can *"entirely satisfy"* the recommended daily intake of vitamins C, E and K.

Fatty Fish: Research suggests eating clean fish like wild-caught salmon, sardines or anchovies once or twice a week may increase your lifespan by more than two years and reduce your risk of dying from cardiovascular disease by 35%. *"Fatty fish contain omega-3 fatty acids that are necessary for optimal brain function,"* said Barry Sears, a scientist and president of the Inflammation Research Foundation.

Garlic: Has played an important dietary and medicinal role throughout the history of mankind. In some Western countries, the sale of garlic preparations ranks with those of leading prescription drugs. The therapeutic efficacy of garlic encompasses a wide variety of ailments, including cardiovascular, blood pressure, cholesterol, cancer, liver disorders, and microbial infections to name but a few. Reactive oxygen species *(ROS)* seem to be at the core of many disease processes, and it is an attractive and convenient hypothesis that garlic might exert its activities through modulatory effects on ROS. Various preparations of garlic, mainly aged garlic extract *(AGE)* have been shown to have promising antioxidant potential. Raw garlic homogenate is the major preparation of garlic hat has been subjected to intensive scientific study because it is the normal manner of garlic consumption. Raw garlic homogenate is the same as an aqueous extract of garlic. Allicin is the major thiosulfinate compound found in garlic homogenate. [440]

The use of garlic was well-documented by many major civilizations, including the Egyptians, Babylonians, Greeks, Romans and Chinese. Scientists now know that most of its health benefits are caused by sulfur compounds formed when a garlic clove is chopped, crushed or chewed. Garlic compounds alliin, allyl cysteine, allyl disulfide, and allicin contribute to various health benefits and exhibit different patterns of antioxidant activities as protective compounds against free radical damage. [441, 442]

Broccoli: Research shows this cruciferous veggie may reduce your risk for many common diseases, including arthritis, cancer, heart disease and more. When you eat fresh broccoli, you're getting dozens of super-nutrients that support optimal, body-wide health, including fiber, the anticancer compounds sulforaphane and glucoraphanin, anti-inflammatory and free radical quenching phenolic compounds and immune-boosting diindolylmethane *(DIM)*.

Three servings of broccoli per week may reduce your risk of prostate cancer by more than 60%. Sulforaphane also helps raise testosterone levels, inhibits the retention of body fat, helps detox carcinogens, and helps protect your muscles against exercise-induced damage. Ideally, choose raw broccoli, as frozen broccoli has diminished ability to produce sulforaphane. Even better, opt for broccoli sprouts, which can contain 20 to 50 times more chemoprotective compounds than mature broccoli. When using raw broccoli, steaming it for three to four minutes will optimize the sulforaphane content. Do not go past five minutes.

Onions: Another potent anti-inflammatory, anticancer food. Recent research shows people with the highest consumption of onions have a lower risk of several different types of cancer. Research has also revealed that the stronger the flavor of the onion, the better its cancer-fighting potential. In one analysis, shallots, Western yellow, and pungent yellow onions were the most effective against liver cancer. The latter two were also particularly effective against colon cancer.

Onions also contain compounds known to protect against cardiovascular disease and neurological dysfunction or decline. They also help prevent obesity and diabetes, in part by inhibiting certain enzymes in your digestive tract, and by supporting healthy blood sugar control. Antioxidants are most concentrated in the outer layers of the onion, so peel off only the outermost paper-like layer. Over-peeling can reduce important antioxidants and chemoprotective compounds by as much as 75%.

Spinach: Rich in cancer-fighting antioxidants, vitamin K1 *(good for your veins and arteries),* magnesium and folate, the latter of which is important for short-term memory and helps lower your risk for heart disease and cancer by slowing down wear and tear on your DNA. It also contains more potassium than banana. One caveat and contraindication: If you have calcium oxalate kidney stones, spinach is on the list of foods to strictly avoid, as it is high in oxalate. Also keep in mind that boiling the spinach will leach valuable nutrients like vitamin C into the water. After 10 minutes of boiling, three-quarters of the phytonutrients in spinach will be lost, so you're better off eating it raw, or lightly steamed or sautéed.

Cabbage: Tends to be inexpensive, and you can supercharge its health benefits by fermenting it, (making sauerkraut) thereby also significantly extending its shelf life. Do not buy off the shelf unless refrigerated. Chances are that it has preservatives and other chemicals in it. The fermenting process produces copious quantities of beneficial microbes that are extremely important for your health, as they help balance your intestinal flora and boost your immunity. These beneficial bacteria can even help to normalize your weight and play a significant role in the prevention of type 2 diabetes, depression, and other mood disorders.

Free-Range or Pastured Eggs: Relatively inexpensive and amazing source of high-quality nutrients, especially protein and fat. A single egg also contains nine essential amino acids, lutein and zeaxanthin for your eyes, choline for your brain/nervous/cardiovascular systems, and naturally-occurring B12. Ideally, you'll want to eat your eggs as close to raw as possible, such as soft-boiled or poached, or cook at a very low temperature. Scrambled or fried eggs are the worst, as this oxidizes the cholesterol in the egg yolk. If you have kidney damage, you may want to discard the egg white. If you chose to use the egg white, avoid eating it raw unless it's in combination with the yolk. Eating only egg white could potentially lead to biotin deficiency. Besides superior nutrition, pastured chickens are much healthier than factory-farmed chickens and therefore have a far lower risk of producing eggs infected with salmonella.

Keep in mind that eggs sold as *"cage-free"* does not mean the chickens were raised under ideal conditions. They're not raised in cages, but they may still not have access to the outdoors. So, there are still significant differences between cage-free and free range or pastured eggs. To identify better commercial producers and brands, see the Cornucopia Institute's egg report and scorecard, which ranks 136 egg producers according to 28 organic criteria. Organic eggs insure that no GMO feed or pesticides end up in your eggs.

Berries: Loaded with vitamins, minerals, and micronutrients that impart a host of health advantages. Importantly, their antioxidant power helps keep free radicals in check and fights inflammation. Some of the most important antioxidants in berries are anthocyanins, flavanols, ellagic acid and resveratrol, which studies say help protect your cells and fight off disease.

Blueberries, strawberries, raspberries, cranberries, and blackberries are known as some of the world's best dietary sources of bioactive compounds associated with a reduced risk of heart disease, neurodegeneration, diabetes, inflammation and cancer. One way to prevent waste - as berries can get moldy within days if you don't eat them - is to buy frozen berries and simply thaw what you need. Frozen berries also tend to be less expensive pound-for-pound compared to fresh berries. Research also shows that the polyphenols, which are a type of antioxidant found in brightly colored fruits such as berries, may improve memory capabilities and delay the onset of dementia by reducing inflammation and damage caused by toxins called free radicals. Since we have a blueberry farm, I am particularly partial to blueberries. They have been found to be one of the few things they've tested that actually reverses brain aging. Blackberries also dramatically reduced brain aging and can lower blood pressure. They reduce over activation of the general immune system and brain microglial cell activation as well.

Raw Yogurt and Kefir: While most commercial yogurts are little more than glorified desserts loaded with sugar, real yogurt and kefir made from cultured raw, organic grass-fed milk are a real superfood, providing an array of healthy bacteria that support optimal health, along with high-quality protein, calcium, B vitamins, and even cancer-fighting conjugated linoleic acid *(CLA)*.

If you want to know which commercial yogurts are healthy and which are not, refer to The Cornucopia Institute's Yogurt Report. Their investigation found many products being sold as yogurt do not even meet the standards for real yogurt. The report also includes a comparative cost analysis of commercial yogurt brands. The good news is many organic yogurts are actually less expensive, on a price-per-ounce basis, than conventional, heavily processed yogurts *(although some of the organic brands of yogurt actually contained some of the highest amounts of sugar)*. Your absolute best bet - and also your least expensive - is to make your own kefir or yogurt using organic grass-fed milk. It's a simple process requiring nothing more than the milk, some starter granules and a few mason jars. You can even use a good quality probiotic to culture the milk yogurt at room temperature with no heat.

A good source of calcium and protein, yogurt also contains live cultures called probiotics. These *"good bacteria"* can protect the body from other, more harmful bacteria. Try eating more yogurt, but watch out for fruited or flavored yogurts, which contain a lot of added sugar. Buy plain yogurt and add your own fruit. Look for yogurts that have *"live active cultures"* such as Lactobacillus, L. acidophilus, L. bulgaricus, and S. thermophilus. You can use yogurt in place of mayonnaise or sour cream in dips or sauces.

Beef: Organic, grass-fed, glyphosate and pesticide free is the best bet for beef. Swapping grain-fed beef from concentrated animal feeding operations for organic grass-fed beef is well worth the added price, as you get higher quality nutrients and less exposure to steroids, antibiotics, pesticides, herbicides, and pathogenic bacteria. You can save money by buying directly from a farmer and then freezing the meat.

Butter: Organic, grass-fed, no glyphosate butter is rich in conjugated linoleic acid *(CLA),* known to help fight cancer, diabetes and promote weight loss. Butter is also a rich source of easily absorbed vitamin A and other fat-soluble vitamins *(D, E, and K2)* that are often lacking in the modern industrial diet, plus trace minerals such as manganese, chromium zinc, copper and selenium *(a powerful antioxidant).* About 20% of butterfat consists of short- and medium-chain fatty acids, which your body uses right away for quick energy. Real butter also contains Wulzen Factor, a hormone-like substance that prevents arthritis and joint stiffness, ensuring that calcium in your body is put into your bones rather than your joints and other tissues. The Wulzen factor is present only in raw butter and cream; it is destroyed by pasteurization. Healthy butter is a much healthier choice by orders of magnitude than margarines or spreads. Just beware of *"Monsanto Butter,"* meaning butter that comes from cows fed almost entirely genetically engineered grains with high glyphosate levels.

Mushrooms: A number of different mushrooms - including shiitake, maitake, and reishi - are known for their immune-boosting powers. In fact, some of the most potent immunosupportive agents come from mushrooms, and this is one reason why they're so beneficial for both preventing and treating cancer. Long-chain polysaccharides, particularly alpha and beta-glucan molecules, are primarily responsible for the mushrooms beneficial effect on your immune system. They're also rich in protein, fiber, vitamin C, B vitamins, selenium, calcium, minerals, and antioxidants, including some that are unique to mushrooms. When it comes to mushrooms, make sure they're organic, as mushrooms tend to absorb and concentrate toxins from soil, air, and water.

Kale: The nutritional density of kale is virtually unparalleled among green leafy vegetables, boasting all essential amino acids and nine non-essential ones. One-half cup of raw kale provides 100% of your daily requirement of vitamin A, 340% of your vitamin K and 67% of your vitamin C. It's also loaded with both lutein and zeaxanthin, which are important for good eyesight. Gram-for-gram, kale even contains more calcium than milk.

Like many other superfoods on this list, kale contains potent, chemoprotective agents, which have been shown to aid DNA cell repair and slow the growth of cancer cells. Its anti-inflammatory capabilities have also been shown to help prevent arthritis, heart disease, and several autoimmune diseases. But be careful with kale – it is high on the pesticide list so always buy organic or grow your own.

Whey Protein: Whey protein concentrate *(not to be confused with the far inferior whey protein isolate)* is an ideal choice as it's a rich source of amino acids. It's also the best food for maximizing your glutathione levels as it provides all the raw materials for glutathione production *(cysteine, glycine, and glutamate).* Whey protein, a by-product of milk and cheese, has been linked to a variety of health benefits, including helping your insulin work more effectively, which helps maintain your blood sugar level after a meal, helping to promote your optimal intake of proteins, fats, carbohydrates, vitamins, and minerals needed for your overall wellness, supporting your immune system, as it contains immunoglobulins, helping you preserve lean body tissue *(particularly during exercise)* as it delivers bioavailable amino acids and cysteine, promoting healthy insulin secretion, which is imperative for optimal health. When shopping for a whey protein, be sure to look for a product that is cold-pressed, derived from organic grass-fed cows, free of hormones, toxin-free, no artificial sweeteners and sugar. [443, 444]

Cacao: rich in flavonoids when raw. Processing and heating destroy some of the nutritional value. Also mixing with dairy reduces absorption of anti-oxidant value. Get dark chocolate with 70% cacao. Cacao products - such as unsweetened cocoa powder, nibs, and dark chocolate - are rich sources of minerals. Minimally processed, raw cacao products contain little or no added sugar and are higher in antioxidants than more highly processed products. [445, 446]

Cruciferous Vegetables: Cruciferous vegetables like broccoli, cauliflower, Brussels sprouts, and cabbage are rich in sulfur-containing compounds, which may help protect the brain from everyday oxidative stress, Cruciferous vegetables also have been linked to a reduced risk of stroke. Eat cruciferous veggies raw, lightly steamed, or grilled with a small amount of olive oil. Avoid overcooking, which can lower nutrient levels.

Pineapple: A South American native and a cherished part of Hawaiian folk medicine, pineapple is one of the richest sources in the world of the enzyme bromelain. It is composed of several endopeptidases and compounds like phosphatase, glucosidase, peroxidase, cellulase, escharase, and protease inhibitors. Usually *"bromelain"* sold in extract or supplement form refers to enzymes extracted from pineapple stems or cores, rather than from the fruit's flesh. Used widely as a natural remedy to treat everything from indigestion to allergies, pineapple is not only brimming with this enzyme, but also vitamin C, vitamin B1, potassium, manganese, and phytonutrients. While pineapple has many benefits, the real secret to its healing powers is definitely bromelain. But be careful! Pineapples, notably from Costa Rica, can be high in pesticides.

What is bromelain used to treat? In the medical world, this fascinating compound has traditionally been used as a potent anti-inflammatory and anti-swelling agent. Research has also shown that it has fibrinolytic, antiedematous, and antithrombotic properties, meaning it helps prevent blood clots, edema, and swelling. In the past, this enzyme was also used as a meat tenderizer, reason being it helps to soothe and relax tense, inflamed muscles and connective tissue. Additionally, recent studies have found evidence that this enzyme stops lung metastasis in its tracks, which suggests that bromelain can be used to treat a wide variety of diseases, potentially including cancer.

A look at the scientific literature, which includes 1,600-plus articles evaluating the medicinal benefits of bromelain, shows that it has been used to treat a wide range of health problems, including connective tissue injuries, such as ACL tears, sprained ankles tendonitis, allergies, arthritis, joint pain, and osteoarthritis, digestive issues like heartburn or diarrhea, cardiovascular disorders, asthma, autoimmune diseases, cancer, inflammatory bowel disease, sinus infections, such as bronchitis and sinusitis, surgical trauma and slow healing of skin wounds or burns. [447, 448]

Olive oil: Pressed from fresh olives and is made mainly in the Mediterranean, mostly in Italy, Spain and Greece. Just like in winemaking, several factors affect the character of the oil, including climate, soil, and the way the olives are harvested and pressed.

The flavor, smell, and color of olive oil can vary significantly, based on its origin and whether it is extra-virgin (*finest grade)* or not. Generally, the hotter the country, the more robust the oil's flavor will be. There are four general grades noted.

- **Extra virgin olive oil:** The highest-quality olive oil you can get. It is unrefined and contains more nutrients compared to other processed varieties. **Pure olive oil:** Made by combining extra-virgin olive oil and refined olive oil, resulting in a lower-quality product. It is sometimes sold as *"refined olive oil."*

- **Light olive oil:** The word *"light"* is a marketing term that simply refers to the oil's lighter flavor. In truth, light olive oil is simply refined olive oil that has a neutral taste and a higher smoke point.

- **Olive-pomace oil:** This version of olive oil is made from leftover olive pulps, and the remaining liquid is extracted using chemical solvents. Avoid this type of olive oil at all costs. [449]

Olive oil has been well-researched, and the benefits are extensive. High-quality extra virgin olive oil has anti-inflammatory compounds, antioxidants, and numerous heart-healthy macronutrients. Extra virgin olive oil benefits include lowering rates of inflammation, heart disease, depression, dementia, obesity, and helps fight cancer all of which support longevity. But, not even all of the *"extra virgin"* olive oils have all the desired benefits!

Something that many people don't realize is that it's common for *"extra virgin olive oil"* purchased in most major grocery stores to be laced with GMO canola and herb flavors. A CBS report found that up to 70% of the extra virgin olive oil sold worldwide is watered down with other oils and enhancers, thanks to the Mafia corruption involved in the production process. Yes, you read that correctly, so do your homework and the best practice is to stay organic. You can strike gold with the health benefits of olive oil if you do a little research. [450]

Medium-Chain Triglycerides *(MCT)*: Medium-chain Triglycerides *(MCTs)* are a unique form of dietary fat that impart a wide range of positive health benefits. Dietary fats are molecules composed of individual carbon atoms linked into chains ranging from 2 to 22 carbon atoms in length. Long-Chain Fatty acids *(LCTs)* ranging from 12 to 18 carbons long are the predominant form of fat in the American diet. MCTs, by contrast, are composed of only 6 to 10 carbon links. Because of their shorter chain length, MCTs have a number of unique properties, which give them advantages over the more common LCTs.

MCTs provide about 10% fewer calories than LCTs, are more rapidly absorbed by the body, and more quickly used as fuel. The result of this accelerated metabolic conversion is that instead of being stored as fat, the calories contained in MCTs are very efficiently converted into fuel for immediate use by organs and muscles. So MCTs seem to offer a triple benefit for weight loss - they have a lower calorie content than other fats, are minimally stored as fat, and contribute to enhanced metabolism to burn even more calories. Calorie-restricted diets are often associated with marked declines in energy. A number of studies support the benefits of using MCTs in weight loss programs, to boost energy levels, to think more clearly, experience better digestion, increase fatty acid metabolism, to have better digestion and to improve your mood. MCTs have also been shown to suppress appetite, prevent atherosclerosis, reduce blood sugar, reduce bad cholesterol, enhance immune system function.

Good sources of MCT are organic butter, coconut oil, palm oil, local fresh dairy products from farms using organic practices, and cheeses. If you purchase MCT oil, make sure it is concentrated with capric and caprylic acids mostly and minimal lauric acid. There are some great recipes using MCT as well. You can make salad dressings, *"fat bombs"* - really tasty healthy chocolate treats, the healthy version of Reese's pieces, mayonnaise, and include MCTs in smoothies. You can also use coconut oil directly as well on skin, hair, in toothpaste, facial masks, sunscreens, shaving creams and as a carrier for essential oils. We use coconut oil or palm oil when making popcorn and include some healthy organic butter. [451, 452]

Why Organic Nutrition Is Important

The foods of nature have provided life on earth with all the nutrition needed for survival. There is a symbiotic relationship that exists - everything that is here on earth is here for a reason, and generally, no matter how remote the association may seem, there is some connection to survival. Beneficial to some, and harmful to others, these relationships are essential to many organisms and ecosystems, and they provide a balance. We are organic beings, and our bodies must have the complementary organic nutrients from nature to survive, while anything else is antagonistic to our body. While there is some capacity of our body to tolerate short-term insults from exposure to man-made chemicals and artificial foods, what we have experienced from the beginning of the industrial revolution is a steady decline in the overall health of all organic life on earth, which has caused genetic and epigenetic changes in gene function.

We are surrounded every day by an invisible sea of synthetic chemicals and our bodies absorb them like sponges until we are toxic. Synthetic chemicals permeate our food chain. Store-bought fruits, vegetables, meats, seafood; all of it is contaminated to some degree. Eating organic is a much better choice, but homegrown foods without the pesticides, fungicides, herbicides and using natural fertilizers are still the best option whenever possible. Local gardening coops are springing up all over the place, so find a way to make one happen in your community if you don't have the space for a garden in your back yard. If you have a family with children, remember, your children's futures are at stake - so, take that into consideration. You will either contribute to the problem or help resolve the problem.

Even if you are consuming fresh fruits and vegetables, the quality can make a huge difference. The chances are that, outside of organic, the nutrient levels are depleted because of mass farming techniques that deplete the soil of essential nutrients that do not get replaced. The growers may put in *(synthetic)* nitrogen, phosphorus, and potassium to make the veggies look pretty in the store, but the nutrient levels can be significantly depleted of nutrients like zinc, magnesium, selenium, manganese, protein, calcium, phosphorus, iron, riboflavin *(vitamin B2)* pyridoxine *(B6),* vitamin E, vitamin C, and others.

How bad is it? Scientific American reported a landmark study on the topic by Donald Davis and his team of researchers from the University of Texas *(UT)* at Austin's Department of Chemistry and Biochemistry, published in December 2004, in the Journal of the American College of Nutrition.

They studied the US Department of Agriculture nutritional data from both 1950 and

1999 for 43 different vegetables and fruits, finding *"reliable declines"* in the amount of protein, calcium, phosphorus, iron, riboflavin, *(vitamin B2)* and vitamin C over the past half-century. Davis and his colleagues chalk up this declining nutritional content to the preponderance of agricultural practices designed to improve traits *(size, growth rate, pest resistance)* other than nutrition. The Organic Consumers Association cites several other studies with similar findings: A Kushi Institute analysis of nutrient data from 1975 to 1997 found that average calcium levels in 12 fresh vegetables dropped 27%; iron levels 37%; vitamin A levels 21%, and vitamin C levels 30%. A similar study of British nutrient data from 1930 to 1980, published in the British Food Journal found that in 20 vegetables the average calcium content had declined 19%, iron 22%, and potassium 14%. Yet another study concluded that one would have to eat eight oranges today to derive the same amount of vitamin A as our grandparents would have gotten from one. That is pretty serious. [453]

The processing of food removes even more nutrients. Consider what happens to canned tuna. The canning process removes 99% of vitamin A found in fresh tuna, 97% of vitamin D, 86% of B2, and 45% of niacin. It also increases the level of oxidized cholesterol in the human body. When whole wheat is refined into white flour for white bread the percentage and range of nutrients lost are extraordinary: fiber 95%, iron 84%, vitamin E 95%, manganese 82%, niacin 80%, and vitamin B 81%. Most foods are also irradiated to neutralize insects and microorganisms and this process further destroys vitamins, other essential nutrients in the food, and eliminates the soil organisms that produce natural antibiotic content. To compensate, the food processors have resorted to synthetic food additives. [454]

It is also a myth that we get all the vitamins we need in our daily diet. Our food loses essential nutrients at every step of the process from their growth to our dining tables. The nutrients have been replaced by synthetic chemical additives. These additives in processed foods interact synergistically in our bodies with other synthetic chemicals absorbed from our water, our air, and our consumer products, which weaken our immune systems. There may also be no real difference between *"natural flavor"* and artificial flavor on any list of food ingredients. Both categories can represent synthetic chemicals produced by slightly different methods. Almost every product labeled sugar- free, "diet," or low-calorie contains chemical additives and artificial sweeteners that fool us into thinking they are somehow healthier and what they replaced.

Nutritional Supplements

In today's toxic world, nutritional supplementation is necessary to combat all stresses put on the body. Whether eating healthy or not, the cold reality is that we all need more than what we get in our diets.

The problem is that most of the vitamins and supplements sold in the United States are junk and a waste of your money. Even the ones that are advertised as natural are actually synthetic chemical concoctions that contain coal tar preservative, artificial coloring, and a vast range of other potentially harmful additives.

You'll find three types of vitamins sold today: the naturally occurring kind, taken directly from plants or fruit sources, the much more numerous synthetic brands, and equally numerous yeast tablets injected with synthetic chemicals. This last category misleads the consuming public because even though the synthetics are labeled as natural under FDA guidelines *(only because they include yeast) they are still synthetic imitations).*

The vast majority of vitamin supplements are made from a handful of manufacturers. These vitamins are made from coal tars and use artificial coloring preservatives, coating materials, and other additives. Synthetic vitamin C is really just ascorbic acid. Yes, it may have some bioactivity, but does it have the same bioactive *"signature"* of natural vitamin C? Vitamin B1 is made from a coal tar derivative, and vitamin E comes from an Eastman Kodak plant where it is a byproduct of the emulsification process used to manufacture film.

After purification, it is sold to the supplement industry. Studies of both vitamin C and vitamin E show that naturally occurring forms are more absorbable by the body and more biologically active than synthetics. The scientific studies demonstrating the superiority of naturally occurring vitamins over synthetics have been published in such journals as the Annals of the New York Academy of Sciences, American Journal of Clinical Nutrition, and Britain's Royal Society of Chemistry. In a 1998 study at Oregon State University six volunteers were given one 150 mg doses of synthetic vitamins E, and later the same dose of vitamin E, from natural sources. Urine tests show conclusively that the human body prefers to retain natural vitamin E by how quickly it excretes the synthetic version. Other studies essentially confirmed these findings. [455 - 458]

Some researchers make a convincing argument that vitamins in nature are a complex mixture of interactive molecular compounds that necessarily must be present for the full benefit. Scott Treadway, Ph.D., an expert on vitamin formulation, writes that synthetic vitamin C is really not vitamin C, nor is alpha-tocopherol vitamin E, retinoid acid vitamin A, and so on with other vitamins. The truth is that natural vitamins are not individual molecular compounds, but rather a whole range of vitamins, minerals, cofactors and enzymes that allow for optimal use by the body. [459 - 461]

With this background in the vitamin industry, let's go over a few of the more important points about vitamins:

Fat-Soluble Vitamins

Vitamin A plays a critical role in maintaining vision, neurological function, healthy skin, immune function, and is very important in bone health, reduces cholesterol, helps lower cancer risk, and more. It has also been shown to minimize and shorten symptoms and mortality associated with measles in those deficient in vitamin A, as many people are today. [462]

Vitamin A is found in two primary forms: active vitamin A *(also called retinol, which results in retinyl esters)* and beta-carotene. Retinol comes from animal-derived foods and is a type of *"pre-formed"* vitamin A that can be used directly by the body. The other type, which is obtained from colorful fruits and vegetables, is in the form of provitamin carotenoids. Beta-carotene and other types of carotenoids found in plant-based products need to first be converted to retinol, the active form of vitamin A, in order to be utilized by the body.

Beta carotene is a precursor the body can convert to vitamin A. Unfortunately, as a supplement, synthetic beta carotene is usually *"stabilized"* in refined vegetable oils. In this trans fatty acid form, oxidation occurs and the chemically *"pure"* beta-carotene can no longer act as a nutrient because it was changed. This form can no longer be converted to vitamin A. [463]

Vitamin D plays several roles in the body. Emerging research supports the possible role of vitamin D in protecting against cancer, heart disease, fractures (by insuring proper levels of calcium), autoimmune diseases, influenza, type 2 diabetes, and depression. Most people can get all they need from just 10 to 20 minutes of daily sun exposure. When the sunlight hits the skin, dietary cholesterol is converted into vitamin D. People with darker skin or those who live further from the equator may need longer exposure to get enough vitamin D. Also, in order to make vitamin D, the skin needs to be directly in the sun and not blocked by sunscreen or cover-ups.

Vitamin D in supplements is found in either the D2 or D3 form. Vitamin D3 is the preferred form and is derived from two sources - fish oil and sheep lanolin. Natural vitamin D3 comes from the skin of fatty fish such as salmon or tuna. Lanolin is a waxy substance secreted by glands found in a sheep's skin. Vitamin D3 from either source is the exact same form of vitamin D found in our bodies and, as a supplement, is absorbed the best.

Vitamin D2 is generally used to fortify milk or other foods and is made from yeast or other plant matter. Many experts believe that D2 is not well absorbed or utilized by the body because it is from plants and not the type of vitamin D the body naturally makes. The body can convert D2 to D3, but it may not be as efficient, especially if you are trying to correct a vitamin D deficiency. If you are a vegetarian or vegan, however, vitamin D2 is the only vegan source of vitamin D.

Vitamin E is a lipid-soluble phenolic cellular antioxidant compound obtained from plant sources in the diet. Vitamin E is not a singular substance. It is a collective term for a family of eight homologue *(stereoisomer)* molecules that are synthesized naturally by plants. The compounds can act as an antioxidant by donating a hydrogen atom to reduce free radicals.

The eight homologues are split into two groups: tocopherols and tocotrienols. Both the tocopherols and tocotrienols have four homologues each, named: alpha, beta, gamma, and delta. Each form has slightly different biological activity. All of these various derivatives with vitamin E activity are technically referred to collectively as *"vitamin E."*

Historically, only one of those eight, d-alpha-tocopherol, appeared to have the most nutritional importance, the d-alpha-tocopherol isomer form. It is what is commonly called vitamin E on nutrition/supplement labels. The alpha-tocopherol form constitutes 90% of the tocopherol found in humans, with the largest quantities in blood and tissues and this form has gained the most research attention. However, recent developments warrant a serious reconsideration of this conventional wisdom. Tocotrienols possess powerful neuroprotective, anticancer and cholesterol-lowering properties that are often not exhibited by tocopherols. Current developments in vitamin E research clearly indicate that members of the vitamin E family are not redundant with respect to their biological functions. Alpha-tocotrienol, gamma-tocopherol, and beta-tocotrienol have emerged as vitamin E molecules with functions in health and disease that are clearly distinct from that of alpha-tocopherol. Even at the low concentration seen in the body compared to d-alpha- tocopherol, alpha-tocotrienol prevents neurodegeneration. On a concentration basis, this finding represents the most potent of all biological functions exhibited by any natural vitamin E molecule. Tocotrienols are antioxidants, anti-aging, anticancer, antiplaque, and anti-inflammatory, reduce cholesterol and triglyceride, improves immune function, and reduces harmful effects of diabetes.

The best food sources of vitamin E are vegetable oils *(sunflower and olive)*, nuts, seeds, and fortified cereals. Tocotrienol supplements are available in capsule and tablet form if needed. Crude palm oil extracted from the fruits of Elaeis guineensis contains particularly high amounts of tocotrienols. Annatto seeds are also a superior source of tocotrienols since it is the only natural source that contains only tocotrienols and no tocopherols. Nuts and seeds also have appreciable levels of tocotrienols. [464]

It was also established in the early 1980s that another form of tocopherol *(called alpha-tocopherol succinate)* was the most effective form of vitamin E in comparison to alpha-tocopherol acetate in the inhibition of proliferation and apoptosis *(killing)* of cancer cells. It is now the preferred form of vitamin E to help patients combat breast, prostate, and other cancers. An abundance of research has proven that vitamin E succinate is the most effective form of vitamin E in inducing differentiation, growth inhibition, and programmed cell death *(apoptosis)* in cancer cells. [465]

Whenever someone asks me to take a look at his or her vitamin supplement to check for quality, the first ingredient that I check is vitamin E. If it only says, d-alpha-tocopherol acetate, it is most likely a cheap synthetic vitamin and a waste of your money. If the label says mixed, that may or may not be okay because you do not know what the mix is. If there is a complex containing alpha-tocopherol acetate and succinate, gamma tocopherol, and tocotrienols, it is a nutritional goldmine. [466]

Vitamin K or phylloquinone is present primarily in green leafy vegetables and is the main dietary form of vitamin K. It is then converted to K2. Vitamin K2 includes a range of vitamin K forms collectively referred to as menaquinones. Most menaquinones are synthesized by human intestinal microbiota and found in fermented food *(MK-7)* and in animal products *(MK-4)*. MK-4 is unique in that it is produced by the body from phylloquinone via a conversion process that does not involve bacterial action. Vitamin K functions as a coenzyme for the synthesis of proteins involved in hemostasis *(blood clotting)* and bone metabolism, and other diverse physiological functions.

Food sources of phylloquinone include vegetables, especially green leafy vegetables, vegetable oils, and some fruits. Meat, dairy foods, and eggs contain low levels of phylloquinone but modest amounts of menaquinones. Natto *(a traditional Japanese food made from fermented soybeans)* has high amounts of menaquinones. Other fermented foods, such as cheese, also contain menaquinones. However, the forms and amounts of vitamin K in these foods likely vary depending on the bacterial strains used to make the foods and their fermentation conditions. Animals synthesize MK-4 from menadione *(a synthetic form of vitamin K that can be used in poultry and swine feed)*. Thus, poultry and pork products contain MK-4 if menadione is added to the animal feed. There is a connection with vitamin D in that vitamin D ensures that your blood levels of calcium are high enough to meet your body's demands and vitamin K tells the calcium where to go. [467 - 469]

Water-Soluble Vitamins

Vitamin B Most of the water-soluble B vitamins are readily available in the diets of developed cultures, so deficiencies are not common unless there are some genetic or environmentally induced gene changes. The B vitamins are important in physiologic and metabolic cellular functions throughout the body including cardiovascular, hematological, neurological, immune, skin, and musculoskeletal systems. They play important roles in energy production, the synthesis and repair of DNA and RNA, as well as carbohydrate, protein and fat metabolism. As a routine to cover my bases, I include B supplementation through my multivitamin formula throughout the week. [470 - 471]

Some B vitamins are noteworthy because of an ever-growing incidence of gene mutations, especially B9. I also covered this in part in the epigenetics chapter. Vitamin B9 has been identified in two forms commonly recognized in the general public. They are used interchangeably but are not the same. Folate is the natural pre-vitamin form of B9 while folic acid is the synthetic form. Folic acid goes through an additional step in the liver before entering into the middle of a sequence that converts inactive folate B9 to active B9. Folic acid requires an enzyme that facilitates that conversion. If that gene is mutated, then folic acid can accumulate in the blood with high supplement doses. Also, if the MTHFR gene *(which converts inactive folate B9 to active B9)* is mutated, there can be a whole host of health problems including mental, cardiovascular, bone, and pregnancy problems.

Vitamin C, also known as L-ascorbic acid, is a water-soluble vitamin that is naturally present in some foods, added to others, and available as a dietary supplement. Humans, unlike most animals, are unable to synthesize vitamin C endogenously, so it is an essential dietary component. Vitamin C is required for the biosynthesis of collagen, L-carnitine, and certain neurotransmitters. Vitamin C is also involved in protein metabolism. Collagen is an essential component of connective tissue, which plays a vital role in wound healing. Vitamin C is also an important physiological antioxidant and has been shown to regenerate other antioxidants within the body, including alpha-tocopherol *(vitamin E).* [472]

As mentioned in the Nutritional Supplements intro, there are those who believe that in nature vitamin C is not a single molecular compound, but a complex of interactive compounds *(flavonoids)* that may affect bioavailability and that consumption of vitamin C should include these associated natural *"bioflavonoids"* which have their own health benefits. Nobel Prize-winning biochemist Albert Szent-Gyorgyi M.D., Ph.D., who was given the credit for discovering vitamin C also coined the term vitamin P, which later became known as flavonoids. Some studies that measure blood and excretion levels of L-ascorbic acid with and without bioflavonoids have not supported the idea that natural is better absorbed or made more available to cells than the synthetic form. That may be just a matter of insufficient testing design, but that is was the literature says at this point. Even the Linus Pauling Institute confirms this. But, is that all there is to the discussion? Scott Treadway mentioned earlier, make a convincing argument that absorption is not the only important factor, but the interactive *"life force"* of the vitamin C complex is immeasurable, and current research protocols cannot measure such a quantum effect. I agree and prefer the natural form to the synthetic L-ascorbic acid. I can appreciate the benefits of L ascorbic acid by itself, but I prefer the natural form with all the other healthy components mixed in - God knows what he is doing. That argument aside, L-ascorbic acid is an essential cofactor in numerous enzymatic reactions, *(e.g., in the biosynthesis of collagen, carnitine, and neuropeptides, and in the regulation of gene expression)* and it is a potent antioxidant and regenerates other antioxidants in the body. It is also associated with lower risks of hypertension, coronary heart disease, and stroke, boosts the immune system, and several studies have shown a positive correlation between increased doses of vitamin C and reduction in the incidence of certain cancers. It is also a critical factor in wound healing. [473 - 477]

PART FOUR

Essential Oils And CBD

Essential Oils - Making Perfect
Scents Of The Journey

When I think about New Beginnings, I think fresh! It makes me feel alive inside - a renewed sense of who I am and where I am going. I am reminded of being a young boy going outside and running like the wind, enjoying the freedom to explore. Lying down in a field of grass just daydreaming, climbing trees, discovering shooting stars, the art of imagination, lightning bugs, and playing hide and seek on a beautiful spring evening. Everything was a new and delightful experience. But my fondest memories are associated with the sweet fragrances of spring that come from the essential oils of plants. Even today, when I smell familiar fresh flowers, I can immediately be taken back to my childhood years. It doesn't matter what the circumstances, I just check out to savor the moment. I guess you could say my experience with the therapeutic power of aromatics goes way back.

My journey with essential oils started in 2006 when my wife came to me one day and said that she was going out with the kids on a field trip. We were homeschooling our children, and her good friend, Karen, was having a class that she wanted to attend. When I got home from work that day, she came to me all excited, telling me about this woo-woo stuff called essential oils, which were helping people with this and that problem, and even helped heal someone who was scheduled for kidney surgery. At the time, I had 23 years as a medical and surgical specialist and espoused the idea that the allopathic medical profession offered the best training and care in the world, with medication being the answer to all life's ills. So, the idea that essential oils were a little genie in a bottle was, well, let's just say that I was respectful and listened on the outside, but I was really rolling my eyes on the inside. But she was excited because she thought there would be some hope for her step-dad who was dying from a rare form of cancer, and they didn't give him much time or hope. He had gone through two rounds of chemotherapy, which actually made things worse, and I believe shortened his life. I agreed to give essential oils a try to see if it would help him, but I was certainly skeptical to say the least. He was not doing well and died a short time after we started with essential oils, but I did notice how helpful they were to help him sleep and take away some of the pain. The gallbladder tumor was so large that it was pressing on several other organs and causing a lot of pain. He passed shortly thereafter, and life went on for us and our family.

But I did not forget what I observed with him. *"How could those essential oils work like that,"* I thought. Then, our five school-aged kids started reading and playing around with the oils and found how well they worked for most anything. I was keeping my eye on all of this but was still not totally convinced. There were two events that completely changed my skepticism about essential oils. The first was when we went with the family on a ski trip during spring break. In the past *(and not anymore thanks to essential oils)* I got fever blisters *(cold sores, Herpes simplex)* on my lips if I got too stressed or was out in the high-altitude sun for long. Well, sure enough, I began to feel one coming on. Normally, I would have used a prescription cream, which would help, especially if I got to it before the blisters started. But even then, I might have some remnant for a couple of weeks. When I felt the symptoms of itching on my lip, I knew I was in trouble, and I didn't have any medication. So, I mentioned it to Angel and she said, *"Well, I DO have some essential oils that may work."* I thought, *"Okay, I can spend the next two weeks with my patients staring at the scab on my lip, or I can try some of the woo-woo oils."* I went for it, and to my surprise, it completely took away all of the symptoms, and there was no blistering. That got my attention!

Not too long after that, one Saturday afternoon I was removing weeds in the backyard with my son. There were some weeds between some pavers, and

I used a small curved knife blade to dig it out. The blade slipped, and I cut my little finger pretty badly. It was an angled cut, and they are hard to heal. I should have gone to the ER and gotten some stitches, but I don't like going to docs so, hey, I just decided to take care of it myself and take my chances. It was bleeding all over the place, but I managed to wash it off, compressed it for a short while to reduce some of the bleeding, put some lavender essential oils on it with a gauze pad and a couple of Band-Aids, and went back to digging in the dirt. I left the Band-Aids on even though they were dirty because I knew if I took them off the wound would open back up.

Monday rolled around, and I was in the shower debating whether or not to remove the dirty, haggard bandage. But, I obviously couldn't see patients with it on, so I decided to take it off. I was shocked at what I saw. The wound that was supposed to take at least three weeks to seal shut was about 90% healed. I was so taken back that I yelled for Angel to come and see it. I told her, *"Hey, I am a surgeon, and this is NOT supposed to happen! These types of cuts just don't heal like this."* From then on I was a true believer, and I started researching oils and many other natural options for healing.

I am a researcher at heart. I want to understand not just the what and how, but more importantly the why. And, why weren't we taught this in medical school? I answered my question as soon as it came out of my mouth. The pharmaceutical industry both actively and passively controls a lot of what is taught in medical school regarding treatment options for patients. I started with PubMed, a public access point into the National Library of Medicine. Unless you have complete access status, what you will see is abstracts, which for most people is all that is needed to get the purpose of the study and the end result. At the time, there were over 5000 articles listed when I searched for the term "essential oils." I was shocked at that as well since this was never mentioned in my training. I went through about 3200 of the abstracts leaving out similar studies and research on the bugs, etc. I was absolutely fascinated by the research having already been done that clearly demonstrated the health benefits of essential oils. I really began to see the light, how nature has provided so much that can heal us. There are now over 19,000 references to essential oils when searching the National Library of Medicine database. That says a whole lot! There is a clear resurgence of interest in essential oils, both in the marketplace and research sectors.

Why not before? Because since the early 1900s the pharmaceutical industry has had such a stranglehold on every part of our daily existence that we cannot see through the glass clearly, but we also don't realize there is a cleaner side of our existence on the other side of the glass. So, we just do as we are told. Natural plants cannot be patented, and the pharmaceutical industry cannot make the big bucks without a patent. So, what can they do instead? They can mimic through synthetic versions or chemically change the beneficial compounds in the plant enough to get it patented. The problem is that when the natural essential oils is changed to the unnatural, major side effects can and do result. Patented medications are not *"alive"* like essential oils and other living forms of nature. Inherently, synthetic medications are unidirectional and do not have the capacity to have "dialogue" with your own DNA life force. Oils know what to do in your body, even when you don't.

Direct observations have shown that some oils for example can either raise or lower blood sugar, depending on the need. My wife was at the mall one day. She ran out of the door without eating anything. As she was exiting the mall, she became dizzy and collapsed on the floor from low blood sugar, which she was prone to experience. Someone walked by in the same moment who knew who she was *(another example of God intervening)* and asked if she was okay. Angel said yes, and that her blood sugar was low. She asked her friend to reach into her purse and get a special blend of oils that contained cinnamon bark. It is known to raise or lower blood sugar as needed. The paramedics got there just after she was helped into JC Penney offices. After putting the blend under her tongue just before they arrived, within minutes she was pretty much back to normal. The paramedics took her blood sugar levels, and they were back to normal and all she did was use her essential oil blend!

There are many stories of how essential oils have helped people with various health problems. Their effects can even be observed through electroencephalogram *(EEG)* studies and other more sophisticated scanning technology. We are electromagnetic beings. Every cell in our body generates a measurable energy frequency. We can have altered frequencies when we are unhealthy. Some measuring devices can be very detailed in identifying what body functions are out of sync. Even unhealthy emotions can alter frequency. The science is relatively young and developing, but is very promising. Understanding the quantum mechanics of cellular communication is an exciting field of science.

What Are Essential Oils?

Simply, essential oils *(sometimes referred to as EOs)* are *"volatile"* aromatic compounds extracted from the bark, flowers, leaves, roots, seeds, stems, and other parts of plants. Volatile means that they evaporate from a liquid to a gas. That is what you smell in the air when you pass by some fragrant flowers. The oils are the lifeblood of the plant and are mixtures of dozens, even hundreds, of constituents. They are the purest and most potent form of an herb, very concentrated, potent antioxidants, and can have both *"anti-this"* as well as *"pro-that"* qualities at the same time. They do what the body needs them to do.

They give a plant its distinct aroma and play a crucial role in the survival of the plant as a whole. Each essential oil has a unique composition based on the variety of its chemical constituents that vary from plant to plant and even species to species. Something as simple as the fertilizer used during the growing season, when the plant was harvested, and the part of it that was picked can dramatically affect the potency and efficacy of the resulting essential oils. Add to that the climate, weather patterns, and geographical region where the plants were grown, and you have a small glimpse into the complexity of essential oil production. Even a lavender plant on one side of my farm can have a somewhat different chemical composition than one planted on the other side. For many who are enjoying the fragrance, that may not be so important, but for those in the therapeutic grade essential oils industry, the difference can be quite profound and may determine if a season's harvest is used for therapeutic purposes or to be sold off to other sectors such as industrial, perfume, or food-grade industries. There are different grades of essential oils depending on the purpose.

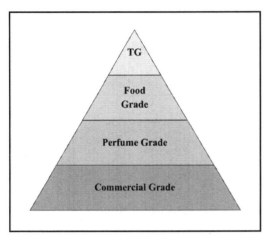

If interested in quality essential oils that provide the highest therapeutic index possible, it is critical that you do not choose a supplier who may be searching the wholesale catalogue for the cheapest price to maximize profits and essentially knows nothing about the chemistry of essential oils, where the oils came from, gas chromatography, mass spectrometry, and Brix results, etc. This is not like buying ibuprofen off the grocery store shelf. You want the best for you and your family. Choose wisely. Choose an essential oils company with a long history of verifiable quality control and safety protocols, and with sustainable farms using organic practices *(no chemical pesticides or herbicides)*. The essential oil company that we use has farms and partner farms to grow their plants and produces the highest quality essential oils possible. Their testing equipment of therapeutic analysis of the oils is unmatched by any other essential oils company. Quality oils are more expensive, period. You can't skimp on this. If you do, you will most likely be getting essential oils with additives such as benzene and other toxic chemicals, as well as synthetic perfume additives, and a therapeutic index that is like comparing a tricycle to a super sports car. And talking about price, the therapeutic grade is a far better price point since you may only need one drop versus five or even ten if the cheaper brands work at all.

Aromatic plants, herbs, barks, resins, incense, and oils have been used for thousands of years in various cultures for medicinal and health purposes.

They are the oldest known medicine, earliest noted at around 4,500 BC. There are over 200 references to aromatics, incense, and ointments in the Bible. In 1922, King Tut's tomb was opened, the contents of which included several thousand items. Fifty alabaster jars, capable of holding approximately 350 liters of fragrant oils, were among those items. Most of the oils were gone, presumably stolen because of their high value. The Ebers Papyrus is arguably the most complete and most beautiful of the medical texts to have survived from ancient Egypt. It contained remedies for a variety of diseases including natural plant ingredients such as myrrh, frankincense, fennel, cassia, thyme, henna, juniper, aloe, linseed and castor oil, and many others. The mid-19th century brought us the brilliance of Rene-Maurice Gattefosse' credited for coining the term *"aromatherapy."* His research took an interesting turn when he accidentally burned himself and successfully treated it topically with lavender essential oil. [478 - 482]

Because of their many documented antitumoral, antioxidant, stimulating, detoxifying, antibacterial, antiviral, antifungal, brain calming and system balancing, anti-inflammatory, muscle relaxing and more properties, essential oils are gaining popularity as a natural, safe, and cost-effective therapy for physical, mental, and emotional health. The side effects of the chemicals in medications are becoming more prominent in the public consciousness and the desire for safe and effective alternatives are taking us full circle back to what has worked for ages. They are also used as a healthy alternative for beauty care and home cleaning. And are known to increase nutrient absorption when consumed with food or supplements.

Essential oils are extracted from plants in two main ways. The process of distillation separates the aromatic oil from a plant by steaming them. Oils can also be removed through expression, also called a "cold-press" process. Citrus oils are generally removed using the cold press process. Essential oils are highly concentrated compounds with distinctive aromas. They can have such high concentrations of therapeutic compounds that only a drop or two may be needed for a desired health effect. People generally think that more is better, but such is not the case with essential oils. It is better to start small and then add more if needed. Why? Because of the tiny molecular structure of the components of an essential oil, they are extremely concentrated. Essential oils are composed of very small molecules that can penetrate your cells, and some compounds in essential oils can even cross the blood-brain barrier. One drop contains approximately 40 million-trillion various molecules. We have an estimated 50-100 trillion cells in our bodies, and that's a lot. One drop of essential oil can provide every cell in our bodies with 40,000 or more molecules. [483]

For example, using one drop of lavender essential oil can help to relax the body from a tension headache instead of taking several pills of an over-the-counter alternative that expires within a few years. Got a headache, a drop of frankincense and peppermint in the hand and smelling the aroma can relieve it. How about sleep? A couple of drops lavender or others in an essential oils diffuser can knock your socks off. For me, I am asleep in about ten minutes. Also, be careful if you use them in cooking. If you are fixing a pot of spaghetti sauce, and you want to add oregano, you may normally use a tablespoon or more of dried herbs. But if you decide to use quality oregano essential oil instead. Just using a drop will be too much. All that is needed in most cases is a toothpick dipped into the oregano oil and swirled into the sauce. If you use a drop, you're done. Start over. It will probably ruin the sauce that you worked so hard to prepare. Quality EOs are that potent.

The Chemistry Of Essential Oils Made Simple

For those of you who want a basic, fairly easy to understand breakdown of EO chemistry, here it is. Based on their chemical compositions, EOs are broadly categorized into oxygenated compounds and hydrocarbons. Oxygenated compounds include esters, aldehydes, ketones, alcohols, phenols, and oxides. Other active groups include aromatics and sulfur-containing components. Hydrocarbon compounds are composed of one specific chemical group called terpenes. These are composed of varying numbers of isoprene units *(C5)*. Monoterpenes *(C10)* and sesquiterpenes *(C15)* are the main terpenes, although the isoprene chains may also include diterpenes *(C20)*. Monoterpenes contribute to 90% of EO overall constituents. Both monoterpenes and sesquiterpenes offer a large variety of structures through adjoining with other biologically active functional groups *(monoterpenoids)*, and chemical rearrangement and addition of oxygenated groups *(sesquiterpenoids)*. Most essential oils are a combination of hydrocarbon and oxygen groups. [484]

When I first started using essential oils in 2006, I was pretty much alone out there in the local medical community. When I talked to others about EOs, I mostly saw blank stares. How things have changed. Most people that I talk to now know about essential oils, many use them or know someone who does. That's encouraging! The average person however knows more about essential oils than most healthcare providers, who by default clearly should know how to use them to help their patients. While the wheels of medicine change very slowly, and EOs are not part of mainstream treatments, they are being recognized and used in many hospital settings and outpatient clinics in the treatment of anxiety and depression. EOs have also been used in pre-op relief from anxiety, and by midwives to help reduce fear and anxiety during childbirth. They are also used in other medical settings. Of course, they were used long before the age of medications. Many oils, when massaged on the skin, can help treat skin conditions, such as burns, cuts, and scrapes. Others may help with insomnia and aid with digestion, improve brain function, reduce blood pressure, reduce cortisol levels, boost energy levels, support the hormone systems, promote sleep, relieve muscle and joint aches and pains, and help repair skin damage, and more.

The Versatility Of Essential Oils

To illustrate how versatile and beneficial essential oils can be to our health, I have chosen to highlight two: frankincense and lavender.

EOs are even being used to help fight cancer, as there is research to support the connection between frankincense *(boswellia) and the reduction of cancer risk or spread* in a laboratory setting. There are also many real-life stories of frankincense being instrumental in healing various forms of cancer. Frankincense has also been used for thousands of years to heighten spiritual awareness and much more from head to toe as the saying goes. This very special essential oil even brought back to consciousness this poor bird *(pictured)* that ran headfirst into our big window in our house. We periodically have birds flying into the window as it reflects the surrounding trees and sky. Most don't survive the trauma. But this time, the family decided to try and revive him. When they heard the classic thump, they grabbed a bottle of frankincense and ran outside. The bird was out cold, and they didn't think there was any chance of survival. But they picked him up and held the bottle of frankincense under its beak. It didn't look good, but all of a sudden, the bird opened his eyes and just stayed there for a couple of moments breathing in the frankincense aroma. They stood him up on the ground, and he was content to stay there and breathe in the aroma from the bottle. After about five or so minutes, he was good to go and flew off.

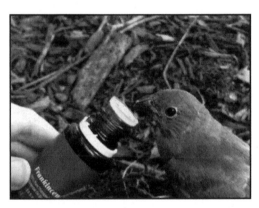

I am partial to frankincense for a number of reasons, and I like to think that it has God's special signature in the world of quantum physics. After all, it was one of the gifts that were given to Jesus sometime shortly after his birth. At the time, it was recognized to have special significance and value. It was expensive, and it is probably fair to assume that most people probably knew about it but could not afford it. Frankincense was associated with kingship and priestly anointing. There were also practical uses for medicinal purposes. Women of the day, I would think, had similar post-delivery issues as many women do today. Stretch marks, postpartum depression, babies not latching on to be fed, etc., and if momma was stressed because a donkey just stepped on her six-year-old's foot, the kids were acting crazy, and the baby needed to be fed, then she might be so stressed that her milk will not let down. You can easily imagine where a mother might burn some frankincense or put some of the resin mixed into a paste or liquid on her chest to breathe to help her relax, let her milk down, and savor the experience while feeding a baby. If a baby was fussy, the frankincense would also help to calm the baby for feeding and snuggling with momma. The value of frankincense in calming the brain has been well established. Both frankincense and myrrh are also good for skin repair such as stretch marks and they have antimicrobial effects and many other health benefits as well.

The gum/resin from frankincense has been used in religious ceremonies for thousands of years because there is a strong spiritual and emotionally sedating connection. Recent research has also identified pathways in the brain that might be involved while in those experiences. Frankincense comes from the genus Boswellia tree and the oil can be sourced from several species including Boswellia Carterii, Boswellia Ferreana or Boswellia Serrata, and Boswellia Dalzielii trees, which are commonly grown in various regions in Africa and Pakistan. Boswellia Sacra is grown in Oman and possibly some other regions. Some have said that it is synonymous with Boswellia Carterii, but studies show that it is a completely different species based on polarity and optical rotation. These characteristics are important in the absorption capacity and overall effect on the body. Each species has its own signature compounds and even within species, depending on growing climate, the levels of the predominant compounds can vary. This is generally true of all plants that produce essential oils. [485 - 488]

Boswellia Papyrifera is another species common in the African Sudan region that has appreciable levels of incensole in its several forms. This compound has recently been studied for its emotional relaxation and for enhancing the spiritual experience as well as anti-inflammatory effects and reducing cortisol levels. Frankincense has been used in religious and cultural ceremonies for eons. The oil is not as common as the resin because of low oil yields, so using it is an incense burner with the resin is probably best to access the incensole. It has also been linked with relieving anxiety and depression and neuroprotective and anti-inflammatory effects, and scientists wonder if it may be useful in treating brain injuries. [489 - 492]

In the present era, frankincense gum/resin/oil has been researched extensively for its health-related benefits, including:

- reduction of anxiety and depression

- enhancing the immune system

- anticancer properties

- antiviral, antibacterial and antifungal properties

- improvement of memory and learning functions

- balancing hormone levels

- relief of constipation, headaches, nausea, fatigue, and mood swings

- healthy gastrointestinal function and sleep

- release joint pain

- relieve headaches

- decreases inflammation and promotes wound healing

- reduce the pain and inflammation from autoimmune disease, and

- promote relaxation and the reduction of stress.

There are many components that contribute to these effects including various boswellic acids, and mono and diterpenes, and sesquiterpenes in the gum/resin and oil, and oxygenated compounds. [493]

Boswellic acids *(major components of frankincense)* are reported to possess anti-inflammatory and antitumor activity due to their cell growth and cancer cell-killing properties in many human cancer cell lines containing meningioma, leukemia, hepatocellular carcinoma, melanoma, fibrosarcoma, colon, and prostate cancer. Moreover, the essential oil of frankincense inhibited proliferation and modulated the death of human cancer cell lines both in vitro and in vivo. Frankincense extracts containing a higher concentration of boswellic acids can be also formulated in several ways to reportedly enhance the cancer fighting effects. Frankincense oil can also be formulated to concentrate some on the cancer-fighting components, or, as I have seen, using B. sacra and B. carterii oils alone have resolved some cancers. Certainly, more research is needed to put all of these pieces together for us, but if you are looking for a natural substance to help prevent or treat cancer, I would include both the oil and the gum/resin/oil extracts. Frankincense truly is an extremely versatile oil with physical, emotional and spiritually enhancing properties. Always have good quality frankincense around. [494 - 504]

Lavender is another essential oil that demonstrates therapeutic versatility. This oil is considered by many as the *"Swiss army knife,"* of essential oils with its therapeutic and curative properties ranging from inducing relaxation to treating parasitic infections, burns, allergies, insect bites, muscle spasm, high blood pressure, and others. Within the psychophysiological properties of aroma, lavender is the most studied plant. The four important Lavandula species are L. angustifolia, L. stoechas, L. latifolia, and L. intermedia. Lavender is mainly used in aromatherapy treatments such as inhalation, aromatherapy massage, and bathing, but is also used topically and is ingested as well. Studies suggest that lavender has anxiolytic, mood stabilizer, sedative, analgesic properties as well as neuroprotective properties that may be helpful in treating Alzheimer's disease, epilepsy, PTSD, attention disorders, and autism. Studies also show significant improvement in the work environment production and contentment when diffusing lavender and even significant improvement in personal orientation related to cognitive function in elderly patients suffering from different forms of dementia. [505]

L. angustifolia aroma can have significant positive impact on brain electrical activity. Studies show that it preferentially stimulates areas of the brain depending on the individual's needs. For example, in sleep studies, decreased alpha activity in the occipital and parietal regions, and increased theta and beta activities in the frontal and occipital regions, respectively, were noted in subjects with good sleep quality. On the other hand, L. angustifolia aroma increased the theta activity in all cranial regions in subjects with poor sleep quality showing a beneficial effect in those with sleep disorders. Further, in another study the inhalation of lavender oil resulted in more active, fresher, and relaxed subjects than those inhaling base oil. Lavender oil increased the theta and alpha wave activities in these subjects. [506]

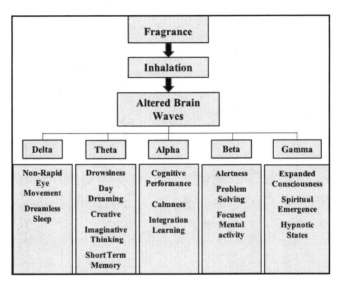

Many other studies have been conducted using lavender. Here is a small sampling:

Aromatic oil massage with essential oils blended with lavender, clary sage, and marjoram in a 2:1:1 ratio in forty-eight outpatients with primary menstrual cramps alleviated the pain and reduced the duration of the cramps. Aromatherapy using lavender essence was also reported as a successful and safe complementary therapy in reduction of pain after the cesarean section in 200 term pregnant women, and after episiotomy in 60 women, as well as in perineal discomfort following normal childbirth in 635 women. It has been shown that lavender aromatherapy through an oxygen face mask with two drops of 2% lavender oil can be used to reduce the demand for opioids in twenty-five patients after immediate postoperative period of breast biopsy surgery and for other analgesics in fifty-four patients undergoing laparoscopic adjustable gastric banding. [507]

How To Use Essential Oils

Okay, so how do you get those wonderfully beneficial molecules of essential oil into your body? There are several routes of entry including breathing in the vapors, absorption through the skin, ingestion, and even rectal and vaginal suppositories when needed, is not only is locally active but also enhances absorption of the oils directly into the bloodstream. Research suggests that essential oil constituents are found in traceable amounts in the bloodstream following topical applications. One study conducted with lavender essential oil tested for linalool and linalyl acetate *(the 2 major constituents of lavender essential oil)* in the blood following a gentle abdominal massage. Amounts of both constituents were identified 15 minutes after the beginning of the massage, with the peak occurring around 30 minutes. [508]

You may be saying, *"I understand the ingestion and breathing routes of entry. But, how does it work that you can get essential oils through the skin?"* That's a common question with an easy answer. There are three mechanisms for transdermal delivery into the bloodstream: the intracellular route - going directly through layers of cells, the intercellular route - going between cells, and the shunt route - going into the dermal support structures such as sweat glands, sebaceous glands, and hair follicles. By disrupting the keratin-rich epidermal layers, these shunt structures allow for a significantly greater relative dermal absorption of molecules. As such, areas on the body that are plentiful in sweat glands, sebaceous glands, and hair follicles *(i.e., scalp, face)* are great locations for absorption. As their name would imply, essential oil constituents are lipophilic *("fat-loving," or fat-soluble)*. This suggests that essential oils mix well with oils, and poorly with water. Since both essential oils and the epidermis are relatively lipophilic, they *"mix"* relatively well together; consequently, essential oils have a greater tendency for transdermal absorption.

My Top 21 Single Essential Oils

We have over 200 different single oils and blends in our home to cover just about any situation. There is a saying with oilers, *"there is an oil for that."* Angel and I have spent years researching and honing our understanding of essential oils. We have many blends of oils, but here are my top 21 single oils to keep around the house for general use: Listed are some main actions, but there are generally many more applications. Purchasing an essential oils desk reference is a great way to learn how to use them.

Basil: powerful antimicrobial and antispasmodic.

Cedarwood: stimulates brain-enhancing focus and relaxation, good for hyperactivity, use with Vetiver for hyperactivity because they calm the brain. Use with rosemary to enhance hair growth.

Chamomile: Roman - calming, anti-inflammatory, antiparasitic.

Cinnamon Bark: anti-inflammatory, antimicrobial, antiviral, circulatory stimulant, balances blood sugar.

Citronella: powerful antioxidant, antimicrobial, insect-repellant, anti-inflammatory, antispasmodic, antiparasitic, relaxant.

Clove: anti-aging, powerful antioxidant, topical anesthetic, analgesic, antimicrobial, ant-viral, anticonvulsant, anticoagulant.

Eucalyptus: expectorant, antimicrobial, antiviral, decongestant, purifying.

Frankincense: antitumoral, anti-inflammatory, immunostimulant, antimicrobial, anti-depressant, relaxant.

Ginger: Anti-nausea, digestion, anti-inflammatory .

Lavender: antimicrobial, anti-inflammatory, antispasmodic, antitumoral, calming.

Lemon: antitumoral, antimicrobial, immune stimulant, improves microcirculation, improves memory, calming.

Myrrh: antitumoral, antimicrobial, antiviral, antioxidant, anti-inflammatory.

Orange: antitumoral, antioxidant, calming, improves microcirculation.

Oregano: powerful antimicrobial, anti-aging, antiviral, antiparasitic, immune stimulant, anti-inflammatory.

Peppermint: anti-inflammatory, analgesic, antitumoral, antiparasitic, antiviral, headaches, digestion, anti-nausea, curbs appetite, is a great decongestant and even anti-ant *(they won't cross the peppermint line to get into your house).*

Quick story here about peppermint. Men, never, ever, carry peppermint in your pants pocket. EVER! I made that mistake early on. The bottle was just a tad open and the peppermint leaked out. Needless to say, I was in a panic when I started *"sensing"* what was happening. I normally move pretty fast anyway, but on this occasion, I headed to the house like a rocket. I must have lost my mind because the only thing I could of think of was to wash it off it with soap and water - wrong thing to do because it spread the effect. I called for my wife, and she told me to dilute it with a carrier oil. I did that and it did help, but I still paid the price for a while longer. Trust me, I learned this lesson the hard way!

Rosemary: antitumoral, antimicrobial, antiparasitic, enhances mental clarity. Do yourself a favor and grow a nice rosemary bush. I have several and when I pass by, I pull some off the branch rub it into my hands and take some deep breaths of it. Very invigorating.

Sandalwood: antitumoral, antiviral, immune stimulant, calming, anti-aging, great for maintaining youthful skin.

Tea Tree: powerful antimicrobial, antiviral, anti-inflammatory, cleansing and purifying.

Wintergreen: anti-inflammatory, analgesic, anesthetic, anticoagulant, vasodilator, lowers blood pressure.

Ylang Ylang: a powerful and exotic aroma. Vasodilator, anti-inflammatory, antispasmodic, emotionally calming, enhances focus on positive thoughts.

There are blends available as well from those who have spent time discovering how oils can interact with others to enhance a specific effect. Or, you can do your own research and DIY to find your perfect blends that are complementary to your body. It is a lot of fun to experiment making bath salts, sunscreens, anti-aging serums and creams, cleaning products, etc. We do in our home! Try making your own peppermint and lavender shampoo, DIY toothpaste and deodorant, and to enhance your intimacy experience with your spouse. If you want to take the edge off the day, have your spouse give you a foot rub with your own relaxing essential oils and fatty oil blend.

Some thoughts on the application of EOs. There are two terms associated with topical application: neat and diluted. Neat application means applying the EOs directly to your skin, which can only be done safely with certain EOs) and for most people. It is always recommended to dilute with a carrier oil first to see how your skin responds. Fair skin individuals are more likely to be sensitive. Carrier oils are fatty vegetable, nut, or seed oils, easily blendable with the EOs, the most commonly used being fractionated coconut oil, but make sure that it is steam distilled and that no chemicals were used during distillation. Other popular carrier oils are jojoba oil, avocado, almond, and argon oils.

To be on the safe side, always, dilute EOs when using them with children. Their skin is sensitive. Certain oils should be diluted with a carrier oil due to their potential to irritate skin. *"Hot"* oils can create a warming or burning sensation, such as with cassia, cinnamon bark, clove, hyssop, and oregano. *"Cooling"* oils create a cooling or tingling sensation such as with camphor, eucalyptus, lemongrass, Ocotea, peppermint, spearmint, thyme, and wintergreen. Also, be aware of oils that cause photosensitivity, mostly citrus oils. They can irritate the skin with a rash or even cause a sunburn reaction, which can be severe in some situations.

When applying, you generally want to apply oils directly to or close to the area of need. For headaches, apply to the temples or wherever your head hurts; for muscle aches, apply directly on the muscles, etc., but for an earache, apply around the ear, never in the ear. There are also certain spots that are more effective than others, such as at your pulse points *(wrists, neck, over your heart, and ankles)*, where pores are bigger; and the bottoms of your feet, following the principles of reflexology. You can also layer the oils systematically but only if you fully understand the effect of each oil and how to layer or blend them together. There are many great and readily available resources that can help you understand the best and safest way to apply essential oils but it is worth mentioning again that having a comprehensive guide such as an essential oils desk reference is critical to having day-to-day successful experiences.[509, 510]

Cannabidiol *(CBD)* And The Endocannabinoid System

I am including cannabidiol *(CBD),* in New Beginnings because the new research supports it being viewed that way. Lives are changing from the new discoveries on the health benefits of CBD. The pulse of excitement is palpable as the research being poured into understanding the very complex endocannabinoid system is demonstrating some very promising results in the treatment of many chronic mental and physical disorders and diseases.

What is the endocannabinoid system *(ES)?* The endocannabinoid system is a biological system, which plays many important roles in the human body to maintain homeostasis. It is considered by some researchers to be the most important regulatory system in the body. Anything that interferes with the function of the ES such as environmental toxins, vaccines, and other epigenetic influences that may lead to gene damage can cause incalculable damage. Endo - stands for endogenous, which means originating within the body. Cannabinoid refers to the group of compounds that activate this system. While it was first discovered in the 1990s, the ES has progressively become a major target of medical research because of its widespread effects and therapeutic potential.

Cannabinoids are the chemical messengers for the endocannabinoid system. While many different cannabinoids exist, they all fall under two categories: endogenous or exogenous. Cannabinoids are distributed throughout the body and are said to be critical to homeostasis through a variety of mechanisms. Low cannabinoids equal disease. Some have created the term Clinical Endocannabinoid Deficiency *(CED)* to describe the epigenetic contributions to low endogenous cannabinoids. Also known as endocannabinoids, these compounds are produced naturally by the human body. They interact with cannabinoid receptors to regulate basic functions including mood, memory, appetite, pain, sleep, and many more. The two main endocannabinoids are anandamide *(primarily peripheral body)* and 2-AG *(primarily brain)*. They are produced *"on demand"* which is consistent with its homeostatic role. Exogenous means originating outside the body. The cannabinoids found in the Cannabis sativa plant, such as the psychoactive tetrahydrocannabinol *(THC)* and the non-psychoactive cannabidiol *(CBD)*, are considered exogenous and are collectively called phytocannabinoids. When consumed, they also interact with cannabinoid receptors to produce physical and psychological effects in the body. The Cannabis sativa plant has many other functional uses such as producing industrial products such as hemp fabric, rope, building materials and is also used in nutritional supplements. Hemp oil is a very nutritious fatty oil from the seeds of the plant. [511, 512]

The endocannabinoid system has two main receptors: CB1 and CB2. Each receptor responds to different cannabinoids, but some cannabinoids can interact with both. The distribution of CB1 and CB2 receptors within the body and brain explains why cannabinoids have certain effects. CB1 receptors are found throughout the body but are mostly present in the brain and spinal cord. They are concentrated in brain regions associated with the behaviors they influence. For example, there are CB1 receptors in the hypothalamus, which is involved with appetite regulation, and the amygdala, which plays a role in memory and emotional processing. CB1 receptors are also found in nerve endings where they act to reduce sensations of pain. CB2 receptors tend to be found in the peripheral nervous system but are present in the brain as well. They are especially concentrated in immune cells. When CB2 receptors are activated, they work to reduce inflammation. Inflammation is an immune response, which is believed to play a role in many diseases and conditions.

CBD attaches to CB2 receptors in the brain and is suggested to also act in some way as antagonists (reducing effects) of CB1 receptors. CBD acts mainly on CB2 receptors in the peripheral organ systems and tissues, especially influencing the immune system. The best sources may come from hybridized cannabis plants that focus on increasing CBD. Research shows no psychoactive (not intoxicating) effects from the consumption of CBD.

CBD has been shown to have some major beneficial effects on the body. It has the highest anti-inflammatory and neuroprotectant properties found in nature. Extensive preclinical research and some clinical studies have shown that CBD has strong antioxidant, anti-inflammatory, anticonvulsant, antidepressant, antipsychotic, antitumoral, and neuroprotective qualities. It can change gene expression and remove beta-amyloid plaque, the hallmark of Alzheimer's, from brain cells.

CBD can eliminate seizure activity, improve mood, and encourage less aggression, less anxiety and obsessiveness, improve fine motor skills, comprehension and sleep, and decreases inflammation in the brain. There are studies using CBD on PTSD, migraines, arthritis, cancer, heart disease, possibly Parkinson's, Alzheimer's, MS, diabetes, autism, ADHD, anxiety, panic, social anxiety, obsessive-compulsive disorder, seizure, and post-traumatic stress disorders. While research is still in its infancy in the grand scheme, the implications are really encouraging! [513]

Charlotte Figi is a girl from Colorado who was diagnosed with Dravet syndrome at the age of three months. Her case drew national attention because of the profound healing that took place using CBD. She suffered from approximately 300 grand mal seizures a week. Charlotte failed to respond to multiple medication treatment regimens , and at five years of age, she had significant cognitive delay and required help with all of her activities of daily living. Her parents sought out a group in Colorado that created an oral, liquid, high-concentration CBD. Once her parents started giving her this strain, dubbed *"Charlotte's Web,"* within three months Charlotte had a > 90% reduction in her seizure frequency and by month 20, Charlotte was able to perform most of her daily activities independently with only two to three nocturnal tonic-clonic seizures per month. Stories like Charlotte's have prompted parents across the country in similar situations to move their families across the country to gain access to these products.

Research studies have also confirmed this positive effect on seizure disorders. It was found that parents of children with severe treatment-resistant epilepsies that are using cannabidiol-enriched cannabis to treat their child's epilepsy report a high rate of success in reducing seizure frequency with CBD, and it is much better tolerated than medications that may not even be effective or minimally so in reducing seizure activity. Beneficial effects of cannabidiol-enriched cannabis other than reduced seizures were also reported including better mood, increased alertness, better sleep, and decreased self-stimulation. Side effects reported while taking other AEDs included rash, vomiting, irritability, dizziness, confusion, and aggressive behavior; none were reported with the use of cannabidiol-enriched cannabis. [514]

Many other jaw-dropping reports have been published as well. Especially prominent in the public consciousness is the out of control incidence of autism. A recent study in the journal Neurology reported some pretty impressive results using CBD in autism spectrum disorder *(ASD)*. Eighty% of parents noted a decrease in problematic behaviors, with 62% reporting significant improvements, 50% of the children experiencing improved communication, and 40% reporting a significant decrease in anxiety in their children. The authors concluded that CBD-based medical cannabis is a promising treatment option for refractory behavioral problems in children with ASD.

Fear and anxiety are adaptive responses essential to coping with threats to survival. Yet excessive or persistent fear may be maladaptive, leading to disability. Symptoms arising from excessive fear and anxiety occur in a number of neuropsychiatric disorders, including generalized anxiety disorder *(GAD)*, panic disorder *(PD)*, post-traumatic stress disorder *(PTSD)*, social anxiety disorder *(SAD)*, and obsessive-compulsive disorder *(OCD)*. Preclinical evidence conclusively demonstrates CBD's efficacy in reducing anxiety behaviors relevant to multiple disorders, including PTSD, GAD, PD, OCD, and SAD, with a notable lack of anxiogenic effects. CBD can be also an awesome weight loss product as well since fear and anxiety can be major contributing factors to weight gain. Think about it, when you are stressed, one of the most common things to do is to go and get something to eat to bring a satisfying experience into your stressed life. [515 - 523]

Cannabigerol *(CBG)* is another phytocannabinoid that holds promise to be a key constituent in the overall medicinal benefits cannabis may provide. It is a minor player, but the concentrations are high is some hemp plants. As cannabis research continues to rapidly evolve, CBG may emerge as one of the most therapeutically applicable and diverse cannabinoids to offer a wide range of possible remedies. CBG is a precursor or stem cell of all the other cannabinoids and supports immune function, skin health, nervous system function, a positive mood, and induces muscle relaxation, antianxiety and anti-depressive effects. [524 - 526]

Research in the endocannabinoid system is ongoing, and momentum is building that the exogenous cannabinoids such as cannabidiol, and the newest kid on the block, cannabigerol, will profoundly help our efforts to heal our broken bodies. I think that the endocannabinoid system will be the most talked-about area of health and fitness over the next decade and the focus of fascinating research findings. While phytocannabinoids are a great help in this time of crisis, what is best is to work backwards and eliminate the things that interfere with our health to begin with - the kinds of things talked about throughout this book. CBD has been proven to be a very promising intervention tool, but ideally it is best to have our own ES system do what it is designed to do. When our body is healthy, free of toxins, chronic stress, and epigenetically induced gene mutations, the ES system produces the cannabinoids that it needs on demand to bring the body into balance.

But if the exogenous cannabinoids are important for your health journey, now or in the future, you may take it up a notch or two by making some complementary additions to your protocol. Essential oils such as clove, rosemary, basil, lavender frankincense, and cinnamon oils, and copaiba oil/resin are all good sources of beta-caryophyllene to enhance the anti-inflammatory effects. Also, adding black pepper resin will help increase absorption of curcumin, CBD, and possibly others. But, as with essential oils, quality makes all the difference. Some CBD is laced with pesticides and other toxic chemicals, and you will never know. Much of it also comes from China, where quality control may be questionable. So, it is best to stick with a CBD oil company with a proven track record of producing high quality natural products, preferably with their own farms or partner farms where a seed to seal quality control monitoring takes place. [527, 528]

PART FIVE

Top Habits Of Satisfied, Gratified, And Highly Accomplished People

> *A smile is the key that fits the lock to everyone's heart.*
> Anthony J. De'angelo

Many times, I am in my head thinking, and I am not aware that I look like I am mad. I'm not mad. I am just intense about my beliefs, and how to help change the world in a loving way. But sometimes it sure doesn't look that way. I will even catch a glimpse of myself in the mirror sometimes and think, no wonder it seems like I am unapproachable. That makes me feel bad sometimes because I really like helping others and listening to their stories.

So, I have had to learn to smile more. It takes practice *(though some of you do it naturally, you Sanguines and E7s in particular)*, but many of us have to work on it! I have to keep in mind that I can't solve the world's problems *(at least not all at once)* and to live in the moment, not in the past. I find that when I put a smile on my face, even when I don't feel like it, it really does make a difference in how I feel about myself and others throughout the day. In addition, when you smile at someone else and purposefully look them straight in the eye, mentally conveying that you love them, it breaks down barriers in an amazing way.

Here are some other benefits to smiling *(in case you need convincing)*.

- Smiling is contagious - Because of complex brain activity that occurs when you see someone smiling, smiles are contagious.

- Smiling lowers stress and anxiety - When recovering from a stressful situation, study participants who were smiling had lower heart rates than those with a neutral facial expression.

- Smiling releases endorphins - Smiling can help you manage stress and anxiety by releasing endorphins.

- You'll be more attractive - A smile suggests that you're personable, easy-going, empathetic, and more attractive to the people you smile at.

- Smiling strengthens your immune system - Smiling makes your immune system stronger by making your body produce white blood cells to help fight illnesses.

- You'll be more approachable - Turn that frown upside-down if you want to make some friends!

- Smiling will make you more comfortable - A study found that smiling can make you more comfortable in situations you would otherwise feel awkward in.

- You'll seem more trustworthy - If you want to improve your credibility, simply smile more. What could be easier than that? Trusting doesn't come easily to many, but smiling at someone may help.

- While smiling is one of the most effective things you can do to enhance your healthy lifestyle, here are my other top habits of satisfied, gratified, and highly accomplished people.

- Guard your heart's input and output.

- Take care of relationships. Forgiveness, laughter, and smiles are some of the best medicines.

- Hug someone daily. Every time people willingly embrace, oxytocin is released. It is appropriately called the *"love hormone"* and is associated with empathy, trust, sexual activity, relationship building, and it reduces depression and anxiety.

- Hang with healthy people whose habits are healthy and will challenge you to grow. Your outside relationships are like the structural parts of a plane that make it fly smoothly. There are four main *"who to hang with"* principles. Lifters are people who make you feel good. Thrusters are those who challenge you and inspire you to become better than you already are. Draggers are those who are always in a crisis and want you to solve their problems. They steal your energy and forward momentum. Weighters, are people who expect you to carry their heavy emotional baggage for them. If you are going to move forward to your destinations in life, limit the drag that slows you down and the weight that requires so much more energy to keep you going and get into God's Jetstream. Say I love you when a family member leaves the house. Believe me, it makes a difference. I don't remember my dad ever saying that to me, and the only time I remember my mom saying it was in her suicide note to me. Start today.

- Plant seeds of love and hope in others. Planting good seeds produces good fruit in them and in future generations. Living a seedless life is like seedless fruit. No seeds are there to plant for others to grow from your own special fruit.

- Your family is like fine china. They need to be treated with special care. Always stand in the gap for your family. If needed in times of trouble, bring in other good people to sit at your table to help heal wounded hearts. But, do not take your family issues out on the street. You have spent years together. Each of you deserves a trusting relationship.

- It takes strength to admit weakness. It doesn't take much to hide weakness. Meekness is different than weakness. We are not all meek, that is a spiritual discipline. Meekness is having the open door and strength to do or say something and choosing not to because wisdom dictates it at the moment. We all are weak in some ways, and it can be turned into a strength when our relationship with God and others is right. Love covers all weaknesses. Don't embarrass people who show weakness.

The same amount of mercy shown to others will be extended to you. You can count on it.

- Be an eagle and rise above all of the turmoil of the crows and storms.

- A true leader can also follow, but a follower can't lead.

- Any viruses destructive to your emotional and spiritual health contaminating your life's computer? Identify, delete, and reset.

- Shed off the many faces of shame. Shame, blame, disrespect, betrayal, and the withholding of affection damage the roots from which love grows. Shame corrodes the very part of us that believes we are capable of change and love can only survive these injuries if they are acknowledged and healed.

- Got junk in your life? That is okay. It doesn't define you. Those scars can give you a beauty and special inner strength if used correctly. You may be a product of your past but you don't have to be a prisoner of it.

- Be vulnerable in the right context. It is not a weakness and can be a powerful emissary of love and healing.

- Guard your heart not with fear but with love, wisdom, and discernment. Don't cast your pearls before those who wallow in the mud. If we can share our story with someone who responds with empathy and understanding, shame can't survive. If we share our shame story with the wrong person, they can easily become one more piece of flying debris in an already dangerous storm.

- Joy and happiness are not a laborious effort but are right in front of you if you are paying attention and practicing gratitude. Living a wholehearted life helps you to experience gratitude. Living a wholehearted life requires that you know in your heart that there is something there bigger than yourself that is all knowing, all good, and all loving.

- Believe the best in others. Love makes allowances. You never know what others are going through.

- Are you a thermostat or a thermometer? A thermostat changes things; a thermometer just monitors them.

- We all are imperfect and wired for struggle. Pain and imperfection are inevitable and necessary for growth. Take the pain that seems pointless and make it productive. Run towards your Goliaths in life and say Make My Day!

- You are worthy of love and belonging. Take heart in that. God's grace is bigger than your background.

- Use your words to encourage others, not tear them down.

- Disappointments are inevitable, misery is optional. Rain falls on everyone, the just and the unjust. Life may seem dreary, but that rain is also life-sustaining and what makes new life grow.

- If you are looking at problems all of the time and they seem bigger than life, that means that you are looking through the telescope of life through the wrong end. Turn it around and you will see that those problems are really a whole lot smaller that you made them out to be. Life can be like a boat on the sand of the beach. The boat has a purpose, but it cannot fulfill its purpose at the moment. It is stuck! The tide comes back in and gives new life to your efforts to get back out there, throw out the nets, and catch your dreams.

- Where you're going is more important than where you've been. Don't look through life through the rear-view mirror - you're destined for a wreck.

- Don't try and fix everyone and don't enable their dysfunction.

- Your belief system is also what you will attract to you. If you focus on despair, then that is what you will draw to you. Focusing on life-giving thoughts like love, joy, peace, patience, kindness, goodness, faithfulness, and self-control, focusing on your dreams, all will bring contentment, clarity of purpose.

- Live your dreams. You are filled with them, and you will deliver at some point. When there are labor pains, that means your dreams are about to give birth. You may feel kicking along the way. The idea is just trying to let you know it is viable.

- Don't put God in a box. He doesn't always show up in the way we expect. But He will show up.

- Focus on a joyful life, not a happy life. Happiness is fickle, shallow and fleeting. It has its origins in the mind and in the moment. Joy is endearing, enduring, and soothes the soul. It connects us to God.

- Don't be afraid to fail. We all make mistakes. Each day is a new day with a fresh start.

Let me end this chapter with this thought from Mark Nepo.

> *What a powerful lesson is the beginning of spring. All around us, everything small and buried surrenders to the process that none of the buried parts can see...*
>
> *By nature, we are all quietly given countless models of how to give ourselves over to what appears dark and hopeless, but which ultimately is an awakening that is beyond all imagining. This moving through the dark into blossom is the threshold to God.*
>
> *As a seed buried into the earth cannot imagine itself as an orchid or hyacinth, neither can a heart packed with hurt imagine itself loved or at peace. The courage of the seed is that once cracking, it cracks all the way.*

Mark Nepo

EPILOGUE

The Call

And so, here we are, in this special place. While we will always be connected through this time together, we will now part and go our separate ways. I hope you have been both inspired and challenged by what you have read. You have added to the story with your own as you think and feel what this all may mean for you. As we walked together on this journey, I have learned so much from you. Does that sound strange? Let me explain why it's not. What you read were not just words on a page; you have experienced my emotions, my passions, my heart and dreams for the future, which are embedded in my words. They were put out there to see who would hear the call. One or 100,000 or more, it doesn't matter. You responded and now we now walk both together and alone - you and me and everyone else who is on the same journey. You have also given me the very special privilege of being summoned into your world. According to the science of quantum physics, we are all connected in that way.

These are difficult times, and none are immune. I wonder how we ever got to this place where life seems messed up and the lines between right and wrong are so blurred? Regardless, we must decide what to do now that we are here. We all have gifts and talents, and they can be used in very powerful ways to make changes. Don't dismiss yourself or your ability to help change the world. Great things are accomplished by a series of small things brought together. You can do this, and it is worth the fight! Don't let anyone else or other distractions tell you that you can't. Stand firmly in your truth, your passions, your purpose, and be brave with it.

When we all do this, both together and alone, in our own special way, we will rock the world! We are BIG and getting bigger! The tide is turning. We have and will continue to make a difference, for ourselves and for our children. Take back what was stolen from you and your ancestors. They may not have had a chance, but you do. And when you do take back what was stolen from you, your children for generations to come will rise up and call you blessed. The stories of your great-grandchildren will be memorials to you, your legacy, and your faithfulness to make a better life for them.

APPENDIX A

Additional Research Showing Connection Between Autism And Vaccines

Vaccines Induce Autistic Disorders

http://unhoodwinked.com/Autism.html

Numerous credible, medical, and scientific journals over the past decade or so have found significant correlations between certain vaccines and autism.

1. "Dr. Peter Fletcher, who was Chief Scientific Officer at the Department of Health (in the U.K.), said if it is proven that the jab causes autism, 'the refusal by governments to evaluate the risks properly will make this one of the greatest scandals in medical history...' He said he has seen a "steady accumulation of evidence" from scientists worldwide that the measles, mumps and rubella jab is causing brain damage in certain children." [529]

2. "Documented causes of autism include genetic mutations and/or deletions, viral infections, and encephalitis [brain damage] following vaccination [emphasis added]. Therefore, autism is the result of genetic defects and/or inflammation of the brain." [530]

3. "Using regression analysis and controlling for family income and ethnicity, the relationship between the proportion of children who received the recommended vaccines by age 2 years and the prevalence of autism (AUT) or speech or language impairment (SLI) in each U.S. state from 2001 and 2007 was determined. A positive and statistically significant relationship was found: The higher the proportion of children receiving recommended

vaccinations, the higher was the prevalence of AUT or SLI." - Journal of Toxicology and Environmental Health, 2011 [531]

4. There was a significant dose-response relationship between the severity of the regressive ASDs (Autism Spectrum Disorder) observed and the total mercury dose children received from Thimerosal-containing vaccines/Rho (D)-immune globulin preparations. Based upon differential diagnoses, 8 of 9 patients examined were exposed to significant mercury from Thimerosal-containing biologic/vaccine preparations during their fetal/ infant developmental periods, and subsequently, between 12 and 24 months of age, these previously normally developing children suffered mercury toxic encephalopathies that manifested with clinical symptoms consistent with regressive ASDs." - Journal of Toxicology and Environmental Health, 2007[532]

5. "From a cellular perspective, it would appear that the existing scientific literature supports the biological plausibility of a Hg-based (mercury) autism pathogenesis. Nevertheless, research studies identifying Hg's effects on glial cells and mitochondria that are consistent with findings in autistic patients, lend further support to the Hg-autism hypothesis." - Environmental Toxicology and Chemistry, 2011. [533]

6. "We studied the effects of thimerosal on cell proliferation and mitochondrial function from B-lymphocytes taken from individuals with autism, their non- autistic twins, and their non-twin siblings...Cells hypersensitive to thimerosal also had higher levels of oxidative stress markers, protein carbonyls, and oxidant generation. This suggests certain individuals with a mild mitochondrial defect may be highly susceptible to mitochondrial specific toxins like the vaccine preservative thimerosal." - Journal of Toxicology, 2013. [534]

7. "It was determined that there were significantly increased odds ratios (ORs) for autism (OR = 1.8, p < .05), mental retardation (OR = 2.6, p < .002), speech disorder (OR = 2.1, p < .02), personality disorders (OR = 2.6, p < .01), and thinking abnormality (OR = 8.2, p < .01) adverse events reported to the VAERS following thimerosal-containing DTaP vaccines in

comparison to thimerosal-free DTaP vaccines." - International Journal of Toxicology, 2004.[535]

8. "Further, linear regression revealed that Varicella (chickenpox) and Hepatitis A immunization coverage was significantly correlated to autistic disorder cases...Autistic disorder change points years are coincident with introduction of vaccines manufactured using human fetal cell lines, containing fetal and retroviral contaminants, into childhood vaccine regimens."

"This pattern was repeated in the US, UK, Western Australia and Denmark. Thus, rising autistic disorder prevalence is directly related to vaccines manufactured utilizing human fetal cells. Increased paternal age and DSM (Diagnostic and Statistical Manual) revisions were not related to rising autistic disorder prevalence." - Journal of Public Health and Epidemiology, 2014

"...the present study provides new epidemiological evidence supporting an association between increasing organic-Hg exposure from Thimerosal-containing childhood vaccines and the subsequent risk of an ASD diagnosis." - Translational Neurodegeneration, 2013. [536]

9. "Thus autistic children have a hyper-immune response to measles virus, which in the absence of a wild-type measles infection might be a sign of an abnormal immune reaction to the vaccine strain or virus reactivation." - Pediatric Neurology, 2003

10. "Measles might be etiologically linked to autism because measles and MMR antibodies (a viral marker) correlated positively to brain autoantibodies (an autoimmune marker) - salient features that characterize autoimmune pathology in autism." - 2009. [538]

11. "An abstract of the study was published in the September, 2009 issue of the respected journal Annals of Epidemiology. In it, Carolyn Gallagher and Melody Goodman of the Graduate Program in Public Health at Stony Brook University Medical Center, NY, wrote that, "Boys who received the

hepatitis B vaccine during the first month of life had 2.94 greater odds for ASD compared to later- or unvaccinated boys." - 2009. [539]

12. "Findings suggest that U.S. male neonates vaccinated with the hepatitis B vaccine prior to 1999 (from vaccination record) had a threefold higher risk for parental report of autism diagnosis compared to boys not vaccinated as neonates during that same time period. Nonwhite boys bore a greater risk." - Journal of Toxicology and Environmental Health, 2010. [540]

13. "Thus the MMR antibody in autistic sera detected measles HA protein, which is unique to the measles subunit of the vaccine. Furthermore, over 90% of MMR antibody-positive autistic sera were also positive for MBP (myelin basic protein) autoantibodies, suggesting a strong association between MMR and CNS (central nervous system) autoimmunity in autism. Stemming from this evidence, we suggest that an inappropriate antibody response to MMR, specifically the measles component thereof, might be related to pathogenesis of autism." - Journal of Biomedical Science, 2002. [541]

14. "The number of dose relationships is linear and statistically significant. You can play with this all you want. They are linear. They are statistically significant." - Dr. Weil from Association of American Physicians and Surgeons, Inc, 2003. [542]

15. When asked about vaccines triggering autism Dr. Bernadine Healy, former head of the National Institutes of Health said, "I think that the public health officials have been too quick to dismiss the hypothesis as irrational." - CBS News, 2008

16. Simpson Meeting - In Norcross, GA on June 7-8, 2000, the CDC hosted a conference using the Vaccine Safety Datalink (VSD) to discuss the possible link between autism and thimerosal. The transcripts of this secret meeting were obtained under the Freedom of Information Act.

17. Dr. Tom Verstraeten, CDC epidemiologist, analyzed the VSD of 100,000 children medical records, and he found what appeared to be the culprit of

the dramatic increase in autism, thimerosal. You can read the whole notes from the meeting at http://www.autismhelpforyou.com/HG%20IN%20 VACCINES%20-%20Simpsonwood%20-%20Internet%20File.pdf.

The below excerpt can be found on page 162, so keep scrolling down.

Dr. Verstraeten said the following during the secret meeting on the mercury caused autism hypothesis, "When I saw this, and I went back through the literature, I was actually stunned by what I saw because I thought it is plausible." He goes on, "Another point is that in many of the studies with animals, it turned out there is quite a different result depending on the doses of mercury. Depending on the route of exposure and depending on the age at which the animals were exposed. Now I don't know how much you can extrapolate that from animal to humans, but that tells me that mercury at one month of age is not the same as mercury at three months, at 12 months, prenatal mercury, later mercury. There is a whole range of plausible outcomes from mercury."

Though many of the various doctors at the conference agree of the strong plausibility of the mercury autism hypothesis, Dr. Weil, on page 187 goes on to say, "Although the data presents a number of uncertainties, there is adequate consistency, biological plausibility, a lack of relationship with phenomenon not expected to be related, and a potential causal role that is as good as any other hypothesized etiology of explanation of the noted associations. In addition, the possibility that the associations could be causal has major significance for public and professional acceptance of Thimerosal containing vaccines. I think that is a critical issue."

Again, these are doctors of the CDC stating these plausibilities in 2000. Did the CDC go on to conduct experiments to determine these plausibilities? Did they recommend spacing out vaccines over time? Did they do anything to explore these plausibilities further for the safety of our children? Nope. They kept it secret and increased the vaccine schedule over time instead.

The period between the last three months of pregnancy to two years old are the brain's growth spurt years. And since mercury gets absorbed into the growing brain and collects there, this can be a major attribution to degenerative diseases of children's brains.

"Thus the MMR antibody in autistic sera detected measles HA protein, which is unique to the measles subunit of the vaccine. Furthermore, over 90% of MMR antibody-positive autistic sera were also positive for MBP (myelin basic protein) autoantibodies, suggesting a strong association between MMR and CNS (central nervous system) autoimmunity in autism. Stemming from this evidence, we suggest that an inappropriate antibody response to MMR, specifically the measles component thereof, might be related to pathogenesis of autism." - Journal of Biomedical Science, 2002

18. The CDC and Merck, one of the major manufacturers of the MMR vaccine, are in very serious hot water for allegedly doctoring their numbers to lower the correlation between the MMR vaccine and the increase in autism. This type of scientific study into the efficacy and safety is what we can expect from a manufacturer fast tracking their own vaccine to get the quick approval of an all to willing FDA. "The scientists (two former Merck employees turned whistleblowers) claim Merck defrauded the U.S. government by causing it to purchase an estimated four million doses of mislabeled and misbranded MMR vaccine per year for at least a decade." - Forbes, 2012. [543]

19. "Hooker said he believes the increased risk for African-American boys he found was not identified in the CDC study because the researchers, including Thompson, deliberately limited the number of participants they included in their analysis, which he said altered the results." "I regret that my co-authors and I omitted statistically significant information in our 2004 article," said William Thompson, senior scientist with the CDC. - CNN, 2014. 544

20. A study published by the Department of Pharmaceutical Sciences at Northeastern University, Boston determined that a novel growth factor signaling pathway that regulates methionine synthase(MS) activity and thereby modulates methylation reactions. The potent inhibition of this pathway by ethanol, lead, mercury, aluminum and thimerosal suggests that it may be an important target of neurodevelopmental toxins. [545]

Additional Studies On Autism

A study published in the American Journal of Clinical Nutrition determined that an increased vulnerability to oxidative stress and decreased capacity for methylation may contribute to the development and clinical manifestation of autism. It's well known that viral infections cause increased oxidative stress. Research suggests that metals, including those found in many vaccines are directly involved in increasing oxidative stress.

http://ajcn.nutrition.org/content/80/6/1611.full

A study published in the Journal of Child Neurology examined the question of what is leading to the apparent increase in autism. They expressed that if there is any link between autism and mercury, it is crucial that the first reports of the question are not falsely stating that no link occurs. Researchers determined that a significant relation does exist between the blood levels of mercury and the diagnosis of an autism spectrum disorder.

http://journals.sagepub.com/doi/abs/10.1177/0883073807307111

A study published in the Journal of Child Neurology noted that autistic spectrum disorders can be associated with mitochondrial dysfunction. Researchers determined that children who have mitochondrial-related dysfunctional cellular energy metabolism might be more prone to undergo autistic regression between 18 and 30 months of age if they also have infections or immunizations at the same time.

http://journals.sagepub.com/doi/abs/10.1177/08830738060210021401

A study conducted by Massachusetts General Hospital at the Centre for Morphometric Analysis by the department of Pediatric Neurology illustrates how autistic brains have a growth spurt shortly after birth and then slow in growth a few short years later. Researchers have determined that neuroinflammation appears to be present in autistic brain tissue from childhood through adulthood. The study excerpt reads:

"Oxidative stress, brain inflammation and microgliosis have been much documented in association with toxic exposures including various heavy metals. The awareness that the brain as well as medical conditions of children with autism may be conditioned by chronic biomedical abnormalities such as inflammation opens the possibility that meaningful biomedical interventions may be possible well past the window of maximal neuroplasticity in early childhood because the basis for assuming that all deficits can be attributed to fixed early developmental alterations in net"

https://www.ncbi.nlm.nih.gov/pubmed/16151044

A study conducted by the Department of Pediatrics at the University of Arkansas determined that thimerosal-induced cytotoxicity was associated with the depletion of intracellular glutathione (GSH) in both cell lines. The study outlines how many vaccines have been neurotoxic, especially to the developing brain. Depletion of GSH is commonly associated with autism. Although thimerosal has been removed from most children's vaccines, it is still present in flu vaccines given to pregnant women, the elderly and to children in developing countries.

https://www.ncbi.nlm.nih.gov/pubmed/15527868

A study published in the Public Library of Science (PLOS) determined that elevation in peripheral oxidative stress is consistent with, and may contribute to more severe functional impairments in the ASD group. We know that oxidative stress is triggered by heavy metals, like the ones contained in multiple vaccines.

http://journals.plos.org/plosone/article?id=10.1371/journal.pone.0068444

A study conducted by the University of Texas Health Science Centre by the Department of Family and Community Medicine determined that for each 1,000 lb of environmentally released mercury, there was a 43% increase in the rate of special education services and a 61% increase in the rate of autism. Researchers emphasized that further research was needed regarding the association between environmentally released mercury and developmental disorders such as autism.

https://www.ncbi.nlm.nih.gov/pubmed/16338635

A study published in the International Journal of Toxicology determined that in light of the biological plausibility of mercury's role in neurodevelopment disorders, the present study provides further insight into one possible mechanism by which early mercury exposures could increase the risk of autism.

https://www.ncbi.nlm.nih.gov/pubmed/12933322

A study published by the US National Library of Medicine conducted by the University of Texas Health Science Centre suspected that persistent low-dose exposures to various environmental toxicants including mercury, that occur during critical windows of neural development among genetically susceptible children, may increase the risk for developmental disorders such as autism.

http://civileats.com/wp-content/uploads/2009/01/palmer2008.pdf

A study conducted by the Department of Obstetrics and Gynecology at University of Pittsburgh's School of Medicine showed that Macaques are commonly used in pre-clinical vaccine safety testing. Collective Evolution does not support animals testing. We feel there is a large amount of evidence and research that already indicated the links to vaccines in which some animals have been used to illustrate. The objective of this study was to compare early infant cognition and behavior with amygdala size and opioid binding in rhesus macaques receiving the recommended childhood vaccines. The animal model, which examines for the first time, behavioral, functional and neuromorphometric consequences of the childhood vaccine regimen, mimics certain neurological abnormalities of autism. These findings raise important safety issues while providing a potential model for examining aspects of causation and disease pathogenesis in acquired disorders of behavior and development.

http://www.ane.pl/pdf/7020.pdf

A study conducted by The George Washington University School of Public. Health from the Department of Epidemiology and Biostatistics determined that significantly increased rate ratios were observed for autism and autism spectrum disorders as a result of exposure to mercury from Thimerosal-containing vaccines.

https://www.ncbi.nlm.nih.gov/pubmed/18482737

A study published in the Journal Cell Biology and Toxicology by Kinki University in Osaka, Japan determined that in combination with the brain pathology observed in patients diagnosed with autism, the present study helps to support the possible biological plausibility for how low-dose exposure to mercury from thimerosal-containing vaccines may be associated with autism.

https://www.ncbi.nlm.nih.gov/pubmed/19357975

A study published in the Journal Neurochemical Research determined that since excessive accumulation of extracellular glutamate is linked with excitotoxicity, data implies that neonatal exposure to thimerosal- containing vaccines might induce excitotoxic brain injuries, leading to neurodevelopmental disorders.

https://www.ncbi.nlm.nih.gov/pmc/articles/PMC3264864/?tool=pubmed

Additional References On Autism

https://childrenshealthdefense.org/wp-content/uploads/2016/11/Truth_Revealed-Scientific_Discoveries_Regarding_Mercury_Medicine_and_Autism.pdf

https://childrenshealthdefense.org/wp-content/uploads/2016/10/
Breakthrough_Discovery_on_the_Causes_of_Autism-Dr.-Mark_Hyman.
pdf

https://childrenshealthdefense.org/wp-content/uploads/thimerosal-autism-
studies-1-12-16.pdf https://childrenshealthdefense.org/wp-content/uploads/
mercury-autism- research-combined.pdf

Vaccine Excipient Summary, Excipients Included in U.S. Vaccines https://
www.cdc.gov/vaccines/pubs/pinkbook/downloads/appendices/B/ excipi-
ent-table-2.pdf

APPENDIX B

Partial Report Of The Connection Between Gun Violence And Psychotropic Medication

A List Of Mass Shooters And The Stark Link To Psychotropic Drugs.

1. Eric Harris age 17 (first on Zoloft then Luvox) and Dylan Klebold aged 18 (Columbine school shooting in Littleton, Colorado), killed 12 students and 1 teacher, and wounded 23 others, before killing themselves. Klebold's medical records have never been made available to the public.

2. Jeff Weise, age 16, had been prescribed 60 mg/day of Prozac (three times the average starting dose for adults!) when he shot his grandfather, his grandfather's girlfriend and many fellow students at Red Lake, Minnesota. He then shot himself. 10 dead, 12 wounded.

3. Cory Baadsgaard, age 16, Wahluke (Washington state) High School, was on Paxil (which caused him to have hallucinations) when he took a rifle to his high school and held 23 classmates hostage. He has no memory of the event.

4. Chris Fetters, age 13, killed his favorite aunt while taking Prozac.

5. Christopher Pittman, age 12, murdered both his grandparents while taking Zoloft.

6. Mathew Miller, age 13, hung himself in his bedroom closet after taking Zoloft for 6 days.

7. Kip Kinkel, age 15, (on Prozac and Ritalin) shot his parents while they slept then went to school and opened fire killing 2 classmates and injuring 22 shortly after beginning Prozac treatment.

8. Luke Woodham, age 16 (Prozac) killed his mother and then killed two students, wounding six others.

9. A boy in Pocatello, ID (Zoloft) in 1998 had a Zoloft-induced seizure that caused an armed stand off at his school.

10. Michael Carneal (Ritalin), age 14, opened fire on students at a high school prayer meeting in West Paducah, Kentucky. Three teenagers were killed, five others were wounded.

11. A young man in Huntsville, Alabama (Ritalin) went psychotic chopping up his parents with an ax and also killing one sibling and almost murdering another.

12. Andrew Golden, age 11, (Ritalin) and Mitchell Johnson, aged 14,

(Ritalin) shot 15 people, killing four students, one teacher, and wounding 10 others.

13. TJ Solomon, age 15, (Ritalin) high school student in Conyers, Georgia opened fire on and wounded six of his class mates.

14. Rod Mathews, age 14, (Ritalin) beat a classmate to death with a bat.

15. James Wilson, age 19, (various psychiatric drugs) from Breenwood, South Carolina, took a .22 caliber revolver into an elementary school killing two young girls, and wounding seven other children and two teachers.

16. Elizabeth Bush, age 13, (Paxil) was responsible for a school shooting in Pennsylvania

17. Jason Hoffman (Effexor and Celexa) - school shooting in El Cajon, California

18. Jarred Viktor, age 15, (Paxil), after five days on Paxil he stabbed his grandmother 61 times.

19. Chris Shanahan, age 15 (Paxil) in Rigby, ID who out of the blue killed a woman.

20. Jeff Franklin (Prozac and Ritalin), Huntsville, AL, killed his parents as they came home from work using a sledge hammer, hatchet, butcher knife and mechanic's file, then attacked his younger brothers and sister.

21. Neal Furrow (Prozac) in LA Jewish school shooting reported to have been court-ordered to be on Prozac along with several other medications.

22. Kevin Rider, age 14, was withdrawing from Prozac when he died from a gunshot wound to his head. Initially it was ruled a suicide, but two years later, the investigation into his death was opened as a possible homicide. The prime suspect, also age 14, had been taking Zoloft and other SSRI antidepressants.

23. Alex Kim, age 13, hung himself shortly after his Lexapro prescription had been doubled.

24. Diane Routhier was prescribed Welbutrin for gallstone problems. Six days later, after suffering many adverse effects of the drug, she shot herself.

25. Billy Willkomm, an accomplished wrestler and a University of Florida student, was prescribed Prozac at the age of 17. His family found him dead of suicide - hanging from a tall ladder at the family's Gulf Shore Boulevard home in July 2002.

26. Kara Jaye Anne Fuller-Otter, age 12, was on Paxil when she hung herself from a hook in her closet. Kara's parents said ".... the damn doctor wouldn't

take her off it and I asked him to when we went in on the second visit. I told him I thought she was having some sort of reaction to Paxil...")

27. Gareth Christian, Vancouver, age 18, was on Paxil when he committed suicide in 2002

28. (Gareth's father could not accept his son's death and killed himself.)

29. Julie Woodward, age 17, was on Zoloft when she hung herself in her family's detached garage.

30. Matthew Miller was 13 when he saw a psychiatrist because he was having difficulty at school. The psychiatrist gave him samples of Zoloft. Seven days later his mother found him dead, hanging by a belt from a laundry hook in his closet.

31. Kurt Danysh, age 18, and on Prozac, killed his father with a shotgun. He is now behind prison bars, and writes letters, trying to warn the world that SSRI drugs can kill.

32. Woody _____, age 37, committed suicide while in his 5th week of taking Zoloft. Shortly before his death his physician suggested doubling the dose of the drug. He had seen his physician only for insomnia. He had never been depressed, nor did he have any history of any mental illness symptoms.

33. A boy from Houston, age 10, shot and killed his father after his Prozac dosage was increased.

34. Hammad Memon, age 15, shot and killed a fellow middle school student. He had been diagnosed with ADHD and depression and was taking Zoloft and "other drugs for the conditions."

35. Matti Saari, a 22-year-old culinary student, shot and killed 9 students and a teacher, and wounded another student, before killing himself. Saari was taking an SSRI and a benzodiazapine.

36. Steven Kazmierczak, age 27, shot and killed five people and wounded 21 others before killing himself in a Northern Illinois University auditorium. According to his girlfriend, he had recently been taking Prozac, Xanax and Ambien. Toxicology results showed that he still had trace amounts of Xanax in his system.

37. Finnish gunman Pekka-Eric Auvinen, age 18, had been taking antidepressants before he killed eight people and wounded a dozen more at Jokela High School - then he committed suicide.

38. Asa Coon from Cleveland, age 14, shot and wounded four before taking his own life. Court records show Coon was on Trazodone.

39. Jon Romano, age 16, on medication for depression, fired a shotgun at a teacher in his New York high school.

Read more here:

https://www.cchrint.org/pdfs/violence-report.pdf

https://www.ammoland.com/2013/04/every-mass-shooting-in-the-last-20-years-shares-psychotropic-drugs/#axzz5vASVxEyT

END NOTES

1. "Industrial Revolution." Wikipedia. April 17, 2019. Accessed April 27, 2019. https://en.wikipedia.org/wiki/Industrial_Revolution.

2. "Diseases in Industrial Cities in the Industrial Revolution." History Learning. Accessed April 27, 2019. http://historylearning.com/great-britain-1700-to-1900/indrevo/diseases-industrial-revolution/.

3. Murray, J. F. "The Industrial Revolution and the Decline in Death Rates ..." Accessed April 27, 2019. https://www.ingentaconnect.com/contentone/iuatld/ijtld/2015/00000019/00000005/art00004.

4. "The Industrial Revolution and the ... - UChicago GeoSci." Accessed April 27, 2019. http://geosci.uchicago.edu/~moyer/GEOS24705/Notes/Lecture6Slides.pdf.

5. Humphries, Suzanne, and Roman Bystrianyk. Dissolving Illusions: Disease, Vaccines and the Forgotten History. United States: CreateSpace, 2015.

6. "BPA and Other Cord Blood Pollutants." EWG. November 23, 2009. Accessed June 15, 2019. https://www.ewg.org/research/minority-cord-blood-report/bpa-and- other-cord-blood-pollutants.

7. "Study Findings." EWG. September 23, 2003. Accessed June 15, 2019. https://www.ewg.org/research/mothers-milk/study-findings.

8. "Nevada Mental Health Counseling Association - Leg.state.nv.us." Accessed April 27, 2019.https://www.leg.state.nv.us/Session/77th2013/Exhibits/Assembly/CL/ACL943C.pdf.

9. Scialla, Mark. "It Could Take Centuries for EPA to Test All the Unregulated Chemicals under a New Landmark Bill." PBS. June 22, 2016. Accessed April 27, 2019. https://www.pbs.org/newshour/science/it-could-take-centuries-for-epa-to-test-all-the-unregulated-chemicals-under-a-new-landmark-bill.

10. "Was Your Baby Born Pre-Polluted?" The Mud Blood. January 02, 2018. Accessed April 27, 2019. http://www.themudblood.com/2017/12/16/babies-born- with-unregulated-toxic-chemicals/.

11. Center for Food Safety and Applied Nutrition. "Cosmetics Labeling "Trade Secret" Ingredients." U.S. Food and Drug Administration. August 8, 2018. Accessed June 15, 2019. https://www.fda.gov/cosmetics/cosmetics-labeling/trade- secret-ingredients.

12. "Hundreds of Cancer-Causing Chemicals Pollute Americans' Bodies." EWG. Accessed April 27, 2019. https://www.ewg.org/release/hundreds-cancer-causing- chemicals-pollute-americans-bodies.

13. Krimsky, Sheldon. "Plastics in Our Diet: The Need for BPA Regulation." Scientific American. September 01, 2008. Accessed April 27, 2019. https://www.scientificamerican.com/article/plastics-in-our-diet/.

14. "Polychlorinated Biphenyl." Wikipedia. March 13, 2019. Accessed April 27, 2019. https://en.wikipedia.org/wiki/Polychlorinated_biphenyl.

15. Sass, Jennifer, Bruce Lanphear, and Maureen Swanson. Projecttendr. com. July 2018. Accessed April 22, 2019. http://projecttendr.com/wp-content/uploads/2018/07/TENDR-ltr-FINAL-July-2018-pdf1.pdf.

16. Kounang, Nadia. "Dangerous Chemicals Hiding in Everyday Products." CNN. July 01, 2016. Accessed April 27, 2019. https://www.cnn.com/2016/07/01/ health/everyday-chemicals-we-need-to-reduce-exposure-to/index.html.

17. Neel, Armon B. "Caution! These 10 Drugs Can Cause Memory Loss." AARP. February 09, 2016. Accessed April 27, 2019. https://www.aarp.org/health/ drugs-supplements/info-2017/caution-these-10-drugs-can-cause-memory-loss.html.

18. Fitzgerald, Randall. The Hundred-year Lie: How to Protect Yourself from the Chemicals That Are Destroying Your Health. New York: Plume, 2007

19. McMillen, Matt. "Banned from Soap, Is Triclosan in Your Toothpaste?" WebMD. July 05, 2018. Accessed April 28, 2019. https://www.webmd.com/beauty/news/20180705/banned-from-soap-triclosan-in-toothpaste.

20. Dinwiddie, Michael T., Paul D. Terry, and Jiangang Chen. "Recent Evidence regarding Triclosan and Cancer Risk." International Journal of Environmental

Research and Public Health. February 21, 2014. Accessed April 28, 2019. https://www.ncbi.nlm.nih.gov/pmc/articles/PMC3945593/.

21. Harrington, Rebecca. "The EPA Has Only Banned These 9 Chemicals - out of Thousands." Business Insider. February 10, 2016. Accessed June 15, 2019. https://www.businessinsider.com/epa-only-restricts-9-chemicals-2016-2.

22. Lunder, Sonya. "Asbestos Kills 12,000-15,000 People per Year in the U.S | Asbestos Nation - EWG Action Fund." Asbestos Nation | EWG Action Fund. Accessed June 15, 2019. http://www.asbestosnation.org/facts/asbestos-kills-12000- 15000-people-per-year-in-the-u-s/.

23. Parker, Laura. "A Whopping 91% of Plastic Isn't Recycled." National Geographic. December 20, 2018. Accessed June 15, 2019. https://news. nationalgeographic.com/2017/07/plastic-produced-recycling-waste-ocean-trash- debris-environment/.

24. Fitzgerald, Randall. The Hundred-year Lie: How to Protect Yourself from the Chemicals That Are Destroying Your Health. New York: Plume, 2007.

25. Westervelt, Amy. "Chemical Enemy Number One: How Bad Are Phthalates Really?" The Guardian. February 10, 2015. Accessed June 15, 2019. https://www. theguardian.com/lifeandstyle/2015/feb/10/phthalates-plastics-chemicals-research- analysis.

26. Kwak, Eun Soo, Allan Just, Robin Whyatt, and Rachel L. Miller. "Phthalates, Pesticides, and Bisphenol-A Exposure and the Development of Nonoccupational Asthma and Allergies: How Valid Are the Links?" The Open Allergy Journal. 2009. Accessed June 15, 2019. https://www.ncbi.nlm.nih.gov/pmc/articles/PMC2901120/.

27. IBID P 150

28. "Banned in 27 Countries, Monsanto's RBGH In Dairy Products." Natural Society. November 07, 2012. Accessed June 15, 2019. http://naturalsociety.com/banned-in-27-countries-monsanto-rbgh-dairy-milk-products/.

29. Gian Carlo Di Renzo, Jeanne A. Conry, Jennifer Blake, Mark S. DeFrancesco, Nathaniel DeNicola, James N. Martin Jr., Kelly A. McCue, David Richmond, Abid Shah, Patrice Sutton, Tracey J. Woodruff, Sheryl Ziemin van der Poel, Linda C. Giudice "International Federation of Gynecology and Obstetrics Opinion on Reproductive Health Impacts of Exposure to Toxic Environmental Chemicals."

Article in Press. October 10, 2016. Accessed June 22, 2019. https://www.figo.org/
sites/default/files/uploads/News/Final%20PDF_8462.pdf

30. "Notorious Cancer-Causing Solvent TCE Taints Tap Water for 14 Million
Americans." EWG. Accessed June 15, 2019. https://www.ewg.org/release/
notorious-cancer-causing-solvent-tce-taints-tap-water-14-million-ameri-
cans#. W4Kykn4nbwc.

31. "Off the Books II: More Secret Chemicals." EWG. Accessed June 15, 2019. https://
www.ewg.org/research/off-the-books-ii-more-secret-chemicals#. W4K1iX4nbwc.

32. "DDT, PCBs Could Affect Polar Bear Hormones." THE
WILDLIFE SOCIETY. Accessed June 15, 2019. http://wildlife.org/
ddt-pcbs-could-affect-polar- bear-hormones/.

33. Rogers, Sherry A. Detoxify or Die. Sarasota, FL: Sand Key Company, 2002.
p. 31-32

34. Schafer, Kristin S. Chemical Trespass: Pesticides in Our Bodies and Corporate
Accountability. San Francisco: Pesticide Action Network North America, 2004.
May 2004. Accessed June 16, 2019. https://www.panna.org/sites/default/files/
ChemTres2004Eng.pdf.

35. "Average UK Woman Wears 515 Chemicals a Day." Reuters. November 19, 2009.
Accessed June 15, 2019. https://www.reuters.com/ article/us-britain-cosmetics/
average-uk-woman-wears-515-chemicals-a-day- idUSTRE5AI3M820091119.

36. Persad, Michelle. "The Average Woman Puts 515 Synthetic Chemicals On
Her Body Every Day." The Huffington Post. March 07, 2016. Accessed June
15, 2019. https://www.huffingtonpost.com/entry/synthetic-chemicals-skin-
care_ us_56d8ad09e4b0000de403d995.

37. Kliff, Sarah. "A Brief History of America's Fluoride Wars." The Washington
Post. May 21, 2013. Accessed June 15, 2019. https://www.washingtonpost.com/
news/wonk/wp/2013/05/21/a-brief-history-of-americas-fluoride-wars/?utm_
term=. c12923aa71ff.

38. "Thyroid." Fluoride Action Network. Accessed June 15, 2019. http:// fluoride-
alert.org/issues/health/thyroid/.

39. "Is Fluoridated Drinking Water Safe?" Harvard Public Health Magazine. June 22, 2018. Accessed June 15, 2019. https://www.hsph.harvard.edu/magazine/ magazine_article/fluoridated-drinking-water/.

40. Connett, Michael, and Tara Blank, PhD. "Fluoride & IQ: The 53 Studies." Fluoride Action Network. September 11, 2016. Accessed June 15, 2019. http:// fluoridealert.org/studies/brain01/.

41. Dwyer, Marge. "Impact Of Fluoride On Neurological Development In Children." Fluoride Action Network. July 25, 2012. Accessed June 15, 2019. http:// fluoridealert. org/articles/hsph_2012/.

42. Fluoride Free Sudbury. ""Fluoridated Water Is Public Murder On A Grand Scale" - Dr. Dean Burk." Welcome to Fluoride Free Sudbury. June 26, 2018. Accessed June 15, 2019. https://fluoridefreesudbury.wordpress.com/2017/12/29/ fluoridated-water-is-public-murder-on-a-grand-scale-dr-dean-burk/.

43. "Is Fluoridated Drinking Water Safe?" Harvard Public Health Magazine. June 22, 2018. Accessed June 15, 2019. https://www.hsph.harvard.edu/magazine/ magazine_article/fluoridated-drinking-water/.

44. Connet, Michael. "Fluoride Intake From Toothpaste VS. Recommended Daily Intake From All Sources." Fluoride Action Network. August 2012. Accessed June 15, 2019. http://fluoridealert.org/content/toothpaste-exposure/.

45. Kheradpisheh, Zohreh, Masoud Mirzaei, Amir Hossein Mahvi, Mehdi Mokhtari, Reyhane Azizi, Hossein Fallahzadeh, and Mohammad Hassan Ehrampoush. "Impact of Drinking Water Fluoride on Human Thyroid Hormones: A Case-Control Study." Scientific Reports. February 08, 2018. Accessed June 15, 2019. https://www.ncbi.nlm.nih.gov/pmc/articles/PMC5805681/.

46. Walden, Rolf U., Avery E. Lindeman, Allison E. Aiello, David Andrews, William A. Arnold, Patricia Fair, Rebecca E. Fuoco, Laura A. Geer, Paula I. Johnson, Rainer Lohmann, Kristopher McNeill, Victoria P. Sacks, Ted Schettler, Roland Weber, R. Thomas Zoeller, and Arlene Blum. "The Florence Statement on Triclosan and Triclocarban." Environmental Health Perspectives. June 20, 2017. Accessed June 15, 2019. https://www.ncbi.nlm.nih.gov/pmc/articles/ PMC5644973/.

47. McMillen, Matt. "Banned from Soap, Is Triclosan in Your Toothpaste?" WebMD. July 05, 2018. Accessed June 15, 2019. https://www.webMD.com/beauty/ news/20180705/banned-from-soap-triclosan-in-toothpaste.

48. "Water Chlorination." Wikipedia. June 01, 2019. Accessed June 15, 2019. https://en.wikipedia.org/wiki/Water_chlorination.

49. Sharp, Renee, and J. Paul Pestano. "Water Treatment Contaminants:." EWG. February 27, 2013. Accessed June 15, 2019. https://www.ewg.org/research/water-treatment-contaminants#.W5e_xn4namw.

50. Sharp, Renee, and J. Paul Pestano. "Water Treatment Contaminants:." EWG. February 27, 2013. Accessed June 15, 2019. https://www.ewg.org/research/water-treatment-contaminants#.W5e_xn4namw.

51. Lum, Gerard T. "Chloramine Facts." Chloramine Facts - Citizens Concerned About Chloramine (CCAC). September 7, 2010. Accessed June 15, 2019. http://www.chloramine.org/chloraminefacts.htm.

52. Sedlak, David L., and Urs Von Gunten. "The Chlorine Dilemma." Science. January 07, 2011. Accessed June 15, 2019. http://science.sciencemag.org/content/331/6013/42.summary.

53. Kirk, Andrea B., P. Kalyani Martinelango, Kang Tian, Aniruddha Dutta, Ernest E. Smith, and Purnendu K. Dasgupta. "Perchlorate and Iodide in Dairy and Breast Milk." Environmental Science & Technology. April 01, 2005. Accessed June 15, 2019. https://www.ncbi.nlm.nih.gov/pubmed/15871231.

54. Center for Food Safety and Applied Nutrition. "Overview of Food Ingredients, Additives & Colors." U.S. Food and Drug Administration. April 2010. Accessed June 15, 2019. https://www.fda.gov/food/ingredientspackaginglabeling/ foodadditivesingredients/ucm094211.htm.

55. "Get Risky Chemicals Out of Food." NRDC. March 16, 2018. Accessed June 15, 2019. https://www.nrdc.org/issues/get-risky-chemicals-out-food.

56. Neltner, Thomas G., Heather M. Alger, Jack E. Leonard, and Maricel V. Maffini. "Data Gaps in Toxicity Testing of Chemicals Allowed in Food in the United States." Reproductive Toxicology. August 13, 2013. Accessed June 15, 2019. https://www.sciencedirect.com/science/article/pii/S0890623813003298.

57. Fitzgerald, Randall. The Hundred-year Lie: How to Protect Yourself from the Chemicals That Are Destroying Your Health. New York: Plume, 2007.

58. http://fortune.com/2018/04/11/strawberries-fruit-vegetables-pesticides- environmental-working-group/

59. Morris, Chris. "Strawberries-And 11 Other Fruits and Vegetables-Are Loaded With Pesticide Residue." Fortune. April 11, 2018. Accessed June 15, 2019. http:// fortune.com/2018/04/11/ strawberries-fruit-vegetables-pesticides-environmental- working-group/.

60. IBID P4

61. onieczna, Aleksandra, Aleksandra Rutkowska, and Dominik Rachoń. "Health Risk of Exposure to Bisphenol A (BPA)." Roczniki Panstwowego Zakladu Higieny. 2015. Accessed June 15, 2019. https://www.ncbi.nlm.nih.gov/pubmed/25813067.

62. Braverman, Jody. "How Much Salt in One Can of Soda?" Healthy Eating | SF Gate. November 19, 2018. Accessed June 15, 2019. https://healthyeating.sfgate. com/much-salt-one-can-soda-4965.html.

63. Naik, Ab Qayoom, Tabassum Zafar, and Vinoy K. Shrivastava. "Health Implications Associated with Aspartame Consumption: A Substantial Review." Pakistan Journal of Biological Sciences : PJBS. 2018. Accessed June 15, 2019. https:// www.ncbi.nlm.nih.gov/pubmed/30187722.

64. "The Growing Crisis of Chronic Disease in the United States." Digital image. FightChronicDisease.org. Accessed June 16, 2019. https://www.fightchronicdisease.org/sites/default/files/docs/ GrowingCrisisofChronicDiseaseintheUSfactsheet_81009.pdf.

65. Laino, Charlene. "Half of Cancer Survivors Die From Other Conditions." WebMD. April 03, 2012. Accessed June 15, 2019. https://www.webmd.com/cancer/ news/20120403/half-cancer-survivors-die-other-conditions.

66. Fitzgerald, Randall. The Hundred-year Lie: How to Protect Yourself from the Chemicals That Are Destroying Your Health. New York: Plume, 2007.

67. Anand, Preetha, Ajaikumar B. Kunnumakkara, Chitra Sundaram, Kuzhuvelil B. Harikumar, Sheeja T. Tharakan, Oiki S. Lai, Bokyung Sung, and Bharat B. Aggarwal. "Cancer Is a Preventable Disease That Requires Major Lifestyle Changes." Pharmaceutical Research. September 25, 2008. Accessed June 15, 2019. https:// www.ncbi.nlm.nih.gov/pmc/articles/PMC2515569/.

68. David, Tanton Ph. D. Dr. Taking the Mystery Out of Cancer: Condensed Version. Vol. 3. Cork: BookBaby, 2013.

69. Cha, Ariana Eunjung. "Study: Up to 90 Percent of Cancers Not 'bad Luck,' but Due to Lifestyle Choices, Environment." The Washington Post. December 17, 2015. Accessed June 15, 2019. https://www.washingtonpost.com/news/to-your- health/ wp/2015/12/17/study-up-to-90-of-cancers-not-bad-luck-but-due-to-lifestyle- choices-environment/?utm_term=.a1ce898b05bd.

70. "Cancer Statistics." National Cancer Institute. April 27, 2018. Accessed June 16, 2019. https://www.cancer.gov/about-cancer/understanding/statistics.

71. "Will You Have Diabetes in 2020?" RN. Accessed June 15, 2019. https:// www. rn.com/Pages/ResourceDetails.aspx?id=3065.

72. Go, Alan S., Dariush Mozaffarian, Véronique L. Roger, Emelia J. Benjamin, Jarett D. Berry, Michael J. Blaha, Shifan Dai, Earl S. Ford, Caroline S. Fox, Sheila Franco, Heather J. Fullerton, Cathleen Gillespie, Susan M. Hailpern, John A. Heit, Virginia J. Howard, Mark D. Huffman, Suzanne E. Judd, Brett M. Kissela, Steven J. Kittner, Daniel T. Lackland, Judith H. Lichtman, Lynda D. Lisabeth, Rachel H. Mackey, David J. Magid, Gregory M. Marcus, Ariane Marelli, David B. Matchar, Darren K. McGuire, Emile R. Mohler, Claudia S. Moy, Michael E. Mussolino, Robert W. Neumar, Graham Nichol, Dilip K. Pandey, Nina P. Paynter, Matthew J. Reeves, Paul D. Sorlie, Joel Stein, Amytis Towfighi, Tanya N. Turan, Salim S. Virani, Nathan D. Wong, Daniel Woo, Melanie B. Turner, and American Heart Association Statistics Committee and Stroke Statistics Subcommittee. "Heart Disease and Stroke Statistics--2014 Update: A Report from the American Heart Association." Circulation. January 21, 2014. Accessed June 15, 2019. https://www. ncbi.nlm.nih.gov/pmc/articles/PMC5408159/.

73. Arthritis By the Numbers / Book of Trusted Facts & Figures. Arthritis Foundation, 2018. Accessed June 16, 2019. https://www.arthritis.org/Documents/ Sections/About-Arthritis/arthritis-facts-stats-figures.pdf.

74. "Environmental Exposure | Cosmetics Trigger Rheumatoid Arthritis." Mercola.com. February 11, 2010. Accessed June 15, 2019. https://articles.mercola. com/sites/articles/archive/2010/02/11/environmental-exposure-to-hairspray-lipstick-and-pollution-can-trigger-arthritis.aspx.

75. Sternberg, Steve, and Geoff Dougherty. "Risks Are High at Low-Volume Hospitals." U.S. News & World Report. May 18, 2015. Accessed June 15, 2019. https://www. usnews.com/news/articles/2015/05/18/risks-are-high-at-low-volume- hospitals.

76. "FastStats - Leading Causes of Death." Centers for Disease Control and Prevention. March 17, 2017. Accessed June 15, 2019. https://www.cdc.gov/nchs/fastats/leading-causes-of-death.htm.

77. Center for Drug Evaluation and Research. "Preventable Adverse Drug Reactions: A Focus on Drug Interactions." U.S. Food and Drug Administration. March 6, 2018. Accessed June 15, 2019. https://www.fda.gov/drugs/ developmentapprovalprocess/developmentresources/druginteractionslabeling/ ucm110632.htm.

78. Allen, Marshall, and Olga Pierce. "Medical Errors Are No. 3 Cause Of U.S Deaths, Researchers Say." NPR. May 03, 2016. Accessed June 15, 2019. https://www.npr.org/sections/health-shots/2016/05/03/476636183/death- certificates-undercount-toll-of-medicalerrors?utm_source=twitter.com&utm_ medium=social&utm_campaign=morningedition&utm_term=nprnews&utm_ content=20160504.

79. Bonn, Dorothy. "Adverse Drug Reactions Remain a Major Cause of Death." The Lancet 351, no. 9110 (April 18, 1998): 1183. Accessed June 16, 2019. doi:10.1016/s0140-6736(98)23016-9.

80. Sternberg, Steve. "Medical Errors Are Third Leading Cause of Death in the U.S." U.S. News & World Report. May 3, 2016. Accessed June 15, 2019. https:// www.usnews.com/news/articles/2016-05-03/ medical-errors-are-third-leading- cause-of-death-in-the-us.

81. Broxmeyer, Lawrence. "Are the Infectious Roots of Alzheimers Buried Deep in the Past?" Journal of MPE Molecular Pathological Epidemiology. February27, 2017. Accessed June 15, 2019. http://molecular-pathological-epidemiology. imedpub.com/are-the-infectious-roots-of-alzheimersburied-deep-in-the-past. php?aid=18399.

82. Icheku, Vincent. "A Review of the Evidence Linking Zika Virus to the Developmental Abnormalities That Lead to Microcephaly in View of Recent Cases of Birth Defects in Africa." Journal of MPE Molecular Pathological Epidemiology 1, no. 1 (October 28, 2016). Accessed June 16, 2019. oai:researchopen.lsbu. ac.uk:514.

83. Richardson, Jason R., Ananya Roy, Stuart L. Shalat, Richard T. Von Stein, Muhammad M. Hossain, Brian Buckley, Marla Gearing, Allan I. Levey, and Dwight C. German. "Elevated Serum Pesticide Levels and Risk for Alzheimer Disease." JAMA Neurology. March 2014. Accessed June 15, 2019. https://www. ncbi.nlm. nih.gov/pmc/articles/PMC4132934/.

84. Bisht, Kanchan, Kaushik Sharma, and Marie-Ève Tremblay. "Chronic Stress as a Risk Factor for Alzheimer's Disease: Roles of Microglia-mediated Synaptic Remodeling, Inflammation, and Oxidative Stress." Neurobiology of Stress. May 19, 2018. Accessed June 15, 2019. https://www.ncbi.nlm.nih.gov/ pubmed/29992181.

85. Calderón-Garcidueñas, Lilian, William Reed, Robert R. Maronpot, Carlos Henríquez-Roldán, Ricardo Delgado-Chavez, Ana Calderón-Garcidueñas, Irma Dragustinovis, Maricela Franco-Lira, Mariana Aragón-Flores, Anna C. Solt, Michael Altenburg, Ricardo Torres-Jardón, and James A. Swenberg. "Brain Inflammation and Alzheimer's-like Pathology in Individuals Exposed to Severe Air Pollution." Toxicologic Pathology. November/December 2004. Accessed June 15, 2019. https://www.ncbi.nlm.nih.gov/pubmed/15513908.

86. UHN Staff. "Environmental Toxins Can Increase the Risk of Memory Loss, Mild Cognitive Impairment, and Alzheimer's." University Health News. June 22, 2016. Accessed June 15, 2019. https://universityhealthnews.com/daily/memory/ environmental-toxins-can-increase-the-risk-of-memory-loss-mild-cognitive-impairment-and-alzheimers/.

87. Xu, Lin, Wenchao Zhang, Xianchen Liu, Cuili Zhang, Pin Wang, and Xiulan Zhao. "Circulatory Levels of Toxic Metals (Aluminum, Cadmium, Mercury, Lead) in Patients with Alzheimer's Disease: A Quantitative Meta-Analysis and Systematic Review." Journal of Alzheimer's Disease : JAD. 2018. Accessed June 15, 2019. https://www.ncbi.nlm.nih.gov/pubmed/29439342.

88. Xu, Lin, Wenchao Zhang, Xianchen Liu, Cuili Zhang, Pin Wang, and Xiulan Zhao. "Circulatory Levels of Toxic Metals (Aluminum, Cadmium, Mercury, Lead) in Patients with Alzheimer's Disease: A Quantitative Meta-Analysis and Systematic Review." Journal of Alzheimers Disease 62, no. 1 (2018): 361-72. Accessed June 16, 2019. doi:10.3233/jad-170811.

89. Bourgeois, Florence T., Michael W. Shannon, Clarissa Valim, and Kenneth D. Mandl. "Adverse Drug Events in the Outpatient Setting: An 11-year National Analysis." Pharmacoepidemiology and Drug Safety. September 2010. Accessed June 15, 2019. https://www.ncbi.nlm.nih.gov/pmc/articles/PMC2932855/.

90. "Nearly 7 in 10 Americans Take Prescription Drugs, Mayo Clinic, Olmsted Medical Center Find." Mayo Clinic. June 19, 2013. Accessed June 15, 2019. https:// newsnetwork.mayoclinic.org/discussion/nearly-7-in-10-americans-take- prescription-drugs-mayo-clinic-olmsted-medical-center-find/?src=email-release.

91. Tyson, Peter. "The Hippocratic Oath Today." PBS. March 26, 2001. Accessed June 15, 2019. https://www.pbs.org/wgbh/nova/article/hippocratic-oath-today/.

92. Baccarelli, Andrea, and Valentina Bollati. "Epigenetics and Environmental Chemicals." Current Opinion in Pediatrics. April 2009. Accessed June 15, 2019. https://www.ncbi.nlm.nih.gov/pmc/articles/PMC3035853/.

93. Weinhold, Bob. "Epigenetics: The Science of Change." Environmental Health Perspectives. March 2006. Accessed June 15, 2019. https://www.ncbi.nlm. nih.gov/ pmc/articles/PMC1392256/.

94. Smeester, Lisa, Andrew E. Yosim, Monica D. Nye, Cathrine Hoyo, Susan K. Murphy, and Rebecca C. Fry. "Imprinted Genes and the Environment: Links to the Toxic Metals Arsenic, Cadmium, Lead and Mercury." Genes. June 11, 2014. Accessed June 15, 2019. https://www.ncbi.nlm.nih.gov/pmc/articles/ PMC4094944/.

95. Jirtle, Randy L., and Michael K. Skinner. "Environmental Epigenomics and Disease Susceptibility." Nature Reviews Genetics 8, no. 4 (2007): 253-62. doi:10.1038/nrg2045.

96. Waterland, R. A., and R. L. Jirtle. "Transposable Elements: Targets for

Early Nutritional Effects on Epigenetic Gene Regulation." Molecular and Cellular Biology 23, no. 15 (August 2003): 5293-300. Accessed June 16, 2019. doi:10.1128/ mcb.23.15.5293-5300.2003.

97. "Human Genome Project FAQ." Genome.gov. November 12, 2018. Accessed June 15, 2019. https://www.genome.gov/11006943/ human-genome-project- completion-frequently-asked-questions/.

98. University, Quantum. YouTube. June 26, 2016. Accessed June 15, 2019. https:// www.youtube.com/watch?v=G4T0LzU_rv0.

99. Charles Q Choi. "How Epigenetics Affects Twins." Genome Biology. July 08, 2005. Accessed June 15, 2019. https://genomebiology.biomedcentral.com/ articles/10.1186/gb-spotlight-20050708-02.

100. Choi, Charles. "How Epigenetics Affects Twins." The Scientist Magazine®. July 7, 2005. Accessed June 15, 2019. https://www.the-scientist.com/research- round-up/ how-epigenetics-affects-twins-48565.

101. TranJul, Cathy, Kai KupferschmidtJun, Jocelyn KaiserJun, Jon CohenJun, Herton EscobarJun, and David MalakoffJun. "Identical Twins Not So Identical." Science. December 10, 2017. Accessed June 15, 2019. http://www.sciencemag.org/news/2005/07/identical-twins-not-so-identical.

102. Segal, Nancy L., Yesika S. Montoya, Yuk J. Loke, and Jeffery M. Craig. "Identical Twins Doubly Exchanged at Birth: A Case Report of Genetic and Environmental Influences on the Adult Epigenome." Identical Twins Doubly Exchanged at Birth: A Case Report of Genetic and Environmental Influences on the Adult Epigenome | Epigenomics. December 12, 2016. Accessed June 15, 2019. https://www.future-medicine.com/doi/10.2217/epi-2016-0104.

103. Bell, Jordana T., and Tim D. Spector. "A Twin Approach to Unraveling Epigenetics." Trends in Genetics : TIG. March 2011. Accessed June 15, 2019. https://www.ncbi.nlm.nih.gov/pmc/articles/PMC3063335/.

104. Carr, Flora. "Scott Kelly's DNA Differs From Twin Mark's After NASA Study." Time. March 15, 2018. Accessed June 15, 2019. http://time.com/5201064/scott-kelly-mark-nasa-dna-study/.

105. "Dutch Famine of 1944-45." Wikipedia. June 03, 2019. Accessed June 15, 2019. https://en.wikipedia.org/wiki/Dutch_famine_of_1944-45.

106. Knopik, Valerie S., Matthew A. Maccani, Sarah Francazio, and John E. McGeary. "The Epigenetics of Maternal Cigarette Smoking during Pregnancy and Effects on Child Development." Development and Psychopathology. November 2012. Accessed June 15, 2019. https://www.ncbi.nlm.nih.gov/pmc/articles/PMC3581096/.

107. Talks, TEDx. YouTube. January 10, 2014. Accessed June 15, 2019. https:// www.youtube.com/watch?v=Udlz7CMLuLQ.

108. Knopik, Valerie S., Matthew A. Maccani, Sarah Francazio, and John E. McGeary. "The Epigenetics of Maternal Cigarette Smoking during Pregnancy and Effects on Child Development." Development and Psychopathology. November 2012. Accessed June 18, 2019. https://www.ncbi.nlm.nih.gov/pmc/articles/PMC3581096/.

109. Thielen, Anja, Hubert Klus, and Lutz Müller. "Tobacco Smoke: Unraveling a Controversial Subject." Experimental and Toxicologic Pathology 60, no. 2-3 (2008): 141-56. doi:10.1016/j.etp.2008.01.014.

110. Talks, TEDx. "Epigenetic Transformation -- You Are What Your Grandparents Ate: Pamela Peeke at TEDxLowerEastSide." YouTube. January 10, 2014. Accessed June 18, 2019. https://www.youtube.com/ watch?v=Udlz7CMLuLQ.

111. Knopik, Valerie S., Matthew A. Maccani, Sarah Francazio, and John E. McGeary. "The Epigenetics of Maternal Cigarette Smoking during Pregnancy and Effects on Child Development." Development and Psychopathology. November 2012. Accessed June 15, 2019. https://www.ncbi.nlm.nih.gov/pmc/articles/ PMC3581096/.

112. Zacharasiewicz, Angela. "Maternal Smoking in Pregnancy and Its Influence on Childhood Asthma." ERJ Open Research. July 29, 2016. Accessed June 15, 2019. https://www.ncbi.nlm.nih.gov/pmc/articles/PMC5034599/.

113. Moosavi, Azam, and Ali Motevalizadeh Ardekani. "Role of Epigenetics in Biology and Human Diseases." Iranian Biomedical Journal. November 2016. Accessed June 15, 2019. https://www.ncbi.nlm.nih.gov/pmc/articles/ PMC5075137/.

114. Hamza, M., S. Halayem, R. Mrad, S. Bourgou, F. Charfi, and A. Belhadj. "Epigenetics' Implication in Autism Spectrum Disorders: A Review." L'Encephale. August 2017. Accessed June 15, 2019. https://www.ncbi.nlm.nih. gov/ pubmed/27692350.

115. "Evaluation of Five Organophosphate Insecticides and Herbicides." International Agency for Research on Cancer 112 (March 20, 2015). Accessed June 16, 2019. https://www.iarc.fr/wp-content/uploads/2018/07/ MonographVolume112-1.pdf.

116. James, Mike, and Jorge L. Ortiz. "Jury Orders Monsanto to Pay $289 Million to Cancer Patient in Roundup Lawsuit." USA Today. August 11, 2018. Accessed June 15, 2019. https://www.usatoday.com/story/news/2018/08/10/jury- orders-monsanto-pay-289-million-cancer-patient-roundup-lawsuit/962297002/.

117. Gori, Randy L. "Roundup Lawsuits." ConsumerSafety.org. April 29, 2019. Accessed June 15, 2019. https://www.consumersafety.org/legal/roundup-lawsuit/.

118. Gonzales, Richard. "California Jury Awards $2 Billion To Couple In Roundup Weed Killer Cancer Trial." NPR. May 14, 2019. Accessed June 15, 2019. https://www.npr.org/2019/05/13/723056453/ california-jury-awards-2-billion-to- couple-in-roundup-weed-killer-cancer-trial.

119. Romano RM, Romano MA, Bernardi MM, Furtado PV, Oliveira CA. Prepubertal exposure to commercial formulation of the herbicide Glyphosate alters testosterone levels and testicular morphology. Arch Toxicol. 2010;84:309-317.

120. Gasnier C, Dumont C, Benachour N, Clair E, Chagnon MC, Séralini GE. Glyphosate-based herbicides are toxic and endocrine disruptors in human cell lines. Toxicology. 2009;262:184-191. doi:10.1016/j.tox.2009.06.006.

121. Hokanson R, Fudge R, Chowdhary R, Busbee D. Alteration of estro- gen- regulated gene expression in human cells induced by the agricultural and horticultural herbicide glyphosate. Hum Exp Toxicol. 2007;26:747-752. doi:10.1177/0960327107083453.

122. Thongprakaisang S, Thiantanawat A, Rangkadilok N, Suriyo T, Satayavivad J. Glyphosate induces human breast cancer cells growth via estrogen receptors. Food Chem Toxicol. 2013;59:129-136. doi:10.1016/j.fct.2013.05.057.

123. "BRCA1 & BRCA2 Genes: Risk for Breast & Ovarian Cancer." Memorial Sloan Kettering Cancer Center. Accessed June 15, 2019. https://www.mskcc.org/cancer-care/risk-assessment-screening/hereditary-genetics/genetic-counseling/brca1-brca2-genes-risk-breast-ovarian.

124. Ornish, Dean, MD. "Nutrition." Ornish Lifestyle Medicine. Accessed June 15, 2019. https://www.ornish.com/proven-program/nutrition/.

125. "How Does the Large Percent of People That Have 'the Gene' Not Get 'the Cancer?'" 2019. Accessed June 15, 2019. https://www.brucelipton.com/blog/how- does-the-large-percent-people-have-the-gene-not-get-the-cancer.

126. V, Rai. "The MTHFR C677T Polymorphism and Hyperuricemia Risk: A Meta-analysis of 558 Cases and 912 Controls." OMICS International. January 29, 2016. Accessed June 15, 2019. https://www.omicsonline.org/open-access/the-mthfr-c677t-polymorphism-and-hyperuricemia-risk-a-metaanalysisof-558-cases-and-912-controls-2153-0769-1000166.php?aid=67596.

127. Calle, E. E., M. J. Thun, J. M. Petrelli, C. Rodriguez, and C. W. Heath. "Body Mass Index and Mortality in a Prospective Cohort of US Adults." Journal of Cardiopulmonary Rehabilitation 20, no. 2 (2000): 131. doi:10.1097/00008483- 200003000-00010.

128. Cheung, Man-ka Marcella, and Giles S.H. Yeo. "FTO Biology and Obesity: Why Do a Billion of Us Weigh 3 Kg More?" Frontiers. February 07, 2011. Accessed June 15, 2019. https://www.frontiersin.org/articles/10.3389/ fendo.2011.00004/full.

129. UCL. "How 'obesity Gene' Triggers Weight Gain." UCL News. November 15, 2018. Accessed June 15, 2019. https://www.ucl.ac.uk/news/news- articles/0713/15072013-How-obesity-gene-triggers-weight-gain-Batterham.

130. Wanjek, Christopher. "How Amish Avoid Obesity." LiveScience. September 16, 2008. Accessed June 15, 2019. https://www.livescience.com/5087-amish-avoid-obesity.html.

131. Gottfried, Sara, MD. "5 Genes That Make It Hard to Lose Weight, and What You Can Do To Combat Them." Sara Gottfried MD. January 11, 2017. Accessed June 15, 2019. https://www.saragottfriedMD.com/five-genes-that-make- it-hard-to-lose-weight-and-what-you-can-do-to-combat-them/.

132. Rampersaud, Evadnie, Braxton D. Mitchell, Toni I. Pollin, Mao Fu, Haiqing Shen, Jeffery R. O'Connell, Julie L. Ducharme, Scott Hines, Paul Sack, Rosalie Naglieri, Alan R. Shuldiner, and Soren Snitker. "Physical Activity and the Association of Common FTO Gene Variants with Body Mass Index and Obesity." Archives of Internal Medicine. September 08, 2008. Accessed June 15, 2019. https:// www.ncbi.nlm.nih.gov/pmc/articles/PMC3635949/.

133. Gottfried, Sara, MD. "5 Genes That Make It Hard to Lose Weight, and What You Can Do To Combat Them." Sara Gottfried MD. January 11, 2017. Accessed June 15, 2019. https://www.saragottfriedMD.com/five-genes-that-make- it-hard-to-lose-weight-and-what-you-can-do-to-combat-them/.

134. "Why Is Vitamin D So Important for Your Health?" MD Magazine. August 20, 2007. Accessed June 15, 2019. https://www.mdmag.com/journals/ internal- medicine-world-report/2007/2007-08/2007-08_47.

135. Gröber, Uwe, and Klaus Kisters. "Influence of Drugs on Vitamin D and Calcium Metabolism." Dermato-endocrinology. April 01, 2012. Accessed June 15, 2019. https://www.ncbi.nlm.nih.gov/pmc/articles/PMC3427195/.

136. Whitehouse A.J., Holt B.J., Serralha M., Holt P.G., Hart P.H., Kusel M.M. Maternal vitamin D levels and the autism phenotype among offspring. J. Autism Devl. Disord. 2013;43:1495-1504. doi: 10.1007/s10803-012-1676-8.

137. Cieślińska, Anna, Elżbieta Kostyra, Barbara Chwała, Małgorzata Moszyńska-Dumara, Ewa Fiedorowicz, Małgorzata Teodorowicz, and Huub F J Savelkoul. "Vitamin D Receptor Gene Polymorphisms Associated with Childhood Autism." Brain Sciences. September 09, 2017. Accessed June 15, 2019. https:// www.ncbi.nlm. nih.gov/pmc/articles/PMC5615256/.

138. Moosavi, Azam, and Ali Motevalizadeh Ardekani. "Role of Epigenetics in Biology and Human Diseases." Iranian Biomedical Journal. November 2016. Accessed June 18, 2019. https://www.ncbi.nlm.nih.gov/pmc/articles/PMC5075137/.

139. Stevens, Aaron J., Julia J. Rucklidge, and Martin A. Kennedy. "Epigenetics, Nutrition and Mental Health. Is There a Relationship?" Nutritional Neuroscience. November 2018. Accessed June 15, 2019. https://www.ncbi.nlm.nih.gov/pubmed/28553986.

140. Weinhold, Bob. "Epigenetics: The Science of Change." Environmental Health Perspectives. March 2006. Accessed June 18, 2019. https://www.ncbi.nlm. nih.gov/pmc/articles/PMC1392256/.

141. "Oxytocin: Pair Bonding." Psychology Today. Accessed June 15, 2019. https:// www.psychologytoday.com/us/basics/oxytocin.

142. Colino, Stacey. "The Health Benefits of Hugging." U.S. News & World Report. February 3, 2016. Accessed June 15, 2019. https://health.usnews.com/ health-news/health-wellness/articles/2016-02-03/the-health-benefits-of-hugging.

143. Higashida, Haruhiro, Shigeru Yokoyama, Mitsuru Kikuchi, and Toshio Munesue. "CD38 and Its Role in Oxytocin Secretion and Social Behavior." Hormones and Behavior. March 2012. Accessed June 15, 2019. https://www.ncbi. nlm.nih.gov/pubmed/22227279.

144. Lopatina, Olga, Alena Inzhutova, Alla B. Salmina, and Haruhiro Higashida. "The Roles of Oxytocin and CD38 in Social or Parental Behaviors." Frontiers in Neuroscience. January 11, 2013. Accessed June 15, 2019. https://www.ncbi.nlm. nih.gov/pmc/articles/PMC3542479/.

145. Munesue, Toshio, Shigeru Yokoyama, Kazuhiko Nakamura, Ayyappan Anitha, Kazuo Yamada, Kenshi Hayashi, Tomoya Asaka, Hong-Xiang Liu, Duo Jin, Keita Koizumi, Mohammad Saharul Islam, Jian-Jun Huang, Wen-Jie Ma, Uh- Hyun Kim, Sun-Jun Kim, Keunwan Park, Dongsup Kim, Mitsuru Kikuchi, Yasuki Ono, Hideo Nakatani, Shiro Suda, Taishi Miyachi, Hirokazu Hirai, Alla Salmina, Yu

A. Pichugina, Andrei A. Soumarokov, Nori Takei, Norio Mori, Masatsugu Tsujii, Toshiro Sugiyama, Kunimasa Yagi, Masakazu Yamagishi, Tsukasa Sasaki, Hidenori Yamasue, Nobumasa Kato, Ryota Hashimoto, Masako Taniike, Yutaka Hayashi, Junichiro Hamada, Shioto Suzuki, Akishi Ooi, Mami Noda, Yuko Kamiyama, Mizuho A. Kido, Olga Lopatina, Minako Hashii, Sarwat Amina, Fabio Malavasi, Eric J. Huang, Jiasheng Zhang, Nobuaki Shimizu, Takeo Yoshikawa, Akihiro Matsushima, Yoshio Minabe, and Haruhiro Higashida. "Two Genetic Variants of CD38 in Subjects with Autism Spectrum Disorder and Controls." Neuroscience Research. June 2010. Accessed June 15, 2019. https://www.ncbi.nlm. nih.gov/pubmed/20435366.

146. Domes, G., Heinrichs, M., Michel, A., Berger, C., and Herpertz, S. C. (2007). Oxytocin improves "mind-reading" in humans. Biol. Psychiatry 61, 731- 733.

147. Bartz, J. A., and Hollander, E. (2008). Oxytocin and experimental therapeutics in autism spectrum disorders. Prog. Brain Res. 170, 451-462.

148. Guastella, A. J., Howard, A. L., Dadds, M. R., Mitchell, P., and Carson, D. S. (2009). A randomized controlled trial of intranasal oxytocin as an adjunct to exposure therapy for social anxiety disorder. Psychoneuroendocrinology 34, 917- 923

149. "What Is Epigenetics?" Better the Future. Accessed June 15, 2019. http://betterthefuture.org/what-is-epigenetics/.

150. TED-Ed. YouTube. October 01, 2015. Accessed June 15, 2019. https:// www.youtube.com/watch?v=oe64p-QzhNE.

151. Seaton, Jean. "Culture - Why Orwell's 1984 Could Be about Now." BBC. May 07, 2018. Accessed June 15, 2019. http://www.bbc.com/culture/story/20180507-why-orwells-1984-could-be-about-now.

152. Leetaru, Kalev. "As Orwell's 1984 Turns 70 It Predicted Much Of Today's Surveillance Society." Forbes. May 06, 2019. Accessed June 15, 2019. https:// www.forbes.com/sites/kalevleetaru/2019/05/06/as-orwells-1984-turns-70-it- predicted-much-of-todays-surveillance-society/#5f63f63811de.

153. Solon, Olivia. "Facebook Has 60 People Working on How to Read Your Mind." The Guardian. April 19, 2017. Accessed June 16, 2019. https://www. theguardian.com/technology/2017/apr/19/facebook-mind-reading-technology-f8.

154. Hoffman, Ronald, Dr. "Are Some Medicines Stealing Your Brain Power?" Default Podcast. May 18, 2018. Accessed June 15, 2019. https://drhoffman.com/ article/are-some-medicines-stealing-your-brain-power/.

155. The National Institute of Mental Health. BRAIN HEALTH: Medications' Effects on Older Adults' Brain Function. July 28, 2014. Accessed June 16, 2019. https://www.nia.nih.gov/sites/default/files/d7/MedAgeBrain-Brochure.pdf.

156. Gerasimov, Vadim. "Information Processing in Human Body." Information Processing in Human Body. 2006. Accessed June 15, 2019. https://vadim. oversigma. com/MAS862/Project.html.

157. Grandjean, Philippe, and Philip J. Landrigan. "Neurobehavioural Effects of Developmental Toxicity." The Lancet Neurology 13, no. 3 (February 15, 2014): 330-38. Accessed June 16, 2019. doi:10.1016/s1474-4422(13)70278-3.

158. Johnson, Sara B., Robert W. Blum, and Jay N. Giedd. "Adolescent Maturity and the Brain: The Promise and Pitfalls of Neuroscience Research in Adolescent Health Policy." The Journal of Adolescent Health : Official Publication of the Society for Adolescent Medicine. September 2009. Accessed June 15, 2019. https:// www. ncbi.nlm.nih.gov/pmc/articles/PMC2892678/

159. Gold, Jenny. "Health Insurers Are Still Skimping On Mental Health Coverage." NPR. November 30, 2017. Accessed June 15, 2019. https://www.npr. org/sections/health-shots/2017/11/29/567264925/ health-insurers-are-still-skimping- on-mental-health-coverage

160. Khan, Arif, Kaysee Fahl Mar, Jim Faucett, Shirin Khan Schilling, and Walter A. Brown. "Has the Rising Placebo Response Impacted Antidepressant Clinical Trial Outcome? Data from the US Food and Drug Administration 1987- 2013." World Psychiatry : Official Journal of the World Psychiatric Association (WPA). June 2017. Accessed June 15, 2019. https://www.ncbi.nlm.nih.gov/pmc/ articles/ PMC5428172/.

161. Kirsch, Irving. "Antidepressants and the Placebo Effect." Zeitschrift Fur Psychologie. 2014. Accessed June 15, 2019. https://www.ncbi.nlm.nih.gov/pmc/ articles/PMC4172306/#c17.

162. Whitaker, Robert. "Do Antidepressants Work? A People's Review of the Evidence." Mad In America. May 04, 2019. Accessed June 15, 2019. https://www. madinamerica.com/2018/03/do-antidepressants-work-a-peoples-review-of-the- evidence/.

163. Corrigan, Michael W. "Lancet Psychiatry Needs to Retract ADHD Brain Scan Study." Mad In America. May 28, 2019. Accessed June 15, 2019. https://www.madinamerica.com/2017/04/lancet-psychiatry-needs-to-retract-the-adhd- enigma-study/.

164. Kirsch, Irving. "Antidepressants and the Placebo Effect." Zeitschrift Fur Psychologie. 2014. Accessed June 18, 2019. https://www.ncbi.nlm.nih.gov/pmc/articles/PMC4172306/.

165. Kirsch, Irving, Brett J. Deacon, Tania B. Huedo-Medina, Alan Scoboria, Thomas J. Moore, and Blair T. Johnson. "Initial Severity and Antidepressant Benefits: A Meta-analysis of Data Submitted to the Food and Drug Administration." PLoS Medicine. February 2008. Accessed June 15, 2019. https://www.ncbi.nlm.nih.gov/pmc/articles/PMC2253608/.

166. Breggin, Peter Roger, and Ginger Ross. Breggin. Talking Back to Prozac: What Doctors Wont Tell You about Todays Most Controversial Drug. New York: Open Road Integrated Media, 2014. P163, p 22-23?

167. Ruiz, Bernalyn. "SSRI Exposure in Pregnancy Alters Fetal Neurodevelopment." Mad In America. April 30, 2019. Accessed June 15, 2019. https://www.madinamerica.com/2018/08/ssri-exposure-pregnancy-alters-fetal- neurodevelopment/.

168. Chung, Seockhoon, Jin Pyo Hong, and Hanik K. Yoo. "Association of the DAO and DAOA Gene Polymorphisms with Autism Spectrum Disorders in Boys in Korea: A Preliminary Study." Psychiatry Research. October 31, 2007. Accessed June 15, 2019. https://preview.ncbi.nlm.nih.gov/pubmed/17629951.

169. Gøtzsche, Peter C. "Antidepressants Increase the Risk of Suicide, Violence and Homicide at All Ages." The BMJ. May 22, 2019. Accessed June 15, 2019. https://www.bmj.com/content/358/bmj.j3697/rr-4.

170. Duke, Selwyn. "From Prozac to Parkland: Are Psychiatric Drugs Causing Mass Shootings?" The New American. February 17, 2018. Accessed June 15, 2019. https://www.thenewamerican.com/usnews/crime/item/28307-from-prozac-to-parkland-are-psychiatric-drugs-causing-mass-shootings.

171. AWARENESS, INTERNATIONAL COALITION FOR DRUG. YouTube. June 11, 2009. Accessed June 15, 2019. https://www.youtube.com/watch?v=3XTNXr5DAOo.

172. Roberts, Dan. "Every Mass Shooting Shares 1 Thing In Common, NOT Guns." AmmoLand.com. August 13, 2018. Accessed June 15, 2019. https:// www.

ammoland.com/2013/04/every-mass-shooting-in-the-last-20-years-shares-psychotropic-drugs/#ixzz5OB186FRC.

174. Olsen, Gwen. Confessions of an Rx Drug Pusher. New York: IUniverse Star, 2009.

175. Olsen, Gwen. Confessions of an Rx Drug Pusher. New York: IUniverse Star, 2009.

176. Healy, David, and Graham Aldred. "Antidepressant Drug Use & the Risk of Suicide." International Review of Psychiatry (Abingdon, England). June 2005. Accessed June 15, 2019. https://www.ncbi.nlm.nih.gov/pubmed/16194787.

177. "Pharm Funded Psychiatrists and Conflicts of Interest." CCHR International. September 06, 2016. Accessed June 15, 2019. https://www.cchrint. org/issues/the-corrupt-alliance-of-the-psychiatric-pharmaceutical-industry/.

178. Patrick. "Depression - The Nutrition Connection." Patrick Holford. March 31, 2009. Accessed June 15, 2019. https://www.patrickholford.com/advice/depression-the-nutrition-connection.

178. Weil, Andrew, MD. "St. John's Wort for Depression? - Ask Dr. Weil." DrWeil.com. December 02, 2016. Accessed June 15, 2019. https://www.drweil. com/health-wellness/body-mind-spirit/mental-health/st-johns-wort-for-depression/.

179. Shivappa, Nitin, James R. Hébert, Nicola Veronese, Maria Gabriella Caruso, Maria Notarnicola, Stefania Maggi, Brendon Stubbs, Joseph Firth, Michele Fornaro, and Marco Solmi. "The Relationship between the Dietary Inflammatory Index (DII®) and Incident Depressive Symptoms: A Longitudinal Cohort Study." Journal of Affective Disorders. August 01, 2018. Accessed June 15, 2019. https:// www.ncbi. nlm.nih.gov/pubmed/29649709.

180. Ruiz, Bernalyn. "Research Emphasizes Association Between Inflammation, Diet, and Depression." Mad In America. August 31, 2018. Accessed June 15, 2019. https://www.madinamerica.com/2018/08/research-emphasizes-association- inflammation-diet-depression/.

181. Lange, Klaus W., Susanne Reichl, Katharina M. Lange, Lara Tucha, and Oliver Tucha. "The History of Attention Deficit Hyperactivity Disorder." Attention Deficit and Hyperactivity Disorders. December 2010. Accessed June 15, 2019. https://www.ncbi.nlm.nih.gov/pmc/articles/PMC3000907/.

182. Foley, Denise. "ADHD & Kids: The Truth About Attention Deficit Hyperactivity Disorder." Time. Accessed June 15, 2019. http://time.com/growing- up-with-adhd/.

183. "Products - Data Briefs - Number 201 - May 2015." Centers for Disease Control and Prevention. May 2015. Accessed June 16, 2019. https://www.cdc.gov/ nchs/ productsdata/databriefs/db201.htm.pdf

184. Mahone, E. Mark, and Martha B. Denckla. "Attention-Deficit/Hyperactivity Disorder: A Historical Neuropsychological Perspective." Journal of the International Neuropsychological Society : JINS. October 2017. Accessed June 15, 2019. https:// www.ncbi.nlm.nih.gov/pmc/articles/PMC5724393/

185. Holland, Kimberly, and Elsbeth Riley. "ADHD by the Numbers: Facts, Statistics, and You." Healthline. May 30, 2018. Accessed June 15, 2019. https:// www.healthline.com/health/adhd/facts-statistics-infographic#fast-facts.

186. "Data and Statistics About ADHD | CDC." Centers for Disease Control and Prevention. September 21, 2018. Accessed June 15, 2019. https://www.cdc.gov/ ncbddd/adhd/data.html.

187. Mahone, E. Mark, and Martha B. Denckla. "Attention-Deficit/Hyperactivity Disorder: A Historical Neuropsychological Perspective." Journal of the International Neuropsychological Society : JINS. October 2017. Accessed June 15, 2019. https:// www.ncbi.nlm.nih.gov/pmc/articles/PMC5724393/

188. Smith, Kyle. "ADHD Does Not Exist." New York Post. July 25, 2018. Accessed June 15, 2019. https://nypost.com/2014/01/04/adhd-does-not-exist/.

189. Sax, Leonard, MD PhD. "Evidence That Stimulant Medications May Damage the Developing Brain, Especially the Nucleus Accumbens." Stimulant Medications and the Nucleus Accumbens - Leonard Sax MD PhD, 2012. 2013. Accessed June 15, 2019. https://www.leonardsax.com/stimulants.html.

190. "Leon Eisenberg "Discovered" ADHD Then Makes a Disturbing Deathbed Confession." HealthFreedoms. February 15, 2017. Accessed June 15, 2019. http:// www.healthfreedoms.org/leon-eisenberg-discovered-adhd-then-makes-a- disturb- ing-deathbed-confession/.

191. Grolle, Johann, and Samiha Shafy. "SPIEGEL Interview with Jerome Kagan: 'What About Tutoring Instead of Pills?' - SPIEGEL ONLINE - International." SPIEGEL ONLINE. August 02, 2012. Accessed June 15, 2019. http://www.spiegel.de/international/world/

child-psychologist-jerome-kagan-on- overprescibing-drugs-to-children-a-847500. html.

192. Gaffney, Adam. "How ADHD Was Sold." The New Republic. September 23, 2016. Accessed June 15, 2019. https://newrepublic.com/article/137066/adhd- sold.

193. Schwarz, Alan. "Royal Statistical Society Publications." Significance. December 05, 2016. Accessed June 15, 2019. https://rss.onlinelibrary.wiley.com/ doi/full/10.1111/j.1740-9713.2016.00979.x.

194. Cook, Gareth. "Big Pharma's Manufactured Epidemic: The Misdiagnosis of ADHD." Scientific American. October 11, 2016. Accessed June 15, 2019. https:// www.scientificamerican.com/article/ big-pharma-s-manufactured-epidemic-the- misdiagnosis-of-adhd/.

195. Konofal, Eric, Michel Lecendreux, Isabelle Arnulf, and Marie-Christine Mouren. "Iron Deficiency in Children with Attention-deficit/hyperactivity Disorder." Archives of Pediatrics & Adolescent Medicine. December 2004. Accessed June 15, 2019. https://www.ncbi.nlm.nih.gov/pubmed/15583094.

196. Smith, Kyle. "ADHD Does Not Exist." New York Post. July 25, 2018. Accessed June 15, 2019. https://nypost.com/2014/01/04/adhd-does-not-exist/.

197. Rasmussen, Nicolas. "America's First Amphetamine Epidemic 1929-1971: A Quantitative and Qualitative Retrospective with Implications for the Present." American Journal of Public Health. June 2008. Accessed June 15, 2019. https:// www.ncbi.nlm.nih.gov/pmc/articles/PMC2377281/.

198. Littman, Ellen, PhD. "Never Enough? Why Your Brain Craves Stimulation." ADDitude. January 18, 2019. Accessed June 15, 2019. https://www. additudemag. com/brain-stimulation-and-adhd-cravings-addiction-and-regulation/.

199. Smith, Kyle. "ADHD Does Not Exist." New York Post. July 25, 2018. Accessed June 15, 2019. https://nypost.com/2014/01/04/adhd-does-not-exist/.

200. Chen, Mu-Hong, Wen-Hsuan Lan, Ya-Mei Bai, Kai-Lin Huang, Tung-Ping Su, Shih-Jen Tsai, Cheng-Ta Li, Wei-Chen Lin, Wen-Han Chang, Tai-Long Pan, Tzeng-Ji Chen, and Ju-Wei Hsu. "Influence of Relative Age on Diagnosis and Treatment of Attention-Deficit Hyperactivity Disorder in Taiwanese Children." The Journal of Pediatrics 172 (May 2016): 162-67. Accessed June 16, 2019. doi:10.1016/j. jpeds.2016.02.012.

201. Elder, Todd E. "The Importance of Relative Standards in ADHD Diagnoses: Evidence Based on Exact Birth Dates." Journal of Health Economics. September 2010. Accessed June 15, 2019. https://www.ncbi.nlm.nih.gov/pubmed/20638739.

202. Mahone, E. Mark, and Martha B. Denckla. "Attention-Deficit/Hyperactivity Disorder: A Historical Neuropsychological Perspective." Journal of the International Neuropsychological Society : JINS. October 2017. Accessed June 18, 2019. https://www.ncbi.nlm.nih.gov/pmc/articles/PMC5724393/.

203. Sax, Leonard. "Fewer Prescriptions for A.D.H.D., Less Drug Abuse?" The New York Times. June 9, 2012. Accessed June 15, 2019. https://www.nytimes.com/ roomfordebate/2012/06/09/fewer-prescriptions-for-adhd-less-drug-abuse/adhd- drugs-have-long-term-risks.

204. Robinson, Terry E., and Bryan Kolb. "Structural Plasticity Associated with Exposure to Drugs of Abuse." Neuropharmacology. 2004. Accessed June 15, 2019. https://www.ncbi.nlm.nih.gov/pubmed/15464124.

205. Sax, Leonard, MD PhD. "Evidence That Stimulant Medications May Damage the Developing Brain, Especially the Nucleus Accumbens."

206. Li, Yong, and Julie A. Kauer. "Repeated Exposure to Amphetamine Disrupts Dopaminergic Modulation of Excitatory Synaptic Plasticity and Neurotransmission in Nucleus Accumbens." Synapse (New York, N.Y.). January 2004. Accessed June 15, 2019. https://www.ncbi.nlm.nih.gov/pubmed/14579420.

207. White et al., 1995; Pierce and Kalivas, 1997; Wolf, 1998).

208. Vanderschuren, Louk J. M. J., E. Donné Schmidt, Caroline A. P. Van Moorsel, Fred J.H. Tilders, Anton N. M. Schoffelmeer, and Taco J. De Vries.

"A Single Exposure to Amphetamine Is Sufficient to Induce Long-Term Behavioral, Neuroendocrine, and Neurochemical Sensitization in Rats." Journal of Neuroscience. November 01, 1999. Accessed June 16, 2019. http://www.jneurosci.org/content/19/21/9579.

209. Robinson, Terry E., and Bryan Kolb. "Structural Plasticity Associated with Exposure to Drugs of Abuse." Neuropharmacology. 2004. Accessed June 18, 2019. https://www.ncbi.nlm.nih.gov/pubmed/15464124.

210. Sax, Leonard, MD PhD. "Evidence That Stimulant Medications May Damage the Developing Brain, Especially the Nucleus Accumbens."

211. Sax, Leonard, MD PhD. "Evidence That Stimulant Medications May Damage the Developing Brain, Especially the Nucleus Accumbens."

212. Higgins, Edmund S. "Do ADHD Drugs Take a Toll on the Brain?" Scientific American. July 2009. Accessed June 16, 2019. https://www.scientificamerican. com/article/do-adhd-drugs-take-a-toll/.

213. Simons, Peter. "Large Increase in Poison Control Calls for Children Taking ADHD Drugs." Mad In America. April 30, 2019. Accessed June 16, 2019. https:// www.madinamerica.com/2018/08/ large-increase-poison-control-calls-children- taking-adhd-drugs/.

214. Nevison, Cynthia D. "A Comparison of Temporal Trends in United States Autism Prevalence to Trends in Suspected Environmental Factors." Environmental Health. September 05, 2014. Accessed June 16, 2019. https://ehjournal. biomed-central.com/articles/10.1186/1476-069X-13-73.

215. Blaxill, Mark F. "What's Going On? The Question of Time Trends in Autism." Public Health Reports (Washington, D.C. : 1974). November/December 2004. Accessed June 16, 2019. https://www.ncbi.nlm.nih.gov/pmc/articles/ PMC1497666/.

216. Cone, Marla. "New Study: Autism Linked to Environment." Scientific American. January 09, 2009. Accessed June 16, 2019. https://www. scientificamer-ican.com/article/autism-rise-driven-by-environment/.

217. Li, Huamei, Hui Li, Yun Li, Yujie Liu, and Zhengyan Zhao. "Blood Mercury, Arsenic, Cadmium, and Lead in Children with Autism Spectrum Disorder." Biological Trace Element Research. January 2018. Accessed June 18, 2019. https:// www.ncbi.nlm.nih.gov/pubmed/28480499.

218. Jafari, Tina, Noushin Rostampour, Aziz A. Fallah, and Afshin Hesami. "The Association between Mercury Levels and Autism Spectrum Disorders: A Systematic Review and Meta-analysis." Journal of Trace Elements in Medicine and Biology : Organ of the Society for Minerals and Trace Elements (GMS). December 2017. Accessed June 16, 2019. https://www.ncbi.nlm.nih.gov/pubmed/28965590.

219. Mold, Matthew, Dorcas Umar, Andrew King, and Christopher Exley. "Aluminium in Brain Tissue in Autism." Journal of Trace Elements in Medicine and Biology 46 (March 2018): 76-82. Accessed June 16, 2019. doi:10.1016/j. jtemb.2017.11.012.

220. Theresa, A. Deisher, V. Doan Ngoc, Omaiye Angelica, Koyama Kumiko, and Bwabye Sarah. "Impact of Environmental Factors on the Prevalence of Autistic Disorder after 1979." Journal of Public Health and Epidemiology 6, no. 9 (September 01, 2014): 271-86. Accessed June 16, 2019. doi:10.5897/ jphe2014.0649.

221. Bilbo, Staci, and Beth Stevens. "Microglia: The Brain's First Responders." Cerebrum : The Dana Forum on Brain Science. November 01, 2017. Accessed June 16, 2019. https://www.ncbi.nlm.nih.gov/pmc/articles/PMC6132046/#b12- cer-14-17.

222. Hughes, Virginia. "Brain Imaging Study Points to Microglia as Autism Biomarker | Spectrum | Autism Research News." Spectrum. January 10, 2013. Accessed June 16, 2019. https://www.spectrumnews.org/news/ brain-imaging- study-points-to-microglia-as-autism-biomarker/.

223. Wright, Jessica. "Molecular Mechanisms: Microglia Abnormal in Autism Brains | Spectrum | Autism Research News." Spectrum. June 05, 2012. Accessed June 16, 2019. https://www.spectrumnews.org/news/ molecular-mechanisms- microglia-abnormal-in-autism-brains/.

224. Naltrekson, Düşük Doz. "Microglia and Autism." Mapping Ignorance. January 08, 2018. Accessed June 16, 2019. https://mappingignorance. org/2018/01/08/ microglia-and-autism/.

225. Bilbo, Staci, and Beth Stevens. "Microglia: The Brain's First Responders." Cerebrum : The Dana Forum on Brain Science. November 01, 2017. Accessed June 16, 2019. https://www.ncbi.nlm.nih.gov/pmc/articles/PMC6132046/#b12- cer-14-17.

226. Suzuki, Katsuaki, Genichi Sugihara, Yasuomi Ouchi, Kazuhiko Nakamura, Masami Futatsubashi, Kiyokazu Takebayashi, Yujiro Yoshihara, Kei Omata, Kaori Matsumoto, Kenji J. Tsuchiya, Yasuhide Iwata, Masatsugu Tsujii, Toshirou Sugiyama, and Norio Mori. "Microglial Activation in Young Adults with Autism Spectrum Disorder." JAMA Psychiatry. January 2013. Accessed June 16, 2019. https://www.ncbi.nlm.nih.gov/pubmed/23404112.

227. Hughes, Virginia. "Brain Imaging Study Points to Microglia as Autism Biomarker | Spectrum | Autism Research News."

228. Suzuki, Katsuaki. "Microglial Activation in Young Adults With Autism Spectrum Disorder." JAMA Psychiatry. January 01, 2013. Accessed June 16, 2019. https://jamanetwork.com/journals/jamapsychiatry/fullarticle/1393597.

229. "Brain Inflammation A Hallmark Of Autism, Large-Scale Analysis Shows - 12/10/2014." Johns Hopkins Medicine, Based in Baltimore, Maryland. December 10, 2014. Accessed June 16, 2019. https://www.hopkinsmedicine.org/news/media/ releases/ brain_inflammation_a_hallmark_of_autism_large_scale_analysis_shows.

230. Vargas, Diana L., Caterina Nascimbene, Chitra Krishnan, Andrew W. Zimmerman, and Carlos A. Pardo. "Neuroglial Activation and Neuroinflammation in the Brain of Patients with Autism." Annals of Neurology 57, no. 1 (November 15, 2004): 67-81. Accessed June 16, 2019. doi:10.1002/ana.20315.

231. Takano, Tomoyuki. "Role of Microglia in Autism: Recent Advances." Developmental Neuroscience. May 21, 2015. Accessed June 16, 2019. https://www. ncbi.nlm.nih.gov/pubmed/25998072.

232. Saghazadeh, Amene, and Nima Rezaei. "Systematic Review and Meta- analysis Links Autism and Toxic Metals and Highlights the Impact of Country Development Status: Higher Blood and Erythrocyte Levels for Mercury and Lead, and Higher Hair Antimony, Cadmium, Lead, and Mercury." Progress in Neuro- psychophar-macology & Biological Psychiatry. October 03, 2017. Accessed June 16, 2019. https:// www.ncbi.nlm.nih.gov/pubmed/28716727.

233. Vargas, Diana L., Caterina Nascimbene, Chitra Krishnan, Andrew W. Zimmerman, and Carlos A. Pardo. "Neuroglial Activation and Neuroinflammation in the Brain of Patients with Autism."

234. Chakrabarti, Bhismadev, Antonio Persico, Natalia Battista, and Mauro Maccarrone. "Endocannabinoid Signaling in Autism." SpringerLink. July 28, 2015. Accessed June 16, 2019. https://link.springer.com/article/10.1007/ s13311-015- 0371-9.

235. Li, Qinrui, Ying Han, Angel Belle C Dy, and Randi J. Hagerman. "The Gut Microbiota and Autism Spectrum Disorders." Frontiers in Cellular Neuroscience. April 28, 2017. Accessed June 16, 2019. https://www.ncbi.nlm.nih.gov/pmc/ articles/ PMC5408485/.

236. V, Rai. "The MTHFR C677T Polymorphism and Hyperuricemia Risk: A Meta-analysis of 558 Cases and 912 Controls."

237. Smallwood, Melissa, Ashley Sareen, Emma Baker, Rachel Hannusch, Eddy Kwessi, and Tyisha Williams. "Increased Risk of Autism Development in Children Whose Mothers Experienced Birth Complications or Received Labor and Delivery

Drugs." ASN Neuro. August 09, 2016. Accessed June 16, 2019. https://www.ncbi. nlm.nih.gov/pmc/articles/PMC4984315/.

238. Hubbard, Sylvia Booth. "Dr. Russell Blaylock Warns: Don't Get the Flu Shot - It Promotes Alzheimer's." Newsmax. December 18, 2011. Accessed June 16, 2019. https:// www.newsmax.com/health/headline/flu-shot-promotes- alzheimer-s/2011/12/18/ id/477912/.

239. Broxmeyer, Lawrence. "Are the Infectious Roots of Alzheimers Buried Deep in the Past?" Journal of MPE Molecular Pathological Epidemiology. February 27, 2017. Accessed June 18, 2019. http://molecular-pathological-epidemiology. imedpub.com/ are-the-infectious-roots-of-alzheimersburied-deep-in-the-past. php?aid=18399.

240. Lionetti, Elena, Salvatore Leonardi, Chiara Franzonello, Margherita Mancardi, Martino Ruggieri, and Carlo Catassi. "Gluten Psychosis: Confirmation of a New Clinical Entity." Nutrients. July 08, 2015. Accessed June 16, 2019. https://www. ncbi.nlm.nih.gov/pmc/articles/PMC4517012/.

241. Uhde, Melanie, Mary Ajamian, Giacomo Caio, Roberto De Giorgio, Alyssa Indart, Peter H. Green, Elizabeth C. Verna, Umberto Volta, and Armin Alaedini. "Intestinal Cell Damage and Systemic Immune Activation in Individuals Reporting Sensitivity to Wheat in the Absence of Coeliac Disease." Gut. December 01, 2016. Accessed June 16, 2019. https://gut.bmj.com/content/65/12/1930.full.

242. Hadjivassilou, Marios, MD. "Gluten-Related Disorders: Time to Move from Gut to Brain." The Gluten Summit. Accessed June 16, 2019. http:// theglutensummit. com/team/marios-hadjivassiliou/.

243. Hamblin, James. "This Is Your Brain on Gluten." The Atlantic. August 21, 2018. Accessed June 16, 2019. https://www.theatlantic.com/health/archive/2013/12/ this-is-your-brain-on-gluten/282550/.

244. Meredith, Steven E., Laura M. Juliano, John R. Hughes, and Roland R. Griffiths. "Caffeine Use Disorder: A Comprehensive Review and Research Agenda." Mary Ann Liebert, Inc., Publishers. September 13, 2013. Accessed June 16, 2019. https:// www.liebertpub.com/doi/full/10.1089/jcr.2013.0016.

245. Meredith, Steven E., Laura M. Juliano, John R. Hughes, and Roland R. Griffiths. "Caffeine Use Disorder: A Comprehensive Review and Research Agenda." Journal of Caffeine Research. September 2013. Accessed June 16, 2019. https://www.ncbi. nlm.nih.gov/pmc/articles/PMC3777290/.

246. Addicott, Merideth A., Lucie L. Yang, Ann M. Peiffer, Luke R. Burnett, Jonathan H. Burdette, Michael Y. Chen, Satoru Hayasaka, Robert A. Kraft, Joseph A. Maldjian, and Paul J. Laurienti. "The Effect of Daily Caffeine Use on Cerebral Blood Flow: How Much Caffeine Can We Tolerate?" Human Brain Mapping. October 2009. Accessed June 16, 2019. https://www.ncbi.nlm.nih.gov/pmc/articles/PMC2748160/.

247. "Caffeine Use Disorder: A Comprehensive Review and Research Agenda." Mary Ann Liebert, Inc., Publishers. Accessed June 18, 2019. https://www.liebertpub.com/doi/full/10.1089/jcr.2013.0016.

248. Studeville, George. "Caffeine Addiction Is a Mental Disorder, Doctors Say." Caffeine Addiction Is a Mental Disorder, Doctors Say. January 19, 2005. Accessed June 16, 2019. https://web.archive.org/web/20050209011402/

249. Cappelletti, Simone, Daria Piacentino, Gabriele Sani, and Mariarosaria Aromatario. "Caffeine: Cognitive and Physical Performance Enhancer or Psychoactive Drug?" Current Neuropharmacology. January 2015. Accessed June 16, 2019. https://www.ncbi.nlm.nih.gov/pmc/articles/PMC4462044/.

250. Meredith, Steven E., Laura M. Juliano, John R. Hughes, and Roland R. Griffiths. "Caffeine Use Disorder: A Comprehensive Review and Research Agenda." Journal of Caffeine Research. September 2013. Accessed June 18, 2019. https://www.ncbi.nlm.nih.gov/pmc/articles/PMC3777290/.

251. Nobre, Anna C., Anling Rao, and Gail N. Owen. "L-theanine, a Natural Constituent in Tea, and Its Effect on Mental State." Asia Pacific Journal of Clinical Nutrition. 2008. Accessed June 16, 2019. https://www.ncbi.nlm.nih.gov/pubmed/18296328.

252. Nathan, Pradeep J., Kristy Lu, M. Gray, and C. Oliver. "The Neuropharmacology of L-theanine(N-ethyl-L-glutamine): A Possible Neuroprotective and Cognitive Enhancing Agent." Journal of Herbal Pharmacotherapy. 2006. Accessed June 16, 2019. https://www.ncbi.nlm.nih.gov/ pubmed/17182482.

253. Haskell, Crystal F., David O. Kennedy, Anthea L. Milne, Keith A. Wesnes, and Andrew B. Scholey. "The Effects of L-theanine, Caffeine and Their Combination on Cognition and Mood." Biological Psychology. February 2008. Accessed June 16, 2019. https://www.ncbi.nlm.nih.gov/pubmed/18006208.

254. Kelly, Simon P., Manuel Gomez-Ramirez, Jennifer L. Montesi, and John J. Foxe. "L-theanine and Caffeine in Combination Affect Human Cognition as

Evidenced by Oscillatory Alpha-band Activity and Attention Task Performance." The Journal of Nutrition. August 2008. Accessed June 16, 2019. https://www.ncbi. nlm.nih.gov/pubmed/18641209.

255. "Harvard T.H. Chan School of Public Health." Philippe Grandjean. Accessed June 16, 2019. https://www.hsph.harvard.edu/philippe-grandjean/.

256. "Philip J Landrigan, MD Biography." Mount Sinai Health System. Accessed June 16, 2019. https://www.mountsinai.org/profiles/philip-j-landrigan.

257. Terry, Susan. "A 'silent Pandemic' of Toxic Chemicals Is Damaging Our Children's Brains, Experts Claim." MinnPost. February 17, 2014. Accessed June 16, 2019. https://www.minnpost.com/second-opinion/2014/02/silent-pandemic-toxic-chemicals-damaging-our-children-s-brains-experts-claim/.

258. Walton, Alice G. "11 Toxic Chemicals Affecting Brain Development In Children." Forbes. February 15, 2014. Accessed June 16, 2019. https://www. forbes. com/sites/alicegwalton/2014/02/15/11-toxic-chemicals-afffecting-brain- development-in-children/#2a090d4742a8.

259. Hamblin, James. "The Toxins That Threaten Our Brains." The Atlantic. March 18, 2014. Accessed June 16, 2019. https://www.theatlantic.com/health/ archive/2014/03/the-toxins-that-threaten-our-brains/284466/

260. Kessler, Robert. "Outbreak: Pandemic Strikes." EcoHealth Alliance. June 13, 2018. Accessed June 16, 2019. https://www.ecohealthalliance.org/2018/05/ outbreak-pandemic-strikes?gclid=EAIaIQobChMIpbDG-fS_3gIVD-JyzCh3r6AHB EAAYASAAEgKgx_D_BwE.

261. Gale, Richard, and Gary Null, PhD. "GARY NULL: FLU VACCINES... ARE THEY EFFECTIVE AND SAFE? - Progressive Radio Network." The #1 Radio Station for Progressive Minds! September 29, 2009. Accessed June 16, 2019. http:// prn.fm/gary-null-flu-vaccines-effective-safe/.

262. Gale, Richard, and Gary Null, PhD. "GARY NULL: FLU VACCINES... ARE THEY EFFECTIVE AND SAFE? - Progressive Radio Network." The #1 Radio Station for Progressive Minds! September 29, 2009. Accessed June 16, 2019. http:// prn.fm/gary-null-flu-vaccines-effective-safe/.

263. Deisher, Theresa A., Ngoc V. Doan, Kumiko Koyama, and Sarah Bwabye. "Epidemiologic and Molecular Relationship Between Vaccine Manufacture and

Autism Spectrum Disorder Prevalence." Issues in Law & Medicine. Spring 2015. Accessed June 16, 2019. https://www.ncbi.nlm.nih.gov/pubmed/26103708.

264. ProCon.org. "Vaccine Ingredients and Manufacturer Information." ProConorg Headlines. September 19, 2016. Accessed June 16, 2019. https:// vaccines.procon. org/view.resource.php?resourceID=005206#rotavirus.

265. "Vaccines Contain Human Protein & DNA." Digital image. MPVR. Accessed June 16, 2019. https://bethevoice.typepad.com/vax_info_resources/cdc vaccine ingredients .pdf.

266. Deisher, Theresa, Dr. "Open Letter from Dr. Theresa Deisher to Legislators Regarding Fetal Cell DNA in Vaccines." Sound Choice. May 08, 2019. Accessed June 16, 2019. https://www.soundchoice.org/open-letter-to-legislators/.

267. Miller, Neil Z., and Gary S. Goldman. "Infant Mortality Rates Regressed against Number of Vaccine Doses Routinely Given: Is There a Biochemical or Synergistic Toxicity?" Human & Experimental Toxicology. September

2011. Accessed June 16, 2019. https://www.ncbi.nlm.nih.gov/pmc/articles/ PMC3170075/.

268. Goldman, G. S., and N. Z. Miller. "Relative Trends in Hospitalizations and Mortality among Infants by the Number of Vaccine Doses and Age, Based on the Vaccine Adverse Event Reporting System (VAERS), 1990-2010." Human & Experimental Toxicology. October 2012. Accessed June 16, 2019. https://www. ncbi.nlm.nih.gov/pubmed/22531966.

269. Miller, Neil. "Neil Miller: Why People Choose Not to Vaccinate." AGE OF AUTISM. February 21, 2017. Accessed June 16, 2019. https://www.ageofautism. com/2015/02/neil-miller-why-people-choose-not-to-vaccinate.html.

270. Exley, Chris, Leanne Reynolds, Nisith Sheth, Jerome Burne, Rachel Power, Hippocratic Post, and Hippocratic Post. "Aluminium Adjuvants and Vaccine Safety." The Hippocratic Post. December 02, 2016. Accessed June 16, 2019. https://www. hippocraticpost.com/pharmacy-drugs/aluminium-adjuvants-vaccine- safety/.

271. Caceres, Marco. "Here's Where Aluminum Goes When It's Injected Into Your Body From..." The Vaccine Reaction. October 19, 2017. Accessed June 16, 2019. https://thevaccinereaction.org/2016/05/heres-where-aluminum-goes-when-its-injected-into-your-body-from-a-vaccine/.

272. "High Aluminum Found in Autism Brain Tissue: New Study Indicates That Widespread Exposure to Aluminum Is Setting the Stage for Catastrophic Neurological Damage." Children's Health Defense. December 07, 2018. Accessed June 16, 2019. https://childrenshealthdefense.org/news/high-aluminum-found- autism-brain-tissue

273. Mold, Matthew, Dorcas Umar, Andrew King, and Christopher Exley. "Aluminium in Brain Tissue in Autism." Journal of Trace Elements in Medicine and Biology: Organ of the Society for Minerals and Trace Elements (GMS). March 2018. Accessed June 18, 2019. https://www.ncbi.nlm.nih.gov/pubmed/29413113.

274. Mold, Matthew, Dorcas Umar, Andrew King, and Christopher Exley. "Aluminium in Brain Tissue in Autism." Journal of Trace Elements in Medicine and Biology: Organ of the Society for Minerals and Trace Elements (GMS). March 2018. Accessed June 18, 2019. https://www.ncbi.nlm.nih.gov/pubmed/29413113.

275. Fisher, S. G., L. Weber, and M. Carbone. "Cancer Risk Associated with Simian Virus 40 Contaminated Polio Vaccine." Anticancer Research. May/June 1999. Accessed June 16, 2019. https://www.ncbi.nlm.nih.gov/pubmed/10472327.

276. "Oral Polio Vaccine May Be Causing Serious Problems." Mercola.com. May 8, 2012. Accessed June 16, 2019. https://articles.mercola.com/sites/articles/archive/2012/05/08/polio-vaccine-ineffective.aspx.

277. Bookchin, Debbie, and Jim Schumacher. "The Virus and the Vaccine." The Atlantic. October 03, 2014. Accessed June 16, 2019. https://www.theatlantic.com/magazine/archive/2000/02/the-virus-and-the-vaccine/377999/.

278. Curtis, Tom. "Monkeys, Viruses, and Vaccines." The Lancet 364, no. 9432 (July 31, 2004): 407-08. Accessed June 16, 2019. doi:10.1016/s0140- 6736(04)16746-9.

279. Qi, Fang, Michele Carbone, Haining Yang, and Giovanni Gaudino. "Simian Virus 40 Transformation, Malignant Mesothelioma and Brain Tumors." Expert Review of Respiratory Medicine. October 2011. Accessed June 16, 2019. https://www.ncbi.nlm.nih.gov/pmc/articles/PMC3241931/.

280. Debbie Bookchin, Jim Schumacher. "The Virus and the Vaccine." The Atlantic. October 03, 2014. Accessed June 18, 2019. https://www.theatlantic.com/ magazine/archive/2000/02/the-virus-and-the-vaccine/377999/.

281. Sender, Ron, Shai Fuchs, and Ron Milo. "Revised Estimates for the Number of Human and Bacteria Cells in the Body." PLOS Biology. August 19, 2016. Accessed

June 16, 2019. https://journals.plos.org/plosbiology/article?id=10.1371/ journal. pbio.1002533.

282. Sutter, R. W., P. A. Patriarca, A. J. Suleiman, S. Brogan, P. G. Malankar, S. L. Cochi, A. A. Al-Ghassani, and M. S. El-Bualy. "Attributable Risk of DTP (diphtheria and Tetanus Toxoids and Pertussis Vaccine) Injection in Provoking Paralytic Poliomyelitis during a Large Outbreak in Oman." The Journal of Infectious Diseases. March 1992. Accessed June 16, 2019. https://www.ncbi.nlm. nih.gov/ pubmed/1538150.

283. Gromeier, M., and E. Wimmer. "Mechanism of Injury-provoked Poliomyelitis." Journal of Virology. June 1998. Accessed June 16, 2019. https:// www.ncbi.nlm. nih.gov/pmc/articles/PMC110068/.

284. Strebel, P. M., N. Ion-Nedelcu, A. L. Baughman, R. W. Sutter, and S. L. Cochi. "Intramuscular Injections within 30 Days of Immunization with Oral Poliovirus Vaccine--a Risk Factor for Vaccine-associated Paralytic Poliomyelitis." The New England Journal of Medicine. February 23, 1995. Accessed June 16, 2019. https:// www.ncbi.nlm.nih.gov/pubmed/7830731.

285. "Paralytic Illness of Franklin D. Roosevelt." Wikipedia. April 18, 2019. Accessed June 16, 2019. https://en.wikipedia.org/wiki/Paralytic_illness_of_ Franklin_D._Roosevelt.

286. "Cutter Laboratories." Wikipedia. March 19, 2019. Accessed June 16, 2019. https://en.wikipedia.org/wiki/Cutter_Laboratories.

287. Fitzpatrick, Michael. "The Cutter Incident: How America's First Polio Vaccine Led to a Growing Vaccine Crisis." Journal of the Royal Society of Medicine. March 2006. Accessed June 16, 2019. https://www.ncbi.nlm.nih.gov/ pmc/articles/ PMC1383764/.

288. Olmstead, Dan, and Mark Blaxill. "The Age of Polio: How an Old Virus and New Toxins Created a Man-made Epidemic -- Part 4, Post-War Epidemics and the Triumph of Vaccination." AGE OF AUTISM. September 22, 2011. Accessed June 16, 2019. https://www.ageofautism.com/2011/09/the-age-of-polio-how-an-old-virus-and-new-toxins-created-a-man-made-epidemic-.html.

289. Di Iorio, Marco C. "DDT and the Rise and Fall of Polio." IDSENT. August 12, 2015. Accessed June 16, 2019. https://idsent.wordpress.com/2015/07/23/ ddt- and-the-rise-and-fall-of-polio/.

290. Alleman, Mary M., PhD, Rohit Chitale, PhD, Cara C. Burns, PhD, Jane Ilber, MSc, Naomi Dybdahl-Sissoko, Qi Chen, MSc, Djo-Roy Van Koko, MD, Raimi Ewetola, MD, Yogolelo Riziki, Hugo Kavunga-Membo, MD, Cheikh Dah, MD, and Rija Andriamihantanirina, MD. "Vaccine-Derived Poliovirus Outbreaks and Events - Three Provinces, Democratic Republic of the Congo, 2017 | MMWR." Centers for Disease Control and Prevention. March 16, 2018. Accessed June 16, 2019. https://www.cdc.gov/mmwr/volumes/67/wr/mm6710a4.htm.

291. Kyral, Shane, PhD. "Polio Outbreak Warnings Issued for 5 Countries." Polio Outbreak Warnings Issued for 5 Countries - Precision Vaccinations. September 3, 2018. Accessed June 16, 2019. https://www.precisionvaccinations. com/cdc-level-2-travel-alerts-issued-five-countries-due-circulating-vaccine- derived-poliovirus-cvdpv.

292. "Oral Polio Vaccine May Be Causing Serious Problems." Mercola. com. Accessed June 18, 2019. https://articles.mercola.com/sites/articles/ archive/2012/05/08/polio-vaccine-ineffective.aspx.

293. "Oral Polio Vaccine May Be Causing Serious Problems." Mercola. com. Accessed June 18, 2019. https://articles.mercola.com/sites/articles/ archive/2012/05/08/polio-vaccine-ineffective.aspx.

294. Cheng, Maria. "Officials Say Drug Caused Nigeria Polio." The Washington Post. October 5, 2007. Accessed June 16, 2019. http://www.washingtonpost.com/wp-dyn/content/article/2007/10/05/AR2007100501193_pf.html.

295. Goldman, Armond S., Elisabeth J. Schmalstieg, Daniel H. Freeman, Daniel A. Goldman, and Frank C. Schmalstieg. "What Was the Cause of Franklin Delano Roosevelt's Paralytic Illness?" Journal of Medical Biography. November 2003. Accessed June 16, 2019. https://www.ncbi.nlm.nih.gov/pubmed/14562158.

296. Malik, Tara. "Exploration of Franklin D. Roosevelt's Paralytic Illness." Lecture, GEORGIA STATE UNDERGRADUATE RESEARCH CONFERENCE, Lucerne, Student Center East B, Atlanta, GA. Accessed June 16, 2019. https:// scholarworks.gsu.edu/cgi/viewcontent.cgi?referer=https://www.google.com/&https redir=1&article=1498&context=gsurc.

297. Canal2ndOpinion. YouTube. October 21, 2014. Accessed June 16, 2019. https:// www.youtube.com/watch?v=SFQQOv-Oi6U.

298. Hooker, Brian, PhD. "Reanalysis of CDC Data on Autism Incidence ... - Jpands.org." Reanalysis of CDC Data on Autism Incidence and Time of First

MMR Vaccination. June 22, 2018. Accessed June 22, 2019. https://www.jpands. org/ vol23no4/hooker.pdf.

299. Hooker, Brian S., Ph.D., P.E. ". "Retraction Note: Measles-mumps- rubella Vaccination Timing and Autism among Young African American Boys: A Reanalysis of CDC Data on Autism Incidence and Time of First MMR Vaccination." Journal of American Physicians and Surgeons 23." Translational Neurodegeneration 3, no. 4 (Winter 2018): 105-09. Accessed June 16, 2019. https1 (2014). doi:10.1186/2047-9158-3-22..

300. Shara V, Vera. "Former Merck Scientists Sue Merck Alleging MMR Vaccine Efficacy Fraud." AHRP. March 5, 2016. Accessed June 16, 2019. http:// ahrp.org/ former-merck-scientists-sue-merck-alleging-mmr-vaccine-efficacy-fraud/.

301. Peter Patriarca - Asleep at the Switch Email." Digital image. Children's Health Defense. Accessed June 16, 2019. and Beth Brockner Ryan to Lawrence Bachorik. July 2, 1999. https://childrenshealthdefense.org/wp-content/uploads/foia- peter-patriarca-asleep-at-the-switch-email.pdf.

302. Leslie Ball, FDA - No Safe Level of Mercury." Digital image. World Mercury Project. Accessed June 16, 2019. https://worldmercuryproject.org/wp- content/ uploads/foia-leslie-ball-fda-no-safe-level-of-mercury.pdf.

303. Liberty Aggregator. "Dr. Andrew Zimmerman's Full Affidavit on Alleged Link between Vaccines and Autism That U.S. Govt. Covered up." NAMELY LIBERTY. January 09, 2019. Accessed June 16, 2019. https://namelyliberty.com/ dr-andrew-zimmermans-full-affidavit-on-alleged-link-between-vaccines-and-autism-that-u-s-govt-covered-up/.

304. Liberty Aggregator. "Dr. Andrew Zimmerman's Full Affidavit on Alleged Link between Vaccines and Autism That U.S. Govt. Covered up." NAMELY LIBERTY. January 09, 2019. Accessed June 16, 2019. https://namelyliberty.com/ dr-andrew-zimmermans-full-affidavit-on-alleged-link-between-vaccines-and-autism-that-u-s-govt-covered-up/.

305. Attkisson, Sharyl. "Dr. Andrew Zimmerman's Full Affidavit on Alleged Link between Vaccines and Autism That U.S. Govt. Covered up." Sharyl Attkisson. January 06, 2019. Accessed June 16, 2019. https://sharylattkisson.com/2019/01/06/ dr-andrew-zimmermans-full-affidavit-on-alleged-link-between-vaccines-and-autism-that-u-s-govt-covered-up. //

306. Simpsonwood Retreat Center. "Scientific Review of Vaccine Safety Datalink Information."Digital image. Review of Vaccine Safety Datalink Information. June 8, 2000. Accessed June 16, 2019. http://fearlessparent.org/wp- content/ uploads/2016/04/Simpsonwood_Transcript_Scan_by_RJK_OCR.pdf

307. Orestein, W. A., P. N. Heseltine, S. J. LaGagnoux, and B. Portnoy. "Rubella Vaccine and Susceptible Hospital Employees. Poor Physician Participation." National Center for Biotechnology Information. February 20, 1981. Accessed June 16, 2019. https://www.ncbi.nlm.nih.gov/pubmed/?term=JAMA vaccinations California obstetrician-gynecologists.

308. Stroller, Kenneth. "CDC - Influenza Deaths: Request for Correction (RFC)." ASPE. November 23, 2015. Accessed June 16, 2019. https://aspe.hhs.gov/ cdc-influenza-deaths-request-correction-rfc.

309. Hooker, Brian, Janet Kern, David Geier, Boyd Haley, Lisa Sykes, Paul King, and Mark Geier. "Methodological Issues and Evidence of Malfeasance in Research Purporting to Show Thimerosal in Vaccines Is Safe." BioMed Research International. 2014. Accessed June 18, 2019. https://www.ncbi.nlm.nih.gov/pmc/ articles/PMC4065774/.

310. "The Growing Crisis of Chronic Disease in the United States." Accessed June 16, 2019. http://www.fightchronicdisease.org/sites/default/files/docs/ GrowingCrisisofChronicDiseaseintheUSfactsheet_81009.pdf.

311. Hinkes, Mark. "Amputation Prevention in Diabetic Patients." Amputation Prevention in Diabetic Patients | American Diabetes Association. January 2008. Accessed June 16, 2019. https://professional.diabetes.org/abstract/ amputation- prevention-diabetic-patients.

312. Caffrey, Mary. "Diabetic Amputations May Be Rising in the United States." AJMC. December 13, 2018. Accessed June 16, 2019. https://www.ajmc.com/ newsroom/diabetic-amputations-may-be-rising-in-the-united-states.

313. "One Lower Limb Lost to Diabetes Every 30 Seconds, UN Agency Says | UN News." United Nations. November 14, 2005. Accessed June 16, 2019. https:// news. un.org/en/story/2005/11/159922-one-lower-limb-lost-diabetes-every-30- seconds- un-agency-says.

314. Parpia, Rishma. "Why Are Americans So Sick?" The Vaccine Reaction. June 6, 2017. Accessed June 16, 2019. https://thevaccinereaction.org/2017/07/ why- are-americans-so-sick/.

315. egley, Sharon. "Records Found in Dusty Basement Undermine Decades of Dietary Advice." Scientific American. April 19, 2017. Accessed June 16, 2019. https://www.scientificamerican.com/article/records-found-in-dusty-basement- undermine-decades-of-dietary-advice/.

316. Ramsden, Christopher E., Daisy Zamora, Boonseng Leelarthaepin, Sharon F. Majchrzak-Hong, Keturah R. Faurot, Chirayath M. Suchindran, Amit Ringel, John M. Davis, and Joseph R. Hibbeln. "Use of Dietary Linoleic Acid for Secondary Prevention of Coronary Heart Disease and Death: Evaluation of Recovered Data from the Sydney Diet Heart Study and Updated Meta-analysis." The BMJ. February 05, 2013. Accessed June 16, 2019. https://www.bmj.com/ content/346/bmj.e8707.

317. O'Connor, Anahad. "A Decades-Old Study, Rediscovered, Challenges Advice on Saturated Fat." The New York Times. April 13, 2016. Accessed June 16, 2019. https://well.blogs.nytimes.com/2016/04/13/a-decades-old-study- rediscovered-challenges-advice-on-saturated-fat/.

318. "Seven Countries Study." Wikipedia. May 22, 2019. Accessed June 16, 2019. https://en.wikipedia.org/wiki/Seven_Countries_Study#Criticism.

319. Financial Post. "Cholesterol: How a Now Discredited Diet Theory Became a National Mania." Financial Post. January 08, 2016. Accessed June 16, 2019. https://business.financialpost.com/opinion/book-excerpt-lipophobia-and-the-bad- science-diet.

320. Hartley, Roman. "Are You Suffering from Fructose Poisoning?" LifeExtension.com. October 2013. Accessed June 16, 2019. https://www. lifeextension.com/magazine/2013/10/Are-You-Suffering-from-Fructose-Poisoning/ Page-02.

321. La Berge, Ann E. "How The Ideology of Low Fat Conquered America- Journal of the History of Medicine and Allied Sciences." Yumpu.com. April 12, 2014. Accessed June 16, 2019. https://www.yumpu.com/en/document/ view/24390695/how-the-ideology-of-low-fat-conquered-america-journal-of-the-/6.

322. Lowette, Katrien, Lina Roosen, Jan Tack, and Pieter Vanden Berghe. "Effects of High-fructose Diets on Central Appetite Signaling and Cognitive Function." Frontiers in Nutrition. March 04, 2015. Accessed June 16, 2019. https:// www.ncbi.nlm.nih.gov/pmc/articles/PMC4429636/.

323. Thorpe, Matthew, MD, PhD. "Healthy Fats vs. Unhealthy Fats: What You Need to Know." Healthline. April 27, 2018. Accessed June 17, 2019. https://www.healthline.com/nutrition/healthy-vs-unhealthy-fats#the-bottom-line.

324. Lowette, Katrien, Lina Roosen, Jan Tack, and Pieter Vanden Berghe. "Effects of High-fructose Diets on Central Appetite Signaling and Cognitive Function." Frontiers in Nutrition. March 04, 2015. Accessed June 16, 2019. https:// www.ncbi. nlm.nih.gov/pmc/articles/PMC4429636/.

325. "LDL-P." Docs Opinion. Accessed June 16, 2019. https://www.docsopinion. com/health-and-nutrition/lipids/ldl-p/

326. Gunnars, Kris, BSc. "Saturated Fat: Good or Bad?" Healthline. June 22, 2017. Accessed June 16, 2019. https://www.healthline.com/nutrition/ saturated-fat- good-or-bad#section4.

327. Balaster, Cavin. "TIME Magazine Has a Change of Heart on Fat." Learn How to Feed a Brain! June 23, 2014. Accessed June 16, 2019. https://feedabrain. com/ change-of-heart-on-fat/.

328. Blakeslee, Sandra, and Special to the New York Times. "SURGEON QUESTIONS CHOLESTEROL ROLE." The New York Times. April 09, 1987. Accessed June 16, 2019. https://www.nytimes.com/1987/04/09/us/surgeon- questions-cholesterol-role.html.

329. Libretexts. "4.3: How Lipids Work." Medicine LibreTexts. June 03, 2019. Accessed June 16, 2019. https://med.libretexts.org/LibreTexts/American_Public_ University/APUS:_An_Introduction_to_Nutrition_(Byerley)/Chapters/05:_ Lipids/4.3:_How_Lipids_Work.

330. Bulletproof Staff. "Learn Your Lipids: A Quick Guide to Bulletproof Fats." Bulletproof. March 20, 2019. Accessed June 16, 2019. https://blog.bulletproof.com/ omega-3-vs-omega-6-fat-supplements/.

331. Meštrović, Tomislav, MD PhD. "Oils Rich in Linoleic Acid." News. February 27, 2019. Accessed June 16, 2019. https://www.news-medical.net/health/ Oils-Rich-in-Linoleic-Acid.aspx.

332. Libretexts. "4.3: How Lipids Work." Medicine LibreTexts. June 03, 2019. Accessed June 18, 2019. https://med.libretexts.org/LibreTexts/American_Public_ University/APUS:_An_Introduction_to_Nutrition_(Byerley)/Chapters/05:_ Lipids/4.3:_How_Lipids_Work.

333. Krans, Brian. "Sugar Addiction: A Serious Medical Problem That's Hijacking Our Health." Healthline. October 24, 2016. Accessed June 16, 2019. https://www. healthline.com/health/sugar/americas-deadly-sugar-addiction#2.

334. Health and Wellness/ Nutrition. "Not So Sweet - The Average American Consumes 150-170 Pounds Of Sugar Each Year." BambooCore Fitness. November 20, 2018. Accessed June 16, 2019. https://bamboocorefitness.com/not-so-sweet-the-average-american-consumes-150-170-pounds-of-sugar-each-year/.

335. "Global Sugar Consumption, 2019/20 | Statistic." Statista. Accessed June 16, 2019. https://www.statista.com/statistics/249681/total-consumption-of-sugar- worldwide/.

336. "Saturated Fat: Good or Bad?" Healthline. Accessed June 18, 2019. https://www.healthline.com/nutrition/saturated-fat-good-or-bad#section4.

337. Fortuna, Jeffrey L. "Sweet Preference, Sugar Addiction and the Familial History of Alcohol Dependence: Shared Neural Pathways and Genes." Journal of Psychoactive Drugs. June 2010. Accessed June 16, 2019. https://www.ncbi.nlm.nih. gov/pubmed/20648910.

338. Ridgeway, Leslie. "Your Soda Has More Fructose than You Think." Futurity. February 07, 2015. Accessed June 16, 2019. https://www.futurity.org/soda-sugar-fructose/.

339. Health and Wellness/ Nutrition. "Not So Sweet - The Average American Consumes 150-170 Pounds Of Sugar Each Year." Accessed June 16, 2019 https://bamboocorefitness.com/not-so-sweet-the-average-american-consumes-150-170-pounds-of-sugar-each-year/

340. Little, Will. "The Science Behind Fat Metabolism." Accessed June 16, 2019 https://ketoschool.com/the-science-behind-fat-metabolism-60f7a3f678d0

341. "Fructose." Wikipedia. June 13, 2019. Accessed June 16, 2019. https://en.wikipedia.org/wiki/Fructose#Synthesis_of_glycogen_from_DHAP_and_glyceraldehyde_3-phosphate.

342. Little, Will. "The Science Behind Fat Metabolism." Accessed June 16, 2019 https://ketoschool.com/the-science-behind-fat-metabolism-60f7a3f678d0

343. "Manage Your Blood Sugar." Www.heart.org. August 30, 2015. Accessed June 16, 2019. http://www.heart.org/en/health-topics/diabetes/about-diabetes.

344. Mayo Clinic Staf. "Diabetes." Mayo Clinic. August 08, 2018. Accessed June 16, 2019. https://www.mayoclinic.org/diseases-conditions/diabetes/symptoms- causes/syc-20371444.

345. "U.S. Leads Developed Nations in Diabetes Prevalence." Endocrine News. December 01, 2015. Accessed June 16, 2019. https://endocrinenews.endocrine. org/u-s-leads-developed-nations-in-diabetes-prevalence/.

346. Morgan, Kate. "5 Facts about Diabetes, the Third Most Common Health Condition in America." USA Today. November 07, 2018. Accessed June 16, 2019. https://www.usatoday.com/story/sponsor-story/blue-cross-blue-shield- association/2018/11/07/5-facts-diabetes-third-most-common-health-condition- america/1896809002/.

347. "Statistics About Diabetes." American Diabetes Association. March 22, 2018. Accessed June 16, 2019. http://www.diabetes.org/diabetes-basics/statistics/.

348. Hu, Frank B. "Globalization of Diabetes: The Role of Diet, Lifestyle, and Genes." Diabetes Care. May 20, 2011. Accessed June 16, 2019. https://www.ncbi. nlm.nih.gov/pmc/articles/PMC3114340/.

349. https://www.ncbi.nlm.nih.gov/pubmed/24529521 De Felice, Fernanda G., Mychael V. Lourenco, and Sergio T. Ferreira. "How Does Brain Insulin Resistance Develop in Alzheimer's Disease?" Alzheimer's & Dementia : The Journal of the Alzheimer's Association. February 2014. Accessed June 16, 2019. https://www. ncbi.nlm.nih.gov/pubmed/24529521.

350. Kornberg, Jim, Dr. "Diabetes in the Old West." True West Magazine. August 21, 2015. Accessed June 16, 2019. https://truewestmagazine.com/ diabetes- in-the-old-west/.

351. Stanhope, Kimber L. "Sugar Consumption, Metabolic Disease and Obesity: The State of the Controversy." Critical Reviews in Clinical Laboratory Sciences. February 2016. Accessed June 16, 2019. https://www.ncbi.nlm.nih.gov/pmc/ articles/PMC4822166/.

352. Bryant, Bill. "Randonneurs USA." RUSA. Accessed June 16, 2019. https:// rusa.org/newsletter/04-02-09.html.

353. Lynch, Rene. "A Brief Timeline Shows How We're Gluttons for Diet Fads." Los Angeles Times. February 28, 2015. Accessed June 16, 2019. https://www. latimes. com/health/la-he-diet-timeline-20150228-story.html.

354. Mayo Clinic Stafff. "Mediterranean Diet: A Heart-healthy Eating Plan." Mayo Clinic. January 26, 2019. Accessed June 16, 2019. https://www.mayoclinic. org/

healthy-lifestyle/nutrition-and-healthy-eating/in-depth/mediterranean-diet/ art- 20047801.

355. Spero, David. "Glycemic Index Confusion - Diabetes Self." Management. July 11, 2012. Accessed June 16, 2019. https://www.diabetesselfmanagement.com/ blog/ glycemic-index-confusion/.

356. Paoli, A., A. Rubini, J. S. Volek, and K. A. Grimaldi. "Beyond Weight Loss: A Review of the Therapeutic Uses of Very-low-carbohydrate (ketogenic) Diets." Nature News. June 26, 2013. Accessed June 16, 2019. https://www.nature.com/ articles/ejcn2013116.

357. Hamzic, Hana. "Keto vs Atkins: Which One Is Better?" Kiss My Keto. Accessed June 16, 2019. https://www.kissmyketo.com/blogs/weight-loss-obesity/ keto-vs-atkins-which-one-is-better.

358. "Everything Sugar (and How to Eliminate It from Your Diet) with Dr. Mark Hyman." Cleveland Clinic. Accessed June 16, 2019. https://my.clevelandclinic.org/ podcasts/health-essentials/everything-sugar-and-how-to-eliminate-it-from-your-diet-with-dr-mark-hyman.

359. Bauer, Meredith Rutland. "Could Keto Be Safe for People With Diabetes Thanks to Telemedicine?" EverydayHealth.com. February 12, 2018. Accessed June 16, 2019. https://www.everydayhealth.com/type-2-diabetes/diet/ trying-keto-with- online-support-may-safely-reverse-diabetes-study/.

360. "The Side Effects of a Low Carb Diet." Ruled Me. October 19, 2018. Accessed June 18, 2019. https://www.ruled.me/side-effects-low-carb-diet/.

361. "The Science Behind Fat Metabolism." KetoSchool. January 02, 2016. Accessed June 18, 2019. https://ketoschool.com/ the-science-behind-fat- metabolism-60f7a3f678d0.

362. "Fructose." Wikipedia. June 13, 2019. Accessed June 18, 2019. https:// en.wikipedia.org/wiki/Fructose#Synthesis_of_glycogen_from_DHAP_and_ glyceraldehyde_3-phosphate.

363. Flynn, Elizabeth, MD, Paul Matz, MD, Alan Woolf, MD, and Robert Wright, MD MPh. Indoor Air Pollutants Effecting Child Health. US Agency for Toxic Substances and Disease Registry, American College of Medical Toxicology. November 2000. Accessed June 15, 2019. https://www.acmt.net/_Library/docs/ IndoorAirPolution.pdf.

364. Sloan, Mark. "Air Pollution a Leading Cause of Cancer, Declares World Health Organization." EndAllDisease. May 21, 2018. Accessed June 16, 2019. https://endalldisease.com/air-pollution-leading-cause-cancer-declares-world-health- organization/.

365. Thomas, John P. "We All Have Pesticides in Our Homes Even If We Don't Use Pesticides." Health Impact News. July 31, 2014. Accessed June 16, 2019. https://healthimpactnews.com/2014/we-all-have-pesticides-in-our-homes-even-if- we-dont-use-pesticides/.

366. Gavigan, Christopher. "3 Shocking Facts About the Air in Your Home « Healthy Begins Here." WebMD. July 29, 2009. Accessed June 17, 2019.https://web.archive.org/web/20170609195741/http://blogs.webmd.com/health- ehome/2009/07/3-shocking-facts-about-the-air-in-your-home.html

367. Becker, Monica, Sally Edwards, and Rachel I. Massey. "Toxic Chemicals in Toys and Children's Products: Limitations of Current Responses and Recommendations for Government and Industry." Toxic Chemicals in Toys and Children's Products: Limitations of Current Responses and Recommendations for Government and Industry | Environmental Science & Technology. February 27, 2010. Accessed June 16, 2019. https://pubs.acs.org/doi/10.1021/es1009407.

368. Kwan, Nicole. "Baby Teethers May Contain Low Levels of BPA, Study Finds." Fox News. December 13, 2016. Accessed June 16, 2019. https://www. foxnews.com/health/baby-teethers-may-contain-low-levels-of-bpa-study-finds.

369. "The Average Woman Puts 168 Chemicals on Her Body Every Day! This Is What Can Happen to Your Cancer Risk." Mercola.com. May 13, 2015. Accessed June 16, 2019. https://articles.mercola.com/sites/articles/archive/2015/05/13/toxic-chemicals-cosmetics.aspx.

370. "The Average Woman Puts 168 Chemicals on Her Body Every Day! This Is What Can Happen to Your Cancer Risk." Mercola.com. May 13, 2015. Accessed June 16, 2019. https://articles.mercola.com/sites/articles/archive/2015/05/13/toxic-chemicals-cosmetics.aspx.

371. Center for Food Safety and Applied Nutrition. "Cosmetics Labeling "Trade Secret" Ingredients." U.S. Food and Drug Administration. August 8, 2018. Accessed June 16, 2019. https://www.fda.gov/Cosmetics/Labeling/ucm414211.htm.

372. "The Average Woman Puts 168 Chemicals on Her Body Every Day! This Is What Can Happen to Your Cancer Risk." Mercola.com. May 13, 2015. Accessed

June 16, 2019. https://articles.mercola.com/sites/articles/archive/2015/05/13/toxic-chemicals-cosmetics.aspx.

373. Hockey, Joel. "Toxic Cosmetics To Avoid (Updated for 2018)." Compare Beauty & Cosmetology Schools with Beauty Schools Directory. May 29, 2018. Accessed June 16, 2019. https://www.beautyschoolsdirectory.com/blog/toxic- cosmetics.

374. "8 Reasons You Need to Throw Away Your Microwave Immediately." Mercola. com. May 18, 2010. Accessed June 16, 2019. https://articles.mercola.com/ sites/articles/archive/2010/05/18/microwave-hazards.aspx.

375. Roberts, Catherine. "Do I Need to Worry About Radiation From WiFi and Bluetooth Devices?" Consumer Reports. March 1, 2018. Accessed June 16, 2019. https://www.consumerreports.org/radiation/do-i-need-to-worry-about-radiation- from-wifi-and-bluetooth-devices/.

376. "Food Dyes: A Rainbow of Risks." Food Dyes: A Rainbow of Risks | Center for Science in the Public Interest. June 1, 2010. Accessed June 16, 2019. https://cspinet.org/resource/food-dyes-rainbow-risks.

377. "Toxic Food Dyes and Dangers of Artificial Food Coloring." Mercola.com. February 24, 2011. Accessed June 16, 2019. https://articles.mercola.com/sites/articles/archive/2011/02/24/are-you-or-your-family-eating-toxic-food-dyes.aspx.

378. "Colors To Die For: The Dangerous Impact of Food Coloring." Special Education Degrees. Accessed June 16, 2019. https://www.special-education-de-gree. net/food-dyes/.

379. Kobylewski, Sarah, and Michael F. Jacobson. "Toxicology of Food Dyes." International Journal of Occupational and Environmental Health. 2012. Accessed June 16, 2019. https://www.ncbi.nlm.nih.gov/pubmed/23026007.

380. "Food Dyes: A Rainbow of Risks." Digital image. Center for Science in the Public Interest. June 1, 2010. Accessed June 16, 2019. https://cspinet.org/sites/default/files/attachment/food-dyes-rainbow-of-risks.pdf.

381. Gunnars, Kris. "27 Health and Nutrition Tips That Are Actually Evidence-Based." Healthline. June 7, 2019. Accessed June 16, 2019. https://www.healthline.com/nutrition/27-health-and-nutrition-tips#section8.

382. Bush, Zach, MD. "Why Probiotics Don't Always Work." Digital image. Zach Bush MD. Accessed June 16, 2019. https://zachbushmd.com/wp-content/uploads/2017/04/Why-Probiotics-Dont-Always-Work-EG-BB-edit.pdf.

383. Wang, Peggy. "21 Little Lifestyle Changes That Will Help You Get Healthier." BuzzFeed. April 09, 2019. Accessed June 16, 2019. https://www. buzzfeed.com/peggy/little-lifestyle-changes-that-will-help-you-be-healthier.

384. Link, Rachael, MS RD. "15 Healthy Foods That Are High in Folate (Folic Acid)." Healthline. May 22, 2018. Accessed June 16, 2019. https://www.healthline.com/nutrition/foods-high-in-folate-folic-acid.

385. "Documentary Reveals: Chemical Exposure Is in Our Daily Lives." Mercola.com. June 5, 2016. Accessed June 16, 2019. https://articles.mercola.com/ sites/articles/archive/2015/06/06/chemical-exposure.aspx.

386. Taughinbaugh, Cathy. "Guilt, Shame, and Vulnerability: 25 Quotes from Dr. Brené Brown." Cathytaughinbaugh.com. Accessed June 16, 2019. https:// cathytaughinbaugh.com/guilt-shame-and-vulnerability-25-quotes-from-dr-brene- brown/.

387. Hall, Crystal Joy. "New Beginnings." Crystal Joy Hall. April 3, 2018. Accessed June 16, 2019. https://crystaljoyhall.com/new-beginnings/.

388. Mahoney, Manda. "The Subconscious Mind of the Consumer (And How To Reach It)." HBS Working Knowledge. January 13, 2003. Accessed June 16, 2019. https://hbswk.hbs.edu/item/the-subconscious-mind-of-the-consumer-and-how-to- reach-it.

389. Marc. "95 Percent of Brain Activity Is beyond Our Conscious Awareness." Neurosciences UX. August 09, 2008. Accessed June 16, 2019. http://www. simplifyinginterfaces.com/2008/08/01/95-percent-of-brain-activity-is-beyond-our-conscious-awareness/.

390. Ferguson, Grace N. "Temperament." Accessed June 17, 2019. https:// gracen-ferguson.com/wp-content/uploads/2016/10/Temperament.pdf

391. O'Hanrahan, Peter, and Enneagram Studies in the Narrative Tradition. A Guide to the Enneagram and the Nine Types. PDF. Enneagram Work, 2007. https:// www.Enneagramworldwide.com/wp-content/uploads/2014/01/Enneagram-Guide. pdf

392. "Enneagram History and Theory." The Enneagram in Business. Accessed June 16, 2019. http://theEnneagraminbusiness.com/the-Enneagram/Enneagram- history-and-theory/.

393. Cloete, Dirk. "Origins and History of the Enneagram." Integrative9. Accessed June 16, 2019. https://www.integrative9.com/Enneagram/history/.

394. "Enneagram of Personality." Wikipedia. May 25, 2019. Accessed June 16, 2019. https://en.wikipedia.org/wiki/Enneagram_of_Personality.

395. "Type Eight." The Enneagram Institute. Accessed June 16, 2019. https:// www. Enneagraminstitute.com/type-8/.

396. Heuertz, Christopher L. The Sacred Enneagram: Finding Your Unique Path to Spiritual Growth. Grand Rapids, MI: Zondervan, 2017.

397. "Religious Involvement, Spirituality, and Medicine: Implications for Clinical Practice." Mayo Clinic Proceedings 76 (December 2001). Accessed June 15, 2019. https://www.mayoclinicproceedings.org/article/S0025-6196(11)62799-7/ pdf.

398. "Is Faith in God a Crutch?" AllAboutGOD.com. Accessed June 16, 2019. https://www.allaboutgod.com/is-faith-in-god-a-crutch-faq.htm.

399. Tong, David. "What Is Quantum Field Theory?" University of Cambridge. Accessed June 16, 2019. http://www.damtp.cam.ac.uk/user/tong/whatisqft.html.

400. Szalay, Jessie. "What Are Free Radicals?" LiveScience. May 27, 2016. Accessed June 16, 2019. https://www.livescience.com/54901-free-radicals.html.

401. Swanson, Joy E. "Antioxidant Nutrients." Antioxidant Nutrients. Accessed June 16, 2019. http://www.theantiagingdoctor.com/antioxidants.htm.

402. Antonio, Jose, PhD. "Reducing Aging Markers with Lipoic Acid." LifeExtension.com. June 2008. Accessed June 16, 2019. https://www.lifeextension.com/magazine/2008/6/Reducing-Aging-Markers-With-Lipoic-Acid/Page-01

403. Blog Contributor. "Ubiquinone vs. Ubiquinol." Qunol. September 27, 2017. Accessed June 16, 2019. https://www.qunol.com/blogs/blog/ubiquinone-vs- ubiquinol.

404. "Ultimate Guide to Antioxidants." Mercola.com. March 24, 2019. Accessed June 16, 2019. https://articles.mercola.com/antioxidants.aspx.

405. Carotenoids." Linus Pauling Institute. January 02, 2019. Accessed June 16, 2019. https://lpi.oregonstate.edu/mic/dietary-factors/phytochemicals/carotenoids.

406. Ambati, Ranga Rao, Siew Moi Phang, Sarada Ravi, and Ravishankar Gokare Aswathanarayana. "Astaxanthin: Sources, Extraction, Stability, Biological Activities and Its Commercial Applications--a Review." Marine Drugs. January 07, 2014. Accessed June 16, 2019. https://www.ncbi.nlm.nih.gov/pmc/articles/PMC3917265/.

407. Superfoodly. " Natural Astaxanthin Foods: 20 Best High Potency Food Sources." Superfoodly. July 28, 2017. Accessed June 16, 2019. https://www. superfoodly.com/natural-astaxanthin-foods-best-high-potency-food-sources/.

408. Superfoodly. "Astaxanthin Supplements." Superfoodly. Accessed June 16, 2019. https://www.superfoodly.com/orac-value/astaxanthin/.

409. Ambati, Ranga Rao, Siew Moi Phang, Sarada Ravi, and Ravishankar Gokare Aswathanarayana. "Astaxanthin: Sources, Extraction, Stability, Biological Activities and Its Commercial Applications--a Review."https://www.ncbi.nlm.nih. gov/pmc/articles/PMC3917265/

410. "Astaxanthin-Nature's Most Powerful Antioxidant." https://articles.mercola.com/sites/articles/archive/2013/02/10/cysewki-discloses-astaxanthin-benefits.aspx

411. "Antioxidants: In Depth." National Center for Complementary and Integrative Health. May 04, 2016. Accessed June 16, 2019. https://nccih.nih.gov/ health/antioxidants/introduction.htm.

412. "Theanine." Wikipedia. February 21, 2019. Accessed June 16, 2019. https://en.wikipedia.org/wiki/Theanine.

413. "Smart Caffeine W/ L-Theanine." Natural Stacks. Accessed June 16, 2019. https://www.naturalstacks.com/pages/the-science-behind-smart-caffeine.

414. Gebely, Tony. "Theanine: A 4000 Year Old Mind-Hack." American Specialty Tea Alliance. May 15, 2018. Accessed June 16, 2019. https:// specialtyteaalliance.org/world-of-tea/caffeine-and-l-theanine/#to-source3.

415. Juneja, L. "L-theanine - a Unique Amino Acid of Green Tea and Its Relaxation Effect in Humans." Trends in Food Science & Technology 10, no. 6-7 (1999): 199-204. Accessed June 16, 2019. doi:10.1016/s0924-2244(99)00044-8.

416. "Flavonoids." The World's Healthiest Foods. Accessed June 16, 2019. http://www.whfoods.com/genpage.php?tname=nutrient&dbid=119.

417. Thilakarathna, Surangi H., and H. P Vasantha Rupasinghe. "Flavonoid Bioavailability and Attempts for Bioavailability Enhancement." Nutrients. August 28, 2013. Accessed June 16, 2019. https://www.ncbi.nlm.nih.gov/pmc/articles/PMC3798909/.

418. Clark, Kateryna. "Polyphenols Vs. Flavonoids." LIVESTRONG. COM. Accessed June 16, 2019. https://www.livestrong.com/article/479645-polyphenols- vs-flavonoids/.

419. Proestos, Charalampos, Konstantina Lytoudi, Olga Konstantina Mavromelanidou, Panagiotis Zoumpoulakis, and Vassileia J. Sinanoglou. "Antioxidant Capacity of Selected Plant Extracts and Their Essential Oils." Antioxidants (Basel, Switzerland). January 04, 2013. Accessed June 16, 2019. https://www.ncbi.nlm.nih.gov/pmc/articles/PMC4665401/.

420. Shoba, G., D. Joy, T. Joseph, M. Majeed, R. Rajendran, and P. S. Srinivas. "Influence of Piperine on the Pharmacokinetics of Curcumin in Animals and Human Volunteers." Planta Medica. May 1998. Accessed June 16, 2019. https://www.ncbi.nlm.nih.gov/pubmed/9619120.

421. De Santi, C., A. Pietrabissa, F. Mosca, and G. M. Pacifici. "Glucuronidation of Resveratrol, a Natural Product Present in Grape and Wine, in the Human Liver." Xenobiotica; the Fate of Foreign Compounds in Biological Systems. November 2000. Accessed June 16, 2019. https://www.ncbi.nlm.nih.gov/pubmed/11197066.

422. Hewlings, Susan J., and Douglas S. Kalman. "Curcumin: A Review of Its' Effects on Human Health." Foods (Basel, Switzerland). October 22, 2017. Accessed June 16, 2019. https://www.ncbi.nlm.nih.gov/pmc/articles/ PMC5664031/.

423. "Curcumin Benefits: How It Helps in Cancer Treatment." Mercola. com. March 2, 2014. Accessed June 16, 2019. https://articles.mercola.com/ sites/articles/archive/2014/03/02/curcumin-benefits.aspx?e_cid=20140302Z1_ SNL_Art_1&utm_source=snl&utm_medium=email&utm_content=art1&utm_campaign=20140302Z1&et_cid=DM40322&et_rid=442339021.

424. Prasad, Sahdeo, Amit K. Tyagi, and Bharat B. Aggarwal. "Recent Developments in Delivery, Bioavailability, Absorption and Metabolism of Curcumin: The Golden Pigment from Golden Spice." Cancer Research and Treatment : Official Journal of

Korean Cancer Association. January 2014. Accessed June 16, 2019. https://www.ncbi.nlm.nih.gov/pmc/articles/PMC3918523/.

425. Karlstetter, Marcus , Elena Lippe, Yana Walczak, Christoph Moehle, Alexander Aslanidis, Myriam Mirza, and Thomas Langmann. "Curcumin Is a Potent Modulator of Microglial Gene Expression and Migration." Journal of Neuroinflammation. September 29, 2011. Accessed June 16, 2019. https:// jneuroinflammation.biomedcentral.com/articles/10.1186/1742-2094-8-125.

426. Marcus Karlstetter, Elena Lippe, Yana Walczak, Christoph Moehle, Alexander Aslanidis, Myriam Mirza, and Thomas Langmann. "Curcumin Is a Potent Modulator of Microglial Gene Expression and Migration." Journal of Neuroinflammation. September 29, 2011. Accessed June 18, 2019. https:// jneuroinflammation.biomedcentral.com/articles/10.1186/1742-2094-8-125.

427. Mishra, Shrikant, and Kalpana Palanivelu. "The Effect of Curcumin (turmeric) on Alzheimer's Disease: An Overview." Annals of Indian Academy of Neurology. Spring 2008. Accessed June 16, 2019. https://www.ncbi.nlm.nih.gov/ pmc/articles/ PMC2781139/.

428. Cheng, Jiang, Zhi-Wei Zhou, Hui-Ping Sheng, Lan-Jie He, Xue-Wen Fan, Zhi-Xu He, Tao Sun, Xueji Zhang, Ruan Jin Zhao, Ling Gu, Chuanhai Cao, and Shu-Feng Zhou. "An Evidence-based Update on the Pharmacological Activities and Possible Molecular Targets of Lycium Barbarum Polysaccharides." Drug Design, Development and Therapy. December 17, 2014. Accessed June 16, 2019. https:// www.ncbi.nlm.nih.gov/pmc/articles/PMC4277126/.

429. Kocyigit, Emine, and Nevin Sanlier. "A Review of Composition and Health Effects of Lycium Barbarum." International Journal of Chinese Medicine. January 24, 2017. Accessed June 16, 2019. http://article.sciencepublishinggroup.com/html/1 0.11648.j.ijcm.20170101.11.html.

430. Juneja, L. "L-theanine - a Unique Amino Acid of Green Tea and Its Relaxation Effect in Humans." Accessed June 16, 2019 http://www.scicompdf.se/ cooldown/ juneja_1999.pdf

431. Wang, Dongxu, Qiang Gao, George Wang, and Frank Qian. "Theanine: The Unique Amino Acid in the Tea Plant as an Oral Hepatoprotective Agent." Asia Pacific Journal of Clinical Nutrition 26, no. 3 (2017): 384-91. Accessed June 16, 2019. doi:10.6133/apjcn.032017.11.

432. Jówko, Ewa. "Green Tea Catechins and Sport Performance." Antioxidants in Sport Nutrition. January 01, 1970. Accessed June 16, 2019. https://www.ncbi. nlm. nih.gov/books/NBK299060/.

433. Srivastava, Janmejai K., Eswar Shankar, and Sanjay Gupta. "Chamomile: A Herbal Medicine of the past with Bright Future." Molecular Medicine Reports. November 01, 2010. Accessed June 16, 2019. https://www.ncbi.nlm.nih.gov/pmc/ articles/PMC2995283/.

434. Bond, Owen. "Panax Ginseng Vs. Siberian Ginseng." LIVESTRONG. COM. Accessed June 16, 2019. https://www.livestrong.com/ article/414544-panax- ginseng-vs-siberian-ginseng/.

435. Dharmananda, Subhuti, and Institute for Traditional Medicine. "GINSENG IN TRADITIONAL CHINESE LITERATURE." The Nature of Ginseng. September 2002. Accessed June 16, 2019. http://www.itmonline.org/journal/arts/ ginseng-nature.htm.

436. Peng, Lu, Shi Sun, Lai-Hua Xie, Sheila M. Wicks, and Jing-Tian Xie. "Ginsenoside Re: Pharmacological Effects on Cardiovascular System." Cardiovascular Therapeutics 30, no. 4 (2011). doi:10.1111/j.1755- 5922.2011.00271.x.

437. Moffat, Denice, Dr. "Ginseng Differences And Benefits." Natural Health Techniques. August 15, 2014. Accessed June 16, 2019. http:// naturalhealthtech-niques.com/diet_nutritionginsengtypesbenefits/.

438. Gussa, Christopher. "Siberian Ginseng: The Almost Forgotten, Perfect Adaptogen and Energy Booster." NaturalNews. September 18, 2008. Accessed June 16, 2019. https://www.naturalnews.com/024235_ginseng_energy_herb.html.

439. "What Is the Best Ginseng You Can Take There Seems so Many?" What Is the Best Ginseng You Can Take There Seems so Many? October 13, 2009. Accessed June 16, 2019. http://3alternative-medicine.blogspot.com/2009/10/what- is-best-ginseng-you-can-take-there.html.

440. Banerjee, S. K., Pulok K. Mukherjee, and S. K. Maulik. "Garlic as an Antioxidant: The Good, the Bad and the Ugly." Phytotherapy Research 17, no. 2 (2003): 97-106. Accessed June 16, 2019. doi:10.1002/ptr.1281.

441. Chung, Lip Yong. "The Antioxidant Properties of Garlic Compounds: Allyl Cysteine, Alliin, Allicin, and Allyl Disulfide." Journal of Medicinal Food. Summer 2006. Accessed June 16, 2019. https://www.ncbi.nlm.nih.gov/pubmed/16822206.

442. Ried, Karin, Nikolaj Travica, and Avni Sali. "The Effect of Kyolic Aged Garlic Extract on Gut Microbiota, Inflammation, and Cardiovascular Markers in Hypertensives: The GarGIC Trial." Frontiers in Nutrition. December 11, 2018. Accessed June 16, 2019. https://www.ncbi.nlm.nih.gov/pmc/articles/PMC6297383/.

443. "Superfoods That Give You the Most Bang for Your Buck." Mercola.com. March 20, 2017. Accessed June 16, 2019. https://articles.mercola.com/sites/articles/archive/2017/03/20/17-superfoods-cost-saving-nutrition-boosting-tips.aspx.

444. "Food & Nutrition Facts." Mercola.com. Accessed June 16, 2019. https://foodfacts.mercola.com/.

445. "Cacao vs Cocoa: What's the Difference?" Healthline. Accessed June 16, 2019. https://www.healthline.com/nutrition/cacao-vs-cocoa#nutrition.

446. Wilson, Sarah. "Raw Cacao vs Cocoa: What's The Difference?" FOOD MATTERS®. May 21, 2019. Accessed June 16, 2019. https://www.foodmatters.com/article/raw-cacao-vs-cocoa-whats-the-difference.

447. Axe, Josh. "7 Bromelain Benefits, Uses & Best Food Sources." Dr. Axe. October 26, 2018. Accessed June 16, 2019. https://draxe.com/bromelain/.

448. Axe, Josh. "7 Bromelain Benefits, Uses & Best Food Sources." Dr. Axe. October 26, 2018. Accessed June 16, 2019. https://draxe.com/bromelain/.

449. "8 Tips to Follow When Buying a New Bottle of Olive Oil." Mercola.com. July 26, 2018. Accessed June 16, 2019. https://articles.mercola.com/herbal-oils/olive-oil.aspx.

450. Levy, Jillian. "Olive Oil Benefits for Your Heart, Brain and More." Dr. Axe. May 21, 2018. Accessed June 16, 2019. https://draxe.com/olive-oil-benefits/.

451. NutritonReview.org, Ward Dean, MD, and Jim English. "Medium Chain Triglycerides (MCTs)." Nutrition Review. June 20, 2016. Accessed June 16, 2019. https://nutritionreview.org/2013/04/medium-chain-triglycerides-mcts/.

452. Levy, Jillian. "What Is MCT Oil? 6 Benefits and How to Use." Dr. Axe. April 18, 2018. Accessed June 16, 2019. https://draxe.com/mct-oil/.

453. Sheer, Robby, and Doug Moss. "Dirt Poor: Have Fruits and Vegetables Become Less Nutritious?" Scientific American. Accessed June 16, 2019. https:// www.scientificamerican.com/article/soil-depletion-and-nutrition-loss/.

454. Fitzgerald, Randall. The Hundred-year Lie: How to Protect Yourself from the Chemicals That Are Destroying Your Health. New York: Plume, 2007.

455. Lang Integrative Health Seminars. "Natural vs. Synthetic Vitamins." Alternative Health Atlanta - Dr. Melodie Billiot. 2003. Accessed June 16, 2019. https://alternativehealthatlanta.com/vitamins-minerals/natural-vs-synthetic- vitamins/.

456. Preedy, Victor R., and Ronald R. Watson. The Encyclopedia of Vitamin E. Wallingford, Oxon, UK: CABI, 2007.

457. Traber, Maret G., Regina Brigelius-Flohé, and Angelika Elsner. "Synthetic as Compared with Natural Vitamin E Is Preferentially Excreted as α-CEHC in Human Urine: Studies Using Deuterated α-tocopheryl Acetates." FEBS Letters. December 02, 1998. Accessed June 16, 2019. https://www.sciencedirect.com/ science/article/ pii/S0014579398012101.

458. C Clement, Brian, NMD PhD, Scott Treadway, PhD, and Shula Gabbay, MA. "Research Paper-The Naturally Occurring Standard." Naturally Occurring Standards Group. Accessed June 16, 2019. https://nosg.org/?page_id=87.

459. Brown, Mary J., PhD. "Synthetic vs Natural Nutrients: Does It Matter?" Healthline. August 17, 2016. Accessed June 16, 2019. https://www.healthline.com/ nutrition/synthetic-vs-natural-nutrients#section7.

460. Link, Rachael, MS RD. "15 Healthy Foods That Are High in Folate (Folic Acid)." Accessed June 16, 2019 https://www.healthline.com/nutrition/ foods-high- in-folate-folic-acid#section15

461. Fitzgerald, Randall. The Hundred-year Lie: How to Protect Yourself from the Chemicals That Are Destroying Your Health. New York: Plume, 2007.

462. D'Souza, R. M., and R. D'Souza. "Vitamin A for Treating Measles in Children." The Cochrane Database of Systematic Reviews. 2002. Accessed June 16, 2019. https://www.ncbi.nlm.nih.gov/pubmed/11869601.

463. Fallon, Sally, and Mary G. Enig. "Vitamin A Saga." The Weston A. Price Foundation. March 30, 2002. Accessed June 16, 2019. https://www.westonaprice. org/health-topics/abcs-of-nutrition/vitamin-a-saga/.

464. Sen, Chandan K., Savita Khanna, and Sashwati Roy. "Tocotrienols: Vitamin E beyond Tocopherols." Life Sciences. March 27, 2006. Accessed June 16, 2019. https://www.ncbi.nlm.nih.gov/pmc/articles/PMC1790869/.

465. Prasad, Kedar N., Bipin Kumar, Xiang-Dong Yan, Amy J. Hanson, and William C. Cole. "Alpha-tocopheryl Succinate, the Most Effective Form of Vitamin E for Adjuvant Cancer Treatment: A Review." Journal of the American College of Nutrition. April 2003. Accessed June 16, 2019. https://www.ncbi.nlm.nih.gov/pubmed/12672706.

466. Meschino, James. "Vitamin E Succinate: The Preferred Form of Vitamin E to Combat Breast, Prostate and Other Cancers." Accessed June 17, 2019. https:// www. researchgate.net/publication/237506732_Vitamin_E_Succinate_The_Preferred_ Form_of_Vitamin_E_to_Combat_Breast_Prostate_and_Other_Cancers.

467. "Office of Dietary Supplements - Vitamin K." NIH Office of Dietary Supplements. September 26, 2018. Accessed June 16, 2019. https://ods.od.nih. gov/ factsheets/VitaminK-HealthProfessional/.

468. "What Is Vitamin K? Everything You Need to Know About Vitamin K1 and K2." Dr Steven Lin. September 22, 2018. Accessed June 16, 2019. https://www. drstevenlin.com/what-is-vitamin-k/.

469. Arnarson, Atli, PhD. "Is Vitamin D Harmful Without Vitamin K?" Healthline. March 4, 2017. Accessed June 16, 2019. https://www.healthline.com/ nutrition/ vitamin-d-and-vitamin-k#section1.

470. Hariri, Mitra, Zahra Maghsoudi, Leila Darvishi, Gholamreza Askari, Maryam Hajishafiee, Shekoofe Ghasemi, Fariborz Khorvash, Bijan Iraj, and Reza Ghiasvand. "B Vitamins and Antioxidants Intake Is Negatively Correlated with Risk of Stroke in Iran." International Journal of Preventive Medicine. May 2013. Accessed June 16, 2019. https://www.ncbi.nlm.nih.gov/pmc/articles/ PMC3678233/.

471. "B Vitamins | Dr. Weil's Guide To B Vitamins | Andrew Weil, M.D." DrWeil.com. October 29, 2017. Accessed June 16, 2019. https://www.drweil.com/ vitamins-supplements-herbs/vitamins/dr-weils-guide-to-b-vitamins/.

472. "Office of Dietary Supplements - Vitamin C." NIH Office of Dietary Supplements. September 18, 2018. Accessed June 16, 2019. https://ods.od.nih. gov/ factsheets/VitaminC-HealthProfessional/.

473. Michels, Alexander, PhD. "Questions about Vitamin C." Linus Pauling Institute Blog. May 28, 2015. Accessed June 16, 2019. http://blogs.oregonstate. edu/ linuspaulinginstitute/2015/05/28/questions-about-vitamin-c/.

474. Les Prix Nobel. "Albert Szent-Györgyi Biographical." NobelPrize.org. Accessed June 16, 2019. https://www.nobelprize.org/prizes/medicine/1937/szent- gyorgyi/ biographical/.

475. Desaulniers, Veronique, Dr. "What Is Vitamin P and How Can It Help Prevent Cancer?" The Truth About Cancer. January 08, 2018. Accessed June 16, 2019. https://thetruthaboutcancer.com/vitamin-p-cancer/.

476. O'Shea, Timothy. "Whole Food Vitamins: Ascorbic Acid Is Not Vitamin C." Living Well Clinical Nutrition Center. August 17, 2011. Accessed June 16, 2019. https:// www.justlivewell.com/whole-food-vitamins-ascorbic-acid-is-not-vitamin-c/

477. Carr, Anitra C., and Margreet C M Vissers. "Synthetic or Food-derived Vitamin C--are They Equally Bioavailable?" Nutrients. October 28, 2013. Accessed June 16, 2019. https://www.ncbi.nlm.nih.gov/pmc/articles/PMC3847730/.

478. Ferguson, John B. "An Interlinear Transliteration and English Translation of Portions of THE EBERS PAPYRUS Possibly Having to Do With Diabetes Mellitus." Digital image. The Bronx High School of Science. 2008. Accessed June 17, 2019. https://bxscience.edu/ourpages/auto/2008/11/10/43216077/egypt medicine.pdf.

479. "Herbal Medicine in Ancient Egypt." Journal of Medicinal Plant Research 4, no. 2 (February 2010): 82-86. Accessed June 17, 2019. https://

480. "History of Essential Oils." Digital image. The Association for the International Research of Aromatic Science and Education (AIRASE). Accessed June 17, 2019. http://airase.com/wp-content/uploads/2014/01/ HistoryOfEssentialOils.pdf.

481. Young, Kac. The Healing Art of Essential Oils: A Guide to 50 Oils for Remedy, Ritual, and Everyday Use. Woodbury, MN: Llewellyn Publications, 2017.

482. "Ancient Egyptian MedicineIn Sickness and in Health: Preventative and Curative Health Care." Ancient Egypt: Medicine. Accessed June 17, 2019. https:// web.archive.org/web/20110306051633/http://www.reshafim.org.il/ad/egypt/ time-lines/topics/medicine.htm.

483. Stewart, David, PhD RA. "THE BLOOD-BRAIN BARRIER - Http://www. oilhealer.com/bloodbrain.cfm." 50megs. Accessed June 16, 2019. http://www. rnoel.50megs.com/pdf/theblood.htm.

484. Stewart, David. THE BLOOD-BRAIN BARRIER - Http://www. Accessed June 18, 2019. http://www.rnoel.50megs.com/pdf/theblood.htm.

485. Frank, Mark Barton, Qing Yang, Jeanette Osban, Joseph T. Azzarello, Marcia R. Saban, Ricardo Saban, Richard A. Ashley, Jan C. Welter, Kar-Ming Fung, and Hsueh-Kung Lin. "Frankincense Oil Derived from Boswellia Carteri Induces Tumor Cell Specific Cytotoxicity." BMC Complementary and Alternative Medicine. March 18, 2009. Accessed June 16, 2019. https://www.ncbi.nlm.nih.gov/ pmc/ articles/PMC2664784/.

486. Woolley, Cole L., Mahmoud M. Suhail, Brett L. Smith, Karen E. Boren, Lindsey C. Taylor, Marc F. Schreuder, Jeremiah K. Chai, Hervé Casabianca, Sadqa Haq, Hsueh-Kung Lin, Ahmed A. Al-Shahri, Saif Al-Hatmi, and D. Gary Young. "Chemical Differentiation of Boswellia Sacra and Boswellia Carterii Essential Oils by Gas Chromatography and Chiral Gas Chromatography-mass Spectrometry." Journal of Chromatography. A. October 26, 2012. Accessed June 16, 2019. https:// www.ncbi.nlm.nih.gov/pubmed/22835693

487. Sikka, Suresh C., and Alma R. Bartolome. "Learn More about Boswellia Sacra Perfumery, Essential Oils, and Household Chemicals Affecting Reproductive and Sexual Health." Science Direct. Accessed June 16, 2019. https://www. sciencedirect. com/topics/biochemistry-genetics-and-molecular-biology/boswellia- sacra.

488. Buckle, Jane. Clinical Aromatherapy: Essential Oils in Healthcare. Edinburgh: Churchill Livingstone, 2015.

489. https://www.ncbi.nlm.nih.gov/pubmed/22545396 Paul, Michael, and Johann Jauch. "Efficient Preparation of Incensole and Incensole Acetate, and Quantification of These Bioactive Diterpenes in Boswellia Papyrifera by a RP-DAD-HPLC Method." Natural Product Communications. March 2012. Accessed June 16, 2019. https:// www.ncbi.nlm.nih.gov/pubmed/22545396.

490. "Boswellia Papyrifera." Wikipedia. June 13, 2019. Accessed June 16, 2019. https://en.wikipedia.org/wiki/Boswellia_papyrifera.

491. Sikka, Suresh C., and Alma R. Bartolome. "Learn More about Boswellia Sacra Perfumery, Essential Oils, and Household Chemicals Affecting

Reproductive and Sexual Health."https://www.sciencedirect.com/topics/ biochemistry-genetics- and-molecular

492. Moussaieff, Arieh, Neta Rimmerman, Tatiana Bregman, Alex Straiker, Christian C. Felder, Shai Shoham, Yoel Kashman, Susan M. Huang, Hyosang Lee, Esther Shohami, Ken Mackie, Michael J. Caterina, J. Michael Walker, Ester Fride, and Raphael Mechoulam. "Incensole Acetate, an Incense Component, Elicits Psychoactivity by Activating TRPV3 Channels in the Brain." FASEB Journal : Official Publication of the Federation of American Societies for Experimental Biology. August 2008. Accessed June 16, 2019. https://www.ncbi.nlm.nih.gov/ pmc/ articles/PMC2493463/.

493. Iram, Farah, Shah Alam Khan, and Asif Husain. "Phytochemistry and Potential Therapeutic Actions of Boswellic Acids: A Mini-review." Asian Pacific Journal of Tropical Biomedicine. May 25, 2017. Accessed June 16, 2019. https:// www.sciencedirect.com/science/article/pii/S2221169117304914.

494. Ren, Peng, Xiang Ren, Lei Cheng, and Lixin Xu. "Frankincense, Pine Needle and Geranium Essential Oils Suppress Tumor Progression through the Regulation of the AMPK/mTOR Pathway in Breast Cancer." Oncology Reports. January 2018. Accessed June 16, 2019. https://www.ncbi.nlm.nih.gov/pmc/articles/ PMC5783593/.

495. Ren, Peng, Xiang Ren, Lei Cheng, and Lixin Xu. "Frankincense, Pine Needle and Geranium Essential Oils Suppress Tumor Progression through the Regulation of the AMPK/mTOR Pathway in Breast Cancer." Oncology Reports, 2017. Accessed June 17, 2019. doi:10.3892/or.2017.6067.

496. Suhail, Mahmoud M., Weijuan Wu, Amy Cao, Fadee G. Mondalek, Kar-Ming Fung, Pin-Tsen Shih, Yu-Ting Fang, Cole Woolley, Gary Young, and Hsueh-Kung Lin. "Boswellia Sacra Essential Oil Induces Tumor Cell-specific Apoptosis and Suppresses Tumor Aggressiveness in Cultured Human Breast Cancer Cells." BMC Complementary and Alternative Medicine. December 15, 2011. Accessed June 16, 2019. https://www.ncbi.nlm.nih.gov/pmc/articles/ PMC3258268/?tool=pmcentrez.

497. Fidyt, Klaudyna, Anna Fiedorowicz, Leon Strządała, and Antoni Szumny. "β-caryophyllene and β-caryophyllene Oxide-natural Compounds of Anticancer and Analgesic Properties." Cancer Medicine. October 2016. Accessed June 16, 2019. https://www.ncbi.nlm.nih.gov/pmc/articles/PMC5083753/.

498. Legault, Jean, and André Pichette. "Potentiating Effect of Beta- caryophyllene on Anticancer Activity of Alpha-humulene, Isocaryophyllene and Paclitaxel." The Journal of Pharmacy and Pharmacology. December 2007. Accessed June 16, 2019. https://www.ncbi.nlm.nih.gov/pubmed/18053325.

499. Tisserand, Robert. "Frankincense Oil and Cancer in Perspective." Tisserand Institute. August 17, 2017. Accessed June 16, 2019. https://tisserandinstitute.org/frankincense-oil-and-cancer-in-perspective/.

500. Paul, Michael, Gerit Brüning, and Johann Jauch. "A Thin-layer Chromatography Method for the Identification of Three Different Olibanum Resins (Boswellia Serrata, Boswellia Papyrifera and Boswellia Carterii, Respectively, Boswellia Sacra) | Scinapse | Academic Search Engine for Paper." Scinapse. March 01, 2012. Accessed June 16, 2019. https://scinapse.io/papers/1580994982.

501. Al-Yasiry, Ali Ridha Mustafa, and Bożena Kiczorowska. "Frankincense - Therapeutic Properties." Postępy Higieny I Medycyny Doświadczalnej 70 (2016): 380-91. Accessed June 16, 2019. doi:10.5604/17322693.1200553. https://www. research-gate.net/publication/292140720_Frankincense_-_therapeutic_properties

502. The Revisionist. "Frankincense Types: Medicinal, Psychoactive, Cognitive, Scent Properties & More." The Revisionist. November 26, 2017. Accessed June 16, 2019. https://therevisionist.org/reviews/frankincense-types-medicinal- psychoactive-cognitive-scent-properties/.

503. Al-Yasiry, Ali Ridha Mustafa, and Bożena Kiczorowska. "Frankincense - Therapeutic Properties." https://www.researchgate.net/publication/292140720_Frankincense_-_therapeutic_properties

504. Axe, Josh. "8 Frankincense Essential Oil Uses and Benefits for Healing." Dr. Axe. June 30, 2018. Accessed June 16, 2019. https://draxe.com/what-is- frankincense/.

505. Axe, Josh. "Essential Oils Guide Best Essential Oils." Dr. Axe. April 23, 2018. Accessed June 16, 2019. https://draxe.com/essential-oils-guide/.

506. Sowndhararajan, Kandhasamy, and Songmun Kim. "Influence of Fragrances on Human Psychophysiological Activity: With Special Reference to Human Electroencephalographic Response." Scientia Pharmaceutica. November 29, 2016. Accessed June 16, 2019. https://www.ncbi.nlm.nih.gov/pmc/articles/PMC5198031/.

507. Kim, In-Hee, Chan Kim, Kayeon Seong, Myung-Haeng Hur, Heon Man Lim, and Myeong Soo Lee. "Essential Oil Inhalation on Blood Pressure and Salivary Cortisol Levels in Prehypertensive and Hypertensive Subjects." Evidence-based Complementary and Alternative Medicine : ECAM. November 19, 2012. Accessed June 16, 2019. https://www.ncbi.nlm.nih.gov/pmc/articles/ PMC3521421/.

508. Editor. "Dermal Absorption of Essential Oils." Naturopathic Doctor News and Review. June 02, 2015. Accessed June 16, 2019. https://ndnr.com/mindbody/ dermal-absorption-of-essential-oils/.

509. Snyder, Mariza. "Your Ultimate Guide To Essential Oils: Uses, Benefits, Extraction & How To Use Them, Explained." Mindbodygreen. November 12, 2018. Accessed June 16, 2019. https://www.mindbodygreen.com/articles/ how-to- use-essential-oils-guide-essential-oil-benefits-and-essential-oil-uses.

510. Villafranco, Sarah. "How To Make Essential Oils." Mindbodygreen. May 18, 2018. Accessed June 16, 2019. https://www.mindbodygreen.com/articles/ how- essential-oils-are-made.

511. Lu, Hui-Chen, and Ken Mackie. "An Introduction to the Endogenous Cannabinoid System." Biological Psychiatry. April 01, 2016. Accessed June 16, 2019. https://www.ncbi.nlm.nih.gov/pmc/articles/PMC4789136/.

512. Leaf Science Editorial Team. "The Endocannabinoid System: A Beginner's Guide." Leaf Science. March 19, 2019. Accessed June 16, 2019. https://www. leaf-science.com/2017/03/17/the-endocannabinoid-system-a-beginners-guide/.

513. Lu, Hui-Chen, and Ken Mackie. "An Introduction to the Endogenous Cannabinoid System." Biological Psychiatry. April 01, 2016. Accessed June 16, 2019. https://www.ncbi.nlm.nih.gov/pmc/articles/PMC4789136/.

514. Porter, Brenda E., and Catherine Jacobson. "Report of a Parent Survey of Cannabidiol-enriched Cannabis Use in Pediatric Treatment-resistant Epilepsy." Epilepsy & Behavior : E&B. December 2013. Accessed June 16, 2019. https:// www. ncbi.nlm.nih.gov/pmc/articles/PMC4157067/.

515. Blessing, Esther M., Maria M. Steenkamp, Jorge Manzanares, and Charles R. Marmar. "Cannabidiol as a Potential Treatment for Anxiety Disorders." Neurotherapeutics : The Journal of the American Society for Experimental NeuroTherapeutics. October 2015. Accessed June 16, 2019. https://www.ncbi. nlm. nih.gov/pmc/articles/PMC4604171/.

516. Arutz Sheva Staff. "Study: Cannabis Oil 80% Successful in Helping Autistic Children." Israel National News. July 26, 2018. Accessed June 16, 2019. http:// www. israelnationalnews.com/News/News.aspx/249591.

517. Aran, Adi, Hanoch Cassuto, and Asael Lubotzky. "Cannabidiol Based Medical Cannabis in Children with Autism- a Retrospective Feasibility Study (P3.318)." Neurology. April 10, 2018. Accessed June 16, 2019. http://n.neurology. org/content/90/15_Supplement/P3.318.

518. Blessing, Esther M., Maria M. Steenkamp, Jorge Manzanares, and Charles R. Marmar. "Cannabidiol as a Potential Treatment for Anxiety Disorders." Neurotherapeutics : The Journal of the American Society for Experimental NeuroTherapeutics. October 2015. Accessed June 16, 2019. https://www.ncbi. nlm. nih.gov/pmc/articles/PMC4604171/.

519. Leimuranta, Pinja, Leonard Khiroug, and Rashid Giniatullin. "Emerging Role of (Endo)Cannabinoids in Migraine." Frontiers. April 24, 2018. Accessed June 16, 2019. https://www.frontiersin.org/articles/10.3389/fphar.2018.00420/full.

520. Siefert, Wade, RPh, ABAAHP, FAARM. "Get to Know CBD Oil." Digital image. 2017. Accessed June 16, 2019. https://acainfo.org/wp-content/ uploads/2017/04/ Get-to-Know-CBD-Oil-Seifert.pdf.

521. Mandolini, G. M., M. Lazzaretti, A. Pigoni, L. Oldani, G. Delvecchio, and P. Brambilla. "Pharmacological Properties of Cannabidiol in the Treatment of Psychiatric Disorders: A Critical Overview." Epidemiology and Psychiatric Sciences. August 2018. Accessed June 16, 2019. https://www.ncbi.nlm.nih.gov/ pubmed/29789034.

522. Hasenoehrl, Carina, Martin Storr, and Rudolf Schicho. "Cannabinoids for Treating Inflammatory Bowel Diseases: Where Are We and Where Do We Go?" Expert Review of Gastroenterology & Hepatology. April 03, 2017. Accessed June 16, 2019. https://www.ncbi.nlm.nih.gov/pmc/articles/PMC5388177/.

523. Guimarães-Santos, Adriano, Diego Siqueira Santos, Ijair Rogério Santos, Rafael Rodrigues Lima, Antonio Pereira, Lucinewton Silva De Moura, Raul Nunes Carvalho, Osmar Lameira, and Walace Gomes-Leal. "Copaiba Oil-resin Treatment Is Neuroprotective and Reduces Neutrophil Recruitment and Microglia Activation after Motor Cortex Excitotoxic Injury." Evidence-based Complementary and Alternative Medicine : ECAM. February 19, 2012. Accessed June 16, 2019. https:// www.ncbi.nlm.nih.gov/pmc/articles/PMC3291111/.

524. Navarro, Gemma, Katia Varani, Irene Reyes-Resina, Verónica Sánchez De Medina, Rafael Rivas-Santisteban, Carolina Sánchez-Carnerero Callado, Fabrizio Vincenzi, Salvatore Casano, Carlos Ferreiro-Vera, Enric I. Canela, Pier Andrea Borea, Xavier Nadal, and Rafael Franco. "Cannabigerol Action at Cannabinoid CB1 and CB2 Receptors and at CB1-CB2 Heteroreceptor Complexes." Frontiers in Pharmacology. June 21, 2018. Accessed June 16, 2019. https://www.ncbi.nlm. nih. gov/pmc/articles/PMC6021502/.

525. Nikkola, Tom. "Hemp, Essential Oils, and the Endocannabinoid System: Your Guide." TOM NIKKOLA. May 23, 2019. Accessed June 16, 2019. https://tomnikkola. com/hemp-essential-oils-and-the-endocannabinoid- system-your-guide/?fbclid=I-wAR2P_LVjWohm48U0sDdJAT9e5a_a9O- u2gGv5jUO6LElKsDc07Jc624jTrw.

526. The Apothecarium. "Cannabinoids 101: CBG." The Apothecarium. July 24, 2018. Accessed June 16, 2019. https://apothecarium.com/blog/nevada/2018/7/24/ cannabinoids-101-cbg.

527. Almeida, Mara Ribeiro, Joana D'Arc Castania Darin, Lívia Cristina Hernandes, Mônica Freiman De Souza Ramos, Lusânia Maria Greggi Antunes, and Osvaldo De Freitas. "Genotoxicity Assessment of Copaiba Oil and Its Fractions in Swiss Mice." Genetics and Molecular Biology. August 2, 2012. Accessed June 16, 2019. https://www.ncbi.nlm.nih.gov/pmc/articles/PMC3459418/.

528. Guimarães-Santos, Adriano, Diego Siqueira Santos, Ijair Rogério Santos, Rafael Rodrigues Lima, Antonio Pereira, Lucinewton Silva De Moura, Raul Nunes Carvalho, Osmar Lameira, and Walace Gomes-Leal https://www.ncbi.nlm.nih. gov/ pmc/articles/PMC3291111/

529. "Former Science Chief: 'MMR Fears Coming True'." Daily Mail Online. May 22, 2016. Accessed June 18, 2019. https://www.dailymail. co.uk/health/article-376203/ Former-science-chief-MMR-fears-coming-true. html#ixzz3S0gDbqzq.

530. Attkisson, Sharyl. "Vaccines and Autism: A New Scientific Review." CBS News. April 01, 2011. Accessed June 18, 2019. https://www.cbsnews.com/news/ vaccines-and-autism-a-new-scientific-review/.

531. Delong, Gayle. "A Positive Association Found between Autism Prevalence and Childhood Vaccination Uptake across the U.S. Population." Journal of Toxicology and Environmental Health. Part A. 2011. Accessed June 18, 2019. https://www. ncbi.nlm.nih.gov/pubmed/21623535.

532. Geier, David A., and Mark R. Geier. "A Case Series of Children with Apparent Mercury Toxic Encephalopathies Manifesting with Clinical Symptoms of Regressive Autistic Disorders." Journal of Toxicology and Environmental Health. Part A. May 15, 2007. Accessed June 18, 2019. https://www.ncbi.nlm.nih.gov/pubmed/17454560.

533. Garrecht, Matthew, and David W. Austin. "The Plausibility of a Role for Mercury in the Etiology of Autism: A Cellular Perspective." Toxicological and Environmental Chemistry. 2011. Accessed June 18, 2019. https://www.ncbi.nlm.nih.gov/pmc/articles/PMC3173748/.

534. Sharpe, Martyn A., Taylor L. Gist, and David S. Baskin. "B-lymphocytes from a Population of Children with Autism Spectrum Disorder and Their Unaffected Siblings Exhibit Hypersensitivity to Thimerosal." Journal of Toxicology. 2013. Accessed June 18, 2019. https://www.ncbi.nlm.nih.gov/ pubmed/23843785.

535. Geier, David, and Mark R. Geier. "Neurodevelopmental Disorders following Thimerosal-containing Childhood Immunizations: A Follow-up Analysis." International Journal of Toxicology. 2004. Accessed June 18, 2019. https://www.ncbi.nlm.nih.gov/pubmed/15764492.

536. Geier, David A., Brian S. Hooker, Janet K. Kern, Paul G. King, Lisa K. Sykes, and Mark R. Geier. "A Two-phase Study Evaluating the Relationship between Thimerosal-containing Vaccine Administration and the Risk for an Autism Spectrum Disorder Diagnosis in the United States." Translational Neurodegeneration. December 19, 2013. Accessed June 18, 2019. https://www. ncbi.nlm.nih.gov/pmc/articles/PMC3878266/.

537. Singh, Vijendra K., and Ryan L. Jensen. "Elevated Levels of Measles Antibodies in Children with Autism." Pediatric Neurology. April 2003. Accessed June 18, 2019. https://www.ncbi.nlm.nih.gov/pubmed/12849883.

538. Singh, Vijendra K. "Phenotypic Expression of Autoimmune Autistic Disorder (AAD): A Major Subset of Autism." Annals of Clinical Psychiatry : Official Journal of the American Academy of Clinical Psychiatrists. 2009. Accessed June 18, 2019. https://www.ncbi.nlm.nih.gov/pubmed/19758536.

539. Kirby, David, and David Kirby. "New Study: Hepatitis B Vaccine Triples the Risk of Autism in Infant Boys." HuffPost. November 17, 2011. Accessed June 18, 2019. https://www.huffpost.com/entry/new-study-hepatitis-b- vac_b_289288?guccounter=1.

540. Gallagher, Carolyn M., and Melody S. Goodman. "Hepatitis B Vaccination of Male Neonates and Autism Diagnosis, NHIS 1997-2002." Journal of Toxicology and Environmental Health. Part A. 2010. Accessed June 18, 2019. https://www.ncbi.nlm.nih.gov/pubmed/21058170.

541. Singh, Vijendra K., Sheren X. Lin, Elizabeth Newell, and Courtney Nelson. "Abnormal Measles-mumps-rubella Antibodies and CNS Autoimmunity in Children with Autism." Journal of Biomedical Science. 2002. Accessed June 18, 2019. https://www.ncbi.nlm.nih.gov/pubmed/12145534.

542. CDC, FDA, Industry Experts on Vaccine Toxicity. Accessed June 18, 2019. http://www.aapsonline.org/vaccines/cdcfdaexperts.htm.

543. Koleva, Gergana. "Merck Whistleblower Suit A Boon to Vaccine Foes Even As It Stresses Importance of Vaccines." Forbes. July 24, 2012. Accessed June 18, 2019. https://www.forbes.com/sites/gerganakoleva/2012/06/27/merck- whistleblower-suit-a-boon-to-anti-vaccination-advocates-though-it-stresses- importance-of-vac-cines/#5c47a0109678.

544. Goldschmidt, Debra. "Autism and Vaccine Study Results Questioned." CNN. August 28, 2014. Accessed June 18, 2019. https://www.cnn.com/2014/08/27/ health/irpt-cdc-autism-vaccine-study/.

545. Waly, M., H. Olteanu, R. Banerjee, S-W Choi, J. B. Mason, B. S. Parker, S. Sukumar, S. Shim, A. Sharma, J. M. Benzecry, V-A Power-Charnitsky, and R. C. Deth. "Activation of Methionine Synthase by Insulin-like Growth Factor-1 and Dopamine: A Target for Neurodevelopmental Toxins and Thimerosal." Molecular Psychiatry. April 2004. Accessed June 18, 2019. https://www.ncbi.nlm.nih.gov/pubmed/14745455.

CONTACT INFORMATION

Message Dr. Reed directly
Through drtomreed.com for the following:

To Order Books and Other Materials and
Products Directly From Dr. Reed
Includes Special Discounted Bulk Pricing and Promo Gifts.

To Subscribe to *Reed Between The Lines* Newsletter
You will also receive special notices about upcoming
events, speaking engagements, timely health-related
topics, and *Have You Heard* Hot Line Notifications.

To be added to our online Your Health Has Been
Hijacked community for additional training, resources,
health related FB Live events and more.

For Information the best sources for Therapeutic Grade
Essential Oils, CBD Oil, Nutritional Products, and other
Healthy Lifestyle Products.